OXFORD MEDICAL PUBLICATIONS

Essential Endocrinology

Essential Endocrinology

Third Edition

JOHN F. LAYCOCK

Senior Lecturer, Department of Physiology, Charing Cross and Westminster Medical School, London

PETER H. WISE

Consultant Endocrinologist, Charing Cross Hospital, London

Oxford New York Tokyo

OXFORD UNIVERSITY PRESS

1996

Oxford University Press, Walton Street, Oxford OX2 6DP
Oxford New York
Athens Auckland Bangkok Bombay
Calcutta Cape Town Dar es Salaam Delhi
Florence Hong Kong Istanbul Karachi
Kuala Lumpur Madras Madrid Melbourne
Mexico City Nairobi Paris Singapore
Taipei Tokyo Toronto
and associated companies in
Berlin Ibadan

Oxford is a trade mark of Oxford University Press

Published in the United States
by Oxford University Press Inc., New York

A catalogue record for this book is available from the British Library

Library of Congress Cataloging in Publication Data
Laycock, John F.
Essential endocrinology / John F. Laycock, Peter H. Wise. — 3rd ed.
(Oxford medical publications)
Includes bibliographical references and index.
1. Endocrine glands—Diseases. 2. Endocrinology. I. Wise, Peter H. II. Title. III. Series.
[DNLM: 1. Endocrine Glands. 2. Endocrine Diseases. WK 100 L427e 1996]
RC648.L325 1996 DNLM/DLC 95–52145

ISBN 0 19 262 472 5 (h/b)
ISBN 0 19 262 471 7 (p/b)

Typeset by EXPO Holdings, Malaysia

Printed in Great Britain by
Bookcraft (Bath) Ltd
Midsomer Norton, Avon.

Dose schedules are being continually revised and new side effects recognized. Oxford University Press makes no representation, express or implied, that the drug dosages in this book are correct. For these reasons the reader is strongly urged to consult the drug company's printed instructions before administering any of the drugs recommended in this book.

Preface to the third edition

After a gap of nearly 13 years since the previous edition of this textbook was published, many aspects of endocrinology have advanced considerably. These advances have occurred both at the basic science and clinical levels. For example, one major area of change has resulted from the application of molecular biology to hormone synthesis and action, and in the foreseeable future to aspects of treatment. Also, there is an increased interest in endocrine-related conditions such as growth and development, lipids and obesity. The consequence of all this has been the need to almost completely rewrite the text including new chapters covering these rapidly expanding areas of interest, and to increase the number of illustrative figures and tables. Furthermore, for the first time, colour photos of selected patients showing specific clinical manifestations of endocrine disease have been included, and we hope that this will be particularly useful to our readers. Nevertheless, we have kept to the main characteristic feature of the previous editions, namely the provision of a basic synopsis of the basic science and the clinical conditions associated with the principal endocrine glands, these two components always being related to each other in a unique way. The necessity to expand this edition has been balanced by the need to keep the book manageable in size, and to keep it as 'essential' as possible for student and doctor alike. We hope that we have been successful in all these aims.

Many people have suported us in updating this edition. In particular, we should like to thank Dr Saffron Whitehead who was very helpful with comments and suggestions for Chapters 1, 2, and 3, Dr Jaime Alaghband-Zadeh and Mr. Graham Carter for many discussions on endocrine matters; and Churchill Livingstone for permission to reproduce some of the photographs from another publication by one of us.

London
January 1996

J.F.L.
P.H.W.

Contents

1

Hormone synthesis, storage, release, and transport

INTRODUCTION

The term 'endocrinology' refers to the study of endocrine glands. Even twenty years ago, the definition of an endocrine gland was quite straightforward, particularly when compared with an exocrine gland. An exocrine gland is a collection of cells secreting chemicals into a duct leading to the exterior of the body (e.g. the salivary glands). In contrast, an endocrine gland consists of cells producing chemicals — called hormones — which are secreted directly into the bloodstream. Therefore, a hormone is a chemical released into the blood which transports it to its specific target cells where it exerts an effect which should be beneficial to the organism as a whole. In other words, a hormone acts as a chemical 'messenger' carried by the blood from its source to stimulate (or 'arouse') its target cells, to produce a specific effect. The word 'hormone' was first used by Bayliss and Starling in 1905 to describe the gastrointestinal molecule secretin. It is believed to have been coined from the Greek word meaning 'urge'.

Nowadays, these simple definitions are no longer adequate to describe the variety of chemicals synthesized by different cells, or groups of cells, throughout the body and which are released into the bloodstream. Many molecules fit the definition so that we still concentrate on the classical endocrine glands and their hormones such as the thyroid and thyroxine, the adrenals and cortisol, and the testes and testosterone. However, we now have to consider tissues that are not obvious as endocrine glands. Examples of these are the heart which produces atrial natriuretic peptides, the liver which is an important source of growth factors, and the brain (specifically the hypothalamus) which produces various neurosecretions from groups of neurones (called nuclei) which are released into the blood. The last example introduces another complication. Neurones in the hypothalamus can release their neurosecretions either across synapses to influence other neurones, in which case they are clearly neurotransmitters, or into the blood which carries them to their target cells, for instance in the pituitary gland, in which case the chemicals are clearly hormones. This important area of interaction between the endocrine and nervous systems has expanded so rapidly that it is designated by its own term — 'neuroendocrinology'.

The idea that all hormones are, by definition, stimulators (arousers) is clearly erroneous since various true hormones actually inhibit specific activities in their target cells. Another historical concept which no longer holds true is that one endocrine cell can produce only one hormone. There are various examples of endocrine cells being the sites of synthesis of more than one hormone (e.g. the gonadotrophic cells of the pituitary). The concept that a hormone acts on 'distant' target cells is also confusing, because some chemicals secreted from cells have an endocrine effect — but on neighbouring cells close by. This local effect is commonly described as 'paracrine' to differentiate it from the true endocrine system described above. Furthermore, we now have examples of classical hormones (such as oestradiol from glomerulosa cells in the ovary) which actually exert effects on their own sites of production — this is called an 'autocrine' effect.

A final difficulty to overcome arises from the original concept of a hormone, which included the important exclusion of all molecules produced by cells as a result of general metabolism (e.g. carbon dioxide, lactic acid) and molecules which act purely as energy substrates (e.g. glucose). The latest newcomers to the ever-expanding field of endocrinology are, in fact, just such molecules: the gases nitric oxide and carbon monoxide, no less!

The one truism which holds for all these biological control systems, whether involving endocrine secretory cells or neurones, whether they act on distant or nearby target cells or even on adjacent neurones, is that they all involve the release of chemical molecules. Furthermore, they are all vital components of the two communication systems which link cells to each other so that the organism functions as a whole: the nervous and the endocrine systems. Despite all these difficulties we shall attempt to describe the principal (classical) endocrine glands and their hormones as well as other endocrine, paracrine, and autocrine systems when relevant or sufficiently important to warrant a mention.

Where do we begin?

The involvement of any hormone in the control of cellular function depends on a series of reactions, beginning with the synthesis of the hormone in its endocrine cell and ending with the feedback control systems acting on that cell. Each stage can be extremely complex since there may be many interactions to consider: for instance, interactions between different stimuli, some positive others negative, acting on an endocrine cell would have to be integrated continuously to monitor the 'correct' (i.e. required) output of hormone from that cell. In addition, there is tremendous variation between individual hormones, and types of hormone, at any stage.

CHEMICAL STRUCTURE OF HORMONES

Hormones can be classified into three general groups:

(1) protein and polypeptide hormones;
(2) steroid hormones; and
(3) a miscellaneous group of hormones which cannot readily be included in either of the other two groups.

Examples of hormones that characterize these three groups are given in Table 1.1.

Table 1.1. A general classification of the major hormones into the three groups described in the text (pp, s, o)*

Name and common abbreviation	Type	Principal source
Gonadotrophin-releasing hormone (GnRH)	pp	Hypothalamus
Thyrotrophin-releasing hormone (TRH)	pp	Hypothalamus
Corticotrophin-releasing hormone (CRH)	pp	Hypothalamus
Somatostatin (SS)	pp	Hypothalamus (pancreatic islet cells)
Follicle-stimulating hormone (FSH)	pp	Adenohypophysis
Luteinizing hormone (LH)	pp	Adenohypophysis
Somatotrophin (GH)	pp	Adenohypophysis
Prolactin	pp	Adenohypophysis
Thyrotrophin (TSH)	pp	Adenohypophysis
Corticotrophin (ACTH)	pp	Adenohypophysis
Vasopressin (VP)	pp	Neurohypophysis
Oxytocin	pp	Neurohypophysis
Triiodothyronine (T_3)	o	Thyroid
Thyroxine (T_4)	o	Thyroid
Calcitonin (CT)	pp	Thyroid
Parathormone (PTH)	pp	Parathyroids
Noradrenaline (Nadr)	o	Adrenal medulla
Adrenaline (Adr)	o	Adrenal medulla
Aldosterone	s	Adrenal cortex
Cortisol	s	Adrenal cortex
17β-Oestradiol	s	Gonads, placenta (adrenal cortex)
Progesterone	s	Gonads, placenta (adrenal cortex)
Testosterone	s	Gonads (adrenal cortex)
Insulin	pp	Pancreatic islets
Glucagon	pp	Pancreatic islets
Gastrin	pp	Stomach
Secretin	pp	Small intestine
Cholecystokinin/Pancreozymin	pp	Small intestine
Atrial natriuretic peptide (ANP)	pp	Heart, brain
Melatonin	o	Pineal
1,25-Dihydroxyvitamin D_3 (1,25$(OH)_2D_3$)	s	Kidneys
Somatomedins (IGF-I, IGF-II)	pp	Liver

* pp, proteins and polypeptides; s, steroids; o, ‘others’.

Protein and polypeptide hormones

These hormones are synthesized from amino acids linked by peptide bonds. Polypeptide hormones are arbitarily designated as those consisting of less than 75 amino acids. Some of the protein hormones contain carbohydrate residues and are then often called glycoproteins.

Steroid hormones

This group includes the hormones produced from the adrenal cortices (the corticosteroids), the gonads (androgens, oestrogens, and progestogens) and the vitamin D_3 (cholecalciferol) metabolites. They are all derived from cholesterol and therefore consist of the cyclopentanoperhydrophenanthrene nucleus with varying side-chains and groups confering specificity to the different hormone molecules (Fig. 1.1).

Miscellaneous hormones

Various hormones can be included in this 'mixed bag' group. Some of these hormones are derived from amino acids, and could perhaps be considered with the protein and polypeptide group. On the other hand, others are lipid-soluble, and could perhaps be included in the steroid hormone group. However, these hormones usually have a range of properties which overlap both of the standard groups and so can be more conveniently considered separately. Hormones derived from amino acids include the iodinated thyronines of the thyroid gland, the catecholamines of the adrenal medulla, and melatonin which is found in particularly high concentrations in the pineal gland. The prostaglandins and their derivatives the thromboxanes consist of long-chain fatty acids, are lipid soluble, and are found throughout the body; these molecules can be considered to be examples of this miscellaneous group, although their inclusion as true hormones is debatable.

Other molecules acting as chemical messengers, such as the locally acting nitric oxide (NO), could also be considered to be part of this collection. This fascinating gaseous molecule (biological half-life $t_{1/2}$, in seconds) is ubiquitous; it has been shown in many different tissues including brain, vascular endothelium, and cells of the immune system such as neutrophils and macrophages. It is synthesized from L-Arginine in the presence of nitric oxide synthase (NOS) enzymes which may be either constitutive (i.e. already present) or inducible (Fig. 1.2). L-Arginine is converted to citrulline with the concomittent production of NO, the latter being rapidly inactivated by conversion to nitrite and nitrate. Its various actions include vascular smooth muscle relaxation following its release from the endothelium (it was shown to be the same molecule as endothelium-derived relaxation factor, EDRF), inhibition of platelet aggregation, and various possible central nervous system actions (including modulation of hypothalamic hormone release). It is also cytotoxic for various invading microorganisms and it is clearly an important component of the body's defence system.

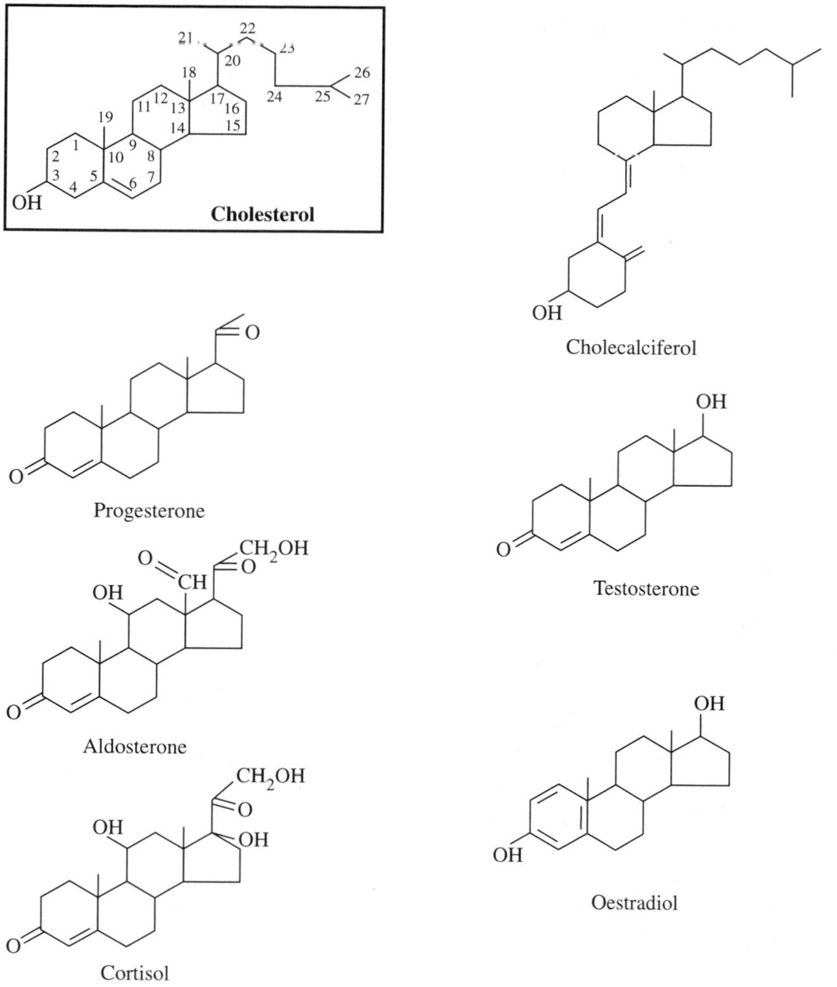

Fig. 1.1. The cyclopentanoperhydrophenanphrene nucleus-based structure of the cholesterol molecule which is related to the structures of many important steroid hormones.

SYNTHESIS

Protein and polypeptide hormones

Various polypeptide hormones are quite small; thyrotrophin-releasing hormone (TRH) is only three amino acids long, for example. These small polypeptide hormones are invariably synthesized initially as part of a much larger protein which subsequently undergoes cleavage to produce the active molecule — or molecules. The initial precursor protein is known as a the prohormone. Thus, the initial prohormone for corticotrophin (called pro-opiomelanocortin, POMC) consists of

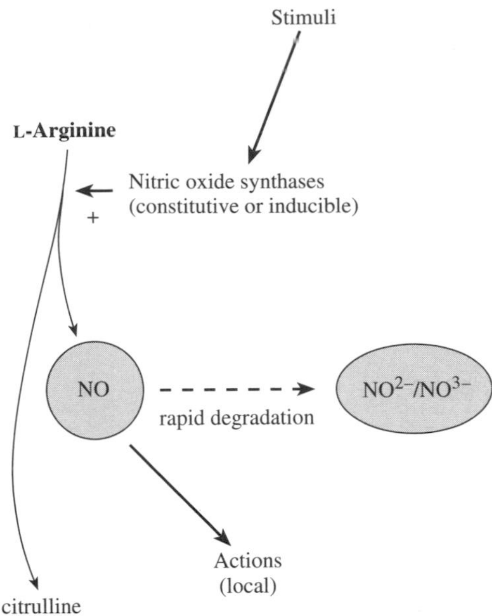

Fig. 1.2. The principal features of nitric oxide (NO) synthesis from the amino acid L-arginine, and its degradation to nitrite (NO^{2-}) and nitrate (NO^{3-}).

241 amino acids which, when processed in the corticotrophe cell of the adenohypophysis (anterior pituitary), produce not only the 39 amino acid polypeptide hormone but also a large protein called β-lipotrophin (β-LPH), a joining polypeptide, and an additional *N*-terminal protein (see Fig. 1.3). To be precise, the actual chain of amino acids initially synthesized is even longer than the prohormone because at the amino end there may be a putative signal (or leader) peptide. This precursor to the prohormone is called the pre-prohormone. The short sequence of amino acids of the signal peptide appears to recognize components on the membranes of the secretory pathway inside the cell. This recognition process is required for the successful transport of prohormone across the membrane of the rough endoplasmic reticulum. From here, the prohormone becomes incorporated into the secretory granules which ultimately release the hormone out of the endocrine cell. The processing of the prohormone can be tissue- (and species-) specific, as exemplified by the POMC molecule. In the adenohypophysis, corticotrophin and β-LPH are released into the circulation but in the intermediate lobe of the pituitary (which is normally vestigial in adults and appears to function only in the fetus or during pregnancy) β-LPH is further cleaved to form β-endorphin while corticotrophin is cleaved to form α-melanocyte-stimulating hormone (α-MSH) and a polypeptide called corticotrophin-like intermediate lobe polypeptide (CLIP).

Synthesis of the pre-prohormone is initiated in the nucleus of the endocrine cell. Active messenger and transfer ribonucleic acid molecules (mRNA and tRNA) are manufactured at specific genes on chromosomes where relevant parts of deoxy-

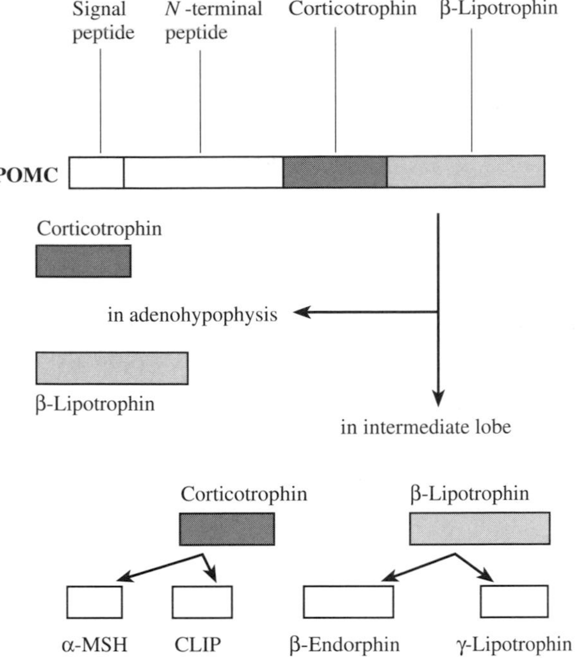

Fig. 1.3. The corticotrophin precursor molecule pro-opiomelanocortin (POMC) and its physiologically active peptide derivatives in the adenohypophysis, and the breakdown products which are possible in the intermediate lobe.

ribonucleic acid (DNA) act as templates. This initial stage, which involves the transferral of appropriate information about the structure of the molecule to be synthesized from the nuclear DNA template to the RNA molecules, is called transcription. The genes for over 200 regulatory protein and polypeptide hormones have now been cloned. The coding sequence of the gene for a polypeptide hormone precursor contains a promoter region and a transcription unit. The promoter region contains a number of short regulatory DNA sequences which can interact with specific DNA-binding proteins. These proteins may act as enhancers or silencers, which allow or prevent gene transcription to proceed respectively. The transcription unit consists of DNA regions called exons, separated by sequences called introns, which are transcribed into the mRNA precursor. The introns are then spliced from this precursor and the exons are joined together. The purpose of the introns is still unclear.

The resulting mRNA then becomes associated with the ribosomes along the rough endoplasmic reticulum in the cytoplasm. The tRNA molecules also enter the cytoplasm where they attach to specific amino acids, and they then migrate to the ribosomes where they link up with the mRNA in a pre-ordained sequence. The amino acids then become linked to each other by peptide bonding to form the new protein or polypeptide molecule. This second stage is called translation.

After synthesis is completed the pre-prohormone molecule migrates through the membrane of the rough endoplasmic reticulum losing its signal peptide sequence in the process. The prohormone then reaches the Golgi complex where it usually becomes incorporated into a vesicle surrounded by a membrane. This granule then dissociates from the Golgi apparatus and moves through the cytoplasm towards the cell membrane (Fig. 1.4). Inside the granule, various specific protease enzymes then split the prohormone into its components.

The above description of prohormones being processed (i.e. altered chemically — or cleaved) within secretory granules to produce the active hormone molecules does not always apply, however. For example, the hormone angiotensin II is an octapeptide which is cleaved from a precursor decapeptide called angiotensin I. Angiotensin I could therefore be considered to be a prohormone. However, angiotensin I is itself only an intermediate molecule, and is not normally present as

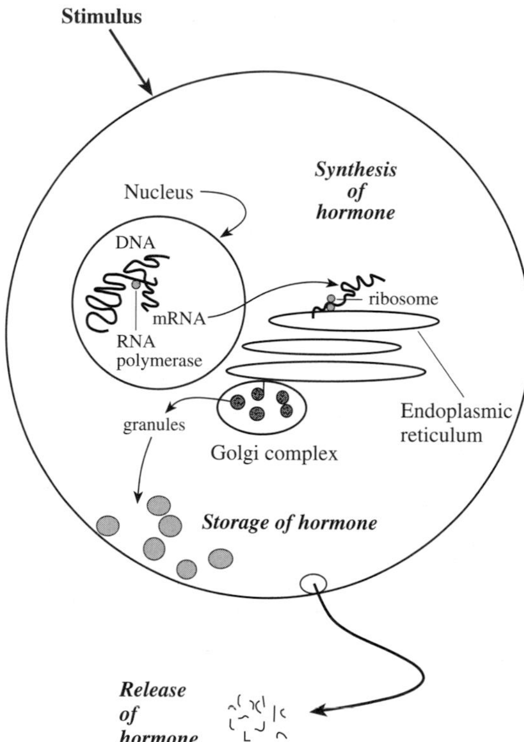

Fig. 1.4. The synthesis of a protein/polypeptide hormone when the endocrine cell is stimulated. The hormone precursor is synthesized on ribosomes associated with the endoplasmic reticulum following the initial nuclear transcription stage. The hormone is incorporated into granules in the Golgi complex, and these act as the intracellular storage form which can be released from the cell by exocytosis. A free hormone component (possibly complexed with another intracellular molecule such as zinc) may also be present in the cytoplasm.

the decapeptide. It is in fact formed by the cleavage of a plasma protein called angiotensinogen, the reaction being catalysed by an enzyme called renin. The protein angiotensinogen could therefore be called the prohormone for angiotensin I, and perhaps the pro-prohormone for angiotensin II!

Steroid hormones

Steroid hormones are lipid-soluble and therefore can diffuse readily through cell membranes. Consequently, they are mainly synthesized when required from various precursor molecules, as the result of specific enzyme-induced reactions within the cell cytoplasm. The synthesis process is therefore determined by the activation of a specific enzyme (or enzymes) following the arrival of some stimulus at the endocrine cell. The initial precursor molecule for steroid hormones is cholesterol which is naturally present in all cells to some extent. Cholesterol can be synthesized by the endocrine cells from acetate or it can reach the cell following its transport in the blood associated with lipoproteins (Fig. 1.5).

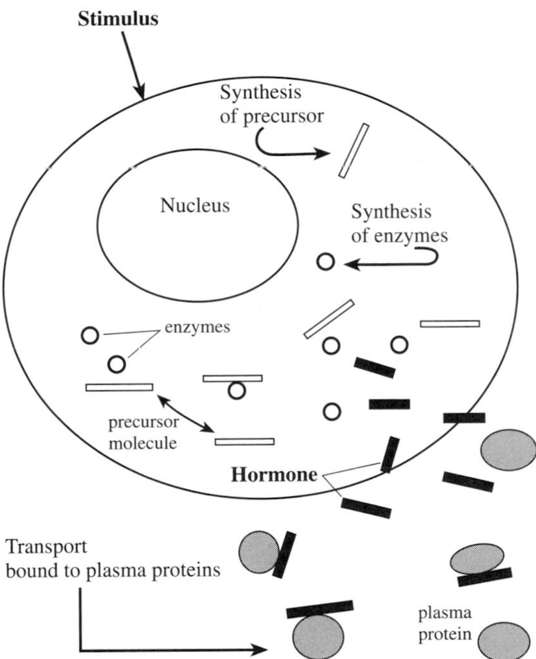

Fig. 1.5. The synthesis of a steroid hormone. Immediate synthesis occurs when specific enzymes are activated within the cytoplasm to act on precursor molecules such as cholesterol. Long-term regulation is directed at the synthesis of the enzymes and precursor molecules. Once the hormone is released from the cell (by diffusion), transport in the blood is accomplished mainly in the bound form to plasma proteins, with only a very small proportion unbound.

Miscellaneous hormones

The synthesis of many hormones in this group also involves enzyme-induced reactions occurring in the cell cytoplasm. For example, the thyroid hormones thyroxine and triiodothyronine are synthesized as the result of iodination of tyrosyl units incorporated in a thyroidal protein called thyroglobulin. This iodination process is catalysed by enzymes within the cytoplasm or located on a cell membrane. The synthesis of nitric oxide is another example of a precursor molecule (L-Arginine) being converted to its components in the presence of specific nitric oxide synthase enzymes.

STORAGE

Protein and polypeptide hormones

These hormones are probably stored exclusively in the secretory granules within the cytoplasm of their respective endocrine cells. However, it is possible that some hormone is always present in a 'free' state in the cytoplasm, but unless it is protected in some way from inactivation by proteolytic enzymes, this component is unlikely to be stable. Storage of the hormone within the granules is probably the principal way in which the hormone is protected from intracellular degradation, but another way could be by association of the hormone with another molecule or element (such as insulin with zinc, for instance), the complex formed then possibly existing within the cytoplasm.

Steroid hormones

The steroid hormones are not believed to be stored to any great extent within the endocrine cells. A stimulus to these cells initiates the synthesis of the hormone which is probably released into the bloodstream as soon as it has been manufactured. It has been suggested, however, that a small pool of steroid hormone may be present in the endocrine cell membranes where, being lipid-soluble, they could be temporarily stored (in the form of its ester for example).

Miscellaneous hormones

The hormones of this group are stored in various ways. For instance the thyroid hormones such as thyroxine are stored in follicles as iodinated components of the precursor thyroglobulin protein, whereas the catecholamines of the adrenal medulla are stored in secretory granules in the cytoplasm. It should be noted that some hormones can be considered to be 'stored' in the form of their circulating precursors. Thus, angiotensin II can be considered to be circulating in a stored form, as the angiotensin I precursor angiotensinogen, while the steroid dihydrotestosterone could conceivably be considered to be stored (at least on a short-term basis) in the form of circulating testosterone.

RELEASE

Protein and polypeptide hormones

The process by which protein and polypeptide hormones stored in secretory granules are released into the blood is called exocytosis. It is a complex process which is still incompletely understood, but it involves the fusion of granule and cell membranes followed by expulsion of the granule contents into the bloodstream (Fig. 1.4).

The process of secretion is associated with the excitation of the endocrine cell by a stimulus, and has been called excitation–secretion coupling. For endocrine cells the process is similar in many respects to the release of neurotransmitters, such as acetylcholine, from a nerve terminal. For instance, both processes generally require the presence of calcium ions, the influx of these cations into the cell being an important stage in the process of exocytosis. The similarities between the secretory process of endocrine cells and the release of neurotransmittors at nerve terminals may be even closer than was originally believed: for instance, the release of insulin from its endocrine cell has been associated with a depolarization of the cell membrane.

Microtubules, which are polymers of an intracellular protein called tubulin, have been observed in various endocrine cells containing secretory granules. Disruption of microtubules with drugs such as colchicine appears to prevent the process of exocytosis, and this had led to the speculation that microtubules are a necessary component of the releasing mechanism.

Steroid hormones

Since steroid hormones are generally synthesized only when the cell is stimulated, these lipid-soluble molecules probably diffuse immediately through the cell membrane into the general circulation.

Miscellaneous hormones

The hormones in this group are secreted by a variety of different releasing mechanisms according to their chemical properties and the forms in which they are stored within the cell. Some hormones are released by exocytosis from secretory granules (e.g. catecholamines), while others diffuse through the cell membrane once they have been synthesized, or once they have been split off from their parent compounds (e.g. thyroxine from the thyroglobulin protein in which it is stored).

TRANSPORT

Certain hormones, particularly steroids and the iodothyronines, once released into the general circulation become bound to plasma proteins. The binding of these hormones to plasma proteins probably serves two purposes: first, the hormone is 'protected' to some extent from inactivating systems present in the blood, and secondly, the hormone is then maintained in a 'stored' circulating form so that hormone is readily available at its target tissues when required. Some plasma proteins have a high affinity for particular hormones, the degree of affinity being a measure of their avidity for these hormones. Such proteins are usually globulins, and include thyronine-binding globulin (TBG) which binds thyroxine and triiodothyronine, transcortin which binds certain steroid hormones such as cortisol, and sex-hormone-binding globulin (SHBG) which binds various sex hormones. Other plasma proteins, particularly albumin, have a low affinity for hormones but a high capacity for binding, this related to the higher concentrations of these proteins in the blood. An example of the differing binding properties of plasma proteins for a particular hormone is given by the transport of throxine in the blood. The bulk of the thyroxine present in the blood is bound to the high-affinity but low-capacity TBG, with another smaller component being transported bound to a medium-affinity, medium-capacity prealbumin fraction. Very little, if any, thyroxine is bound to the albumin fraction under normal conditions, however, because although this protein has a high capacity it has a low affinity for the hormone.

A dynamic equilibrium exists between the concentrations of free (unbound) hormone, plasma protein, and the hormone–plasma protein complex, and this can be expressed by the following relationships:

$$[H] \times [P] \rightleftharpoons [HP]$$

where $[H]$, $[P]$, and $[HP]$ represent the concentrations of free hormone, carrier protein, and protein–bound hormone, respectively.

$$\frac{[H] \times [P]}{[HP]} = K$$

where K is the dissociation constant for the relationship.

The equilibrium state given above indicates that at any instant some hormone will be present in the free (unbound) state, and it is this component which is biologically active both at its target cell and at its own endocrine cells where it may have a feedback-controlling influence on its own production (Fig. 1.6). When target cells require free hormone for increased activity, the equilibrium state is temporarily upset so that more of the protein-bound complex dissociates to increase the concentration of free hormone in the immediate vicinity of the target cells in order to maintain the dissociation constant. A decrease in the free-hormone concentration in the blood then stimulates the endocrine gland to secrete more hormone to restore the free-hormone level to its initial value.

It also follows that if the carrier protein concentration increases, more of the free-hormone component will initially be taken up by the protein. Again, the endocrine gland may be stimulated to produce more hormone until the normal free-hormone level has been restored. In this situation, the total hormone content of the blood may be raised but the active free-hormone level will be normal. An example

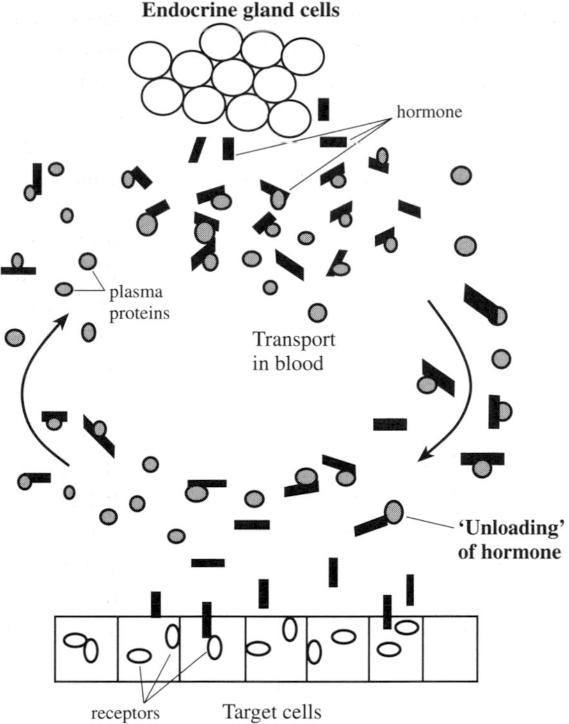

Fig. 1.6. The process of hormone binding to plasma proteins in the blood, and its 'unloading' in the vicinity of its target cells (specifically its receptors).

of this situation is the increase in plasma-protein production which occurs during pregnancy. In this case the total hormone content of the blood may be raised but the free-hormone level is normal, and no clinical abnormalities are observed.

Some hormones may be present in the blood in diverse forms, such as monomers, dimers, and even polymers. Somatotrophin, for example, is present in the circulation as a monomer and as a dimer, the monomer probably being formed by cleavage of the dimeric molecule. The monomer, believed to be the somatotrophin hormone molecule, is much more biologically active than its dimeric 'prohormone'. Such differences between the structures of a hormone and its related molecules and their relative biological potencies probably account for the discrepancies in hormone concentration measurements using different assay techniques. Radioimmunoassays may estimate the total chemical concentration of some part of a molecule which is found in the hormone and its prohormone, while a bioassay method will estimate the total biological activity present in the sample.

PERIPHERAL CONVERSION

Some biologically active hormones are converted to other equally, more or less active hormones in peripheral tissues such as liver, breast, adipose tissue and brain. The term 'peripheral conversion' is used with reference to any tissue which is 'peripheral' to the endocrine gland in question. For example, the androgen testosterone, which is secreted by the testes, is converted to dihydrotestosterone in other tissues. Since both molecules have distinct hormonal activity, testosterone is not simply a prohormone which requires activation by peripheral enzymes. Another example of peripheral conversions, which are of physiological significance, is the deiodination of thyroxine (T_4) to either the more active triiodothyronine (T_3) or to the biologically inactive molecule called reverse triiodothyronine (rT_3).

ECTOPIC HORMONE PRODUCTION

For many years it has been obvious that endocrine disorders can be associated with tumours. For instance, the production of excessive quantities of corticotrophin (ACTH) from a pituitary tumour is the basis for Cushing's disease. An abnormal growth of endocrine secretory tissue is called an adenoma. It is quite possible for an adenoma to produce either peptide or steroid hormones, depending on the endocrine tissue affected. Thus, an excess of glucocorticoids could be due either to increased stimulation of the adrenal cortex by excessive quantities of corticotrophin from the adenohypophysis (giving rise to Cushing's disease, as above) or to excessive production of glucocorticoids due to an adrenal adenoma (giving rise to Cushing's syndrome). More recently, however, it has become clear that the abnormal production of molecules which have the biological activities of well-recognized hormones by non-endocrine tissues is also possible. Indeed, in most cases it is clear that the molecules are identical to the hormones which they mimic. This production of hormones from non-endocrine tissues is called ectopic production, and it occurs in cells which are abnormal (i.e. from tumours). One of the first instances identified was the production of vasopressin from an oat cell carcinoma of the lung. Since then, various hormones produced by tumours have been identified, and in all cases they are polypeptide hormones. It is possible that the cancerous cells have de-repressed genes which consequently transcribe messages for the polypeptide hormone. Ectopic steroid hormone production may be less likely because any steroid hormone requires the activation of sequences of enzymes within the cell.

FURTHER READING

Bredt, D.S. and Snyder, S.H. (1994). Nitric oxide: a physiologic messenger molecule. *Annual Review of Biochemistry*, **63**, 175–96.

Getzenberg, R.H., Pienta, K.J., and Coffey, D.S. (1990). The tissue matrix: cell dynamics and hormone action. *Endocrine Review*, **11**, 399–417.

Lieberman, S. and Prasad, V.V.K. (1990). Heterodox notions on pathways of steroidogenesis. *Endocrine Reviews*, **11**, 469–93.

Pryer, N.K., Wuestehube, L.J., and Schekman, R. (1992). Vesicle-mediated protein sorting. *Annual Review of Biochemistry*, **61**, 471–516.

2

Hormone mechanisms of action

INTRODUCTION

The mechanisms by which different hormones can exert specific effects on their target cells are not yet completely resolved. Originally, it was believed that each hormone produced its characteristic effects by an individual mechanism of action. Thus, parathormone influenced bone resorption by a process which was quite different from the mechanism employed by adrenalin on hepatic glycogenolysis. It now appears that hormonal mechanisms of action have certain common components, but the first stage in which the individual hormones recognize their target cells is quite specific and depends on the presence of receptors. It is therefore necessary to consider first the hormone-receptor binding process.

TARGET CELL RECEPTORS

The characteristic actions of a hormone depend on its recognition of the target cell. This recognition process is essentially a property of the target cell, and it involves the presence of receptor molecules. These receptors are proteins which have specific sites for the binding of that hormone. Other molecules (agonists or antagonists, for example) can bind to the same receptors; molecules which bind to a specific receptor are called ligands for that receptor. The recognition of the receptor by the hormone can simplistically be compared to the way in which a key fits its lock. For any particular lock there is only one true key which will be a perfect fit although others can 'force' their way in. Cellular recognition of hormone molecules can take place at two sites in the cell: at the plasma membrane or within the cell.

Protein and polypeptide hormones are generally unable to penetrate the cell membranes, and for such hormones to influence intracellular events they must first bind to specific receptors on the plasma membrane. The mechanisms by which such hormones can then produce effects within their target cells can be explained on the basis of a 'second messenger' theory which is considered later. Nevertheless, it is increasingly clear that some polypeptide hormones, usually bound to their receptors, can be 'internalized' inside the target cells by endocytosis. This process may be part of the hormone inactivation process.

Fat-soluble hormone molecules, such as the steroids, can penetrate the plasma membranes of their target cells with relative ease by the simple process of diffusion through the lipid component. Presumably, unless the steroids are kept inside by some internal process, they can also diffuse back out of the cells and into the interstitial fluid. For these hormones, the recognition process takes place within the cells and specificity is determined by the presence of cytoplasmic and/or nuclear receptors which have high affinities for the appropriate hormone molecules. Thus, the receptors 'keep' their specific hormone molecules inside the target cells.

Cell membrane receptors

Hormone receptors in the plasma membranes of cells are simply components of quite complex interrelated molecules that span the membranes. Different families of hormone receptors have been identified. For instance, the catecholamine β-receptors (of which there are at least two types) belong to a family the members of which have seven cross-membrane domains as well as extracellular hormone-binding and intracellular protein-binding domains (Fig. 2.1). A novel receptor containing binding sites for two different polypeptide hormones (vasopressin and angiotensin II) has recently been identified. Thus, hormone-receptor interactions may be more complex than has been appreciated hitherto.

The hormone first binds to its receptor to form a complex which subsequently interacts with various nucleotide regulatory proteins within the membrane. Although the precise details of the reaction are still being elucidated, it appears that the hormone-receptor complex undergoes a configurational change which allows it to interact with a regulatory nucleotide protein. The regulatory molecules are guanyl nucleotide regulatory proteins, called G proteins. Two of these proteins either stimulate or inhibit the conversion of guanosine triphosphate to guanosine

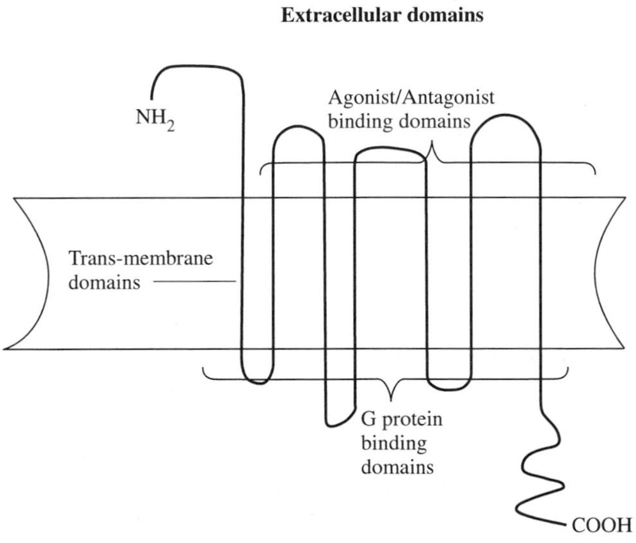

Fig. 2.1. A typical membrane receptor with its transmembrane, extracellular, and intracellular domains which are associated with specific binding characteristics.

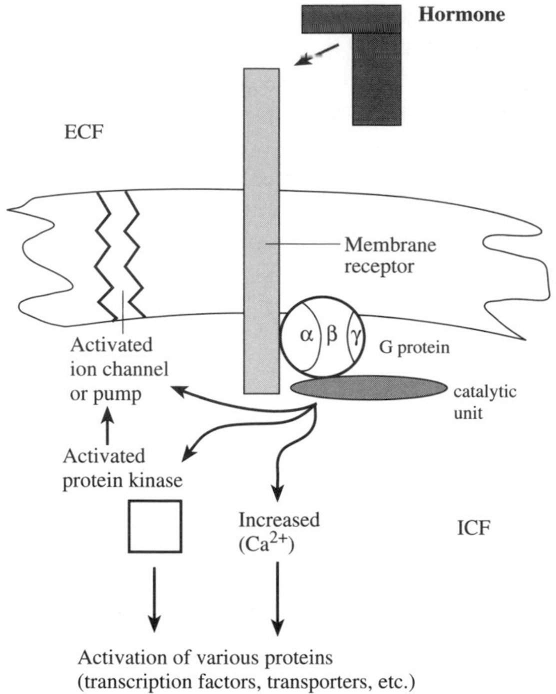

Fig. 2.2. Binding of a hormone to its membrane receptor. The intracellular domains of the receptor are linked to the G protein (α-, β-, and γ-subunits) and its catalytic unit through which various intracellular mechanisms are activated (see text). (ECF and ICF, extracellular and intracellular fluid compartments, respectively.)

diphosphate and are called Gs and Gi, respectively. Each G protein is composed of three subunits, α, ß, and γ. When activated, the subunits dissociate and the α-unit can then either stimulate or inhibit the catalytic unit, depending on whether it comes from the Gs or the Gi protein, respectively. The catalytic units are themselves protein enzymes, such as adenyl cyclase, guanyl cyclase, phospholipase C, and various protein kinases (Fig. 2.2).

Intracellular hormone receptors

For those hormones capable of entering cells, either by diffusion (e.g. steroids) or by other mechanisms, such as by endocytosis or by specific carrier molecules, the receptors allowing for target cell recognition may be intracellular. In general, steroid receptors appear to be located in the nucleus, at least when not bound to a ligand (a molecule which binds to a specific receptor, e.g. the hormone itself or a related molecule). As with membrane-located receptors, nuclear receptors exist in related families with conserved sequences in their structure related to function. Thus, a superfamily of regulatory proteins includes receptors for mineralocorticoids, glucocorticoids, androgens, oestrogens, progesterone, the thyroid iodothyronines, the vitamin D metabolites, and the retinoic acids. The cloning of nuclear receptors has revealed not only receptors for known hormones but also receptors of the same family for which no ligands have yet been identified. These latter receptors have been called, appropriately, orphan receptors.

Each nuclear receptor is composed of different components. The A/B regions have the specific transcription activator components. The C region is highly conserved and corresponds to a DNA-binding domain incorporating two 'zinc fingers', each of which consists of a zinc ion bound to cysteine-histidine structures. The D region, function unclear, links to the E region which is also highly conserved between receptors. This region has multiple functions; in addition to transcription-activating functions it is also the domain for hormone-binding. The final region (F), the function of which is unclear, is not present in all receptors (e.g. progesterone receptors).

Thus nuclear steroid receptors bind their hormones, often as dimers, and then bind to their hormone response elements on the DNA of their target genes. Transcription is then activated (Fig. 2.3).

Receptor regulation

The regulation of hormone receptors is an important feature of any endocrine system, since it can influence the magnitude and duration of a specific hormonal effect. This can be achieved by a change in the number of receptors, which can be increased or decreased (known as up- and down-regulation, respectively) or by an alteration in the affinity of the receptor for its hormone. Relatively little is known about these processes.

MECHANISMS OF ACTION

There are three general mechanisms by which a hormone can exert its specific effects on target cells:

(1) direct membrane effects;

(2) intracellular effects mediated by 'second messenger' systems within the cell; and

(3) intracellular effects mediated by nuclear actions.

Although these three mechanisms form a convenient system for categorizing hormones, it must be emphasized that a hormone can exert its effects by any combination of them. In addition, the mechanisms of action of some hormones have still not been identified and it therefore must be appreciated that other modes of action probably exist and remain to be discovered.

Direct membrane effects

A hormone can have direct effects on plasma membranes such that their permeability to ions or the transport characteristics for particular molecules may be

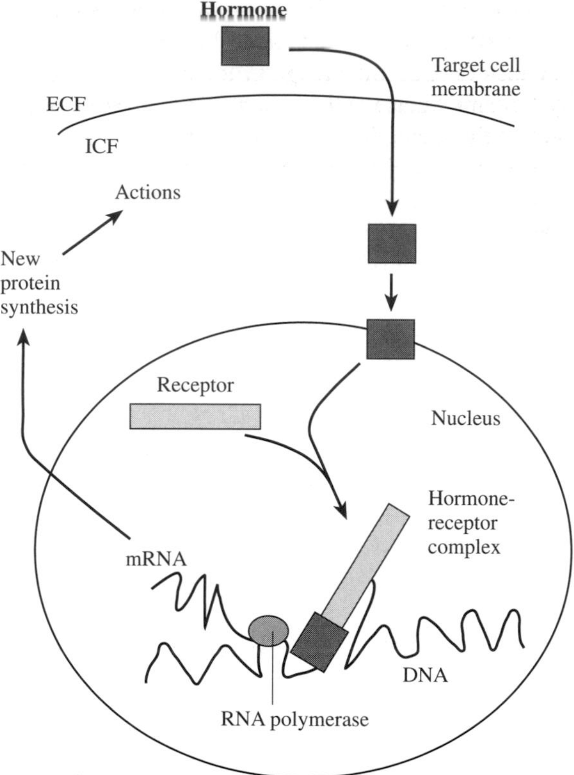

Fig. 2.3. Genomic mechanism of action of hormones. Hormone-receptor binding usually occurs within the nucleus although some binding can also occur in the cytoplasm, with movement of the complex into the nucleus. (ECF and ICF, extracellular and intracellular fluid compartments, respectively.)

altered. This can result from the interaction between hormone and specific membrane receptor such that the structure of the membrane itself is altered (e.g. by the opening up of pores). Alternatively, the activity of some form of carrier molecule is influenced (e.g. by altering its chemical structure, thereby increasing its affinity for the particular solute being transported). Some hormones stimulate the synthesis, and transport to the membrane, of specific 'pores' or 'channels'. Vasopressin, for instance, stimulates the movement of hormone-sensitive water channels to the relevant cell membranes of renal target cells (see Chapter 4). Another possible mechanism is the activation of a specific membrane 'pump' mechanism such as the iodide pump in the follicular cells of the thyroid gland (see Chapter 9).

Receptor tyrosine kinase activity

Some membrane receptors have inherent enzyme (e.g. tyrosine kinase) activity. Consequently, when the appropriate hormone binds to this type of receptor, phosphorylation of specific cytoplasmic proteins occurs. Tyrosine kinase activation is a necessary step in the mediation of the actions of various hormones, including the pancreatic hormone insulin. Our knowledge of the intracellular proteins which are phosphorylated by tyrosine kinase activity is still limited and many of the subsequent steps involved in the mediation of hormone actions remain to be elucidated. Interestingly, one effect invariably associated with activation of tyrosine kinase is phosphorylation of the receptor itself. This auto-phosphorylation may have positive or negative regulatory effects on the inherent receptor tyrosine kinase activity. Adjacent receptors can also be phosphorylated. Finally, other protein kinases can be phosphorylated by receptor tyrosine kinase activity, probably mediating various different actions associated with the hormone itself (Fig. 2.4).

Intracellular second messenger activation

Those hormones ('first messengers') that bind to plasma membrane receptors and yet exert intracellular actions may do so by activating intracellular 'second messengers'. A 'second messenger' system then mediates the various intracellular effects which characterize the actions of such a hormone. This mediation can be

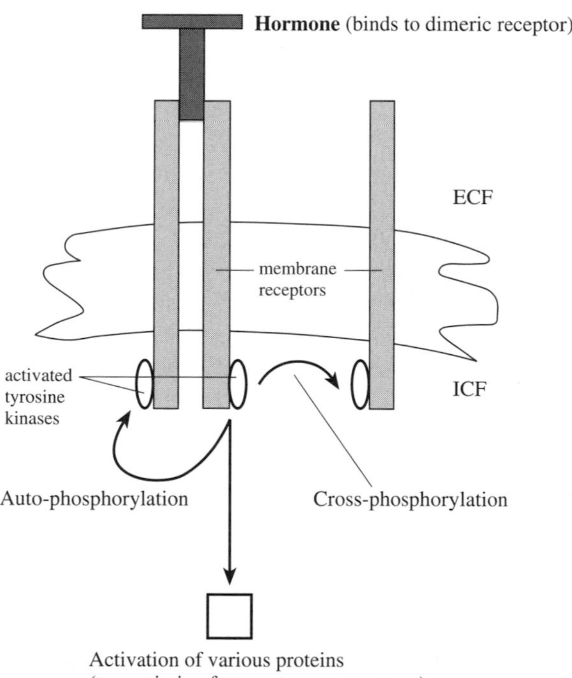

Fig. 2.4. Hormone binding to its membrane receptor is associated with activation of tyrosine kinase which, in turn, can lead to auto-phosphorylation and cross-phosphorylation of nearby receptors (which will potentiate the initial signal) and the activation of various intracellular proteins. (ECF and ICF, extracellular and intracellular fluid compartments, respectively.)

achieved either by influencing previously existing enzyme systems, or by stimulating the synthesis of new protein molecules, or by activating other intracellular mediators. Some membrane effects associated with hormones could in fact be due to the initial activation of intracellular messenger systems which stimulate the formation of enzymes which might then influence the cytoplasmic surface of the cell.

Various 'second messengers' have been identified, and these include the cyclic nucleotides cyclic adenosine 3′,5′-monophosphate (cAMP) and cyclic guanosine 3′,5′-monophosphate (cGMP), inositol triphosphate, diacylglycerol, intracellular calcium ions, and eicosanoids.

Cyclic AMP (cAMP)

In the presence of magnesium or manganese ions, this cyclic nucleotide is formed from adenosine triphosphate (ATP) by the action of an enzyme called adenyl cyclase. In mammalian cells this is the membrane-bound catalytic unit associated with the receptor–G protein complex. Cyclic AMP can then activate specific cytoplasmic enzymes, called protein kinases, by catalysing the transfer of the terminal phosphate of ATP to the kinase. Each protein kinase molecule consists of two regulatory and two catalytic subunits. Cyclic AMP causes the dissociation of catalytic from regulatory subunits, thus allowing the catalytic units to phosphorylate their own substrate proteins. These activated proteins, such as protein kinase A, then induce the intracellular effects associated with the various hormones. Cyclic AMP is degraded by hydrolysis to 5′-adenosine monophosphate (5′-AMP) this reaction being catalysed by phosphodiesterase enzyme (see Fig. 2.5).

The involvement of cAMP as an intracellular mediator of a hormone's action was first shown by Sutherland and Rall in 1958. Their experiments indicated that the formation of this cyclic nucleotide was the intermediate step between the hormone adrenaline and its glycogenolytic action in hepatic tissue. The activation of the protein kinase by cAMP resulted in the subsequent activation of phosphorylase which is an enzyme involved in splitting glycogen down to glucose 1-phosphate resulting ultimately in an increased plasma concentration of glucose.

Some of the actions of other hormones also coincide with increases in intracellular cAMP concentrations and in many cases the administration of this nucleotide can mimic the effects of these hormones. Various hormones which have so far been shown to involve cAMP in at least one of their actions are listed in Table 2.1.

Cyclic GMP (cGMP)

This cylic nucleotide is essentially similar to cAMP. It is formed following activation of a catalytic unit, in this case guanyl cyclase, in the cell membrane. However, whereas adenyl cyclase is linked to the hormone receptor by G proteins, guanyl cyclase resembles receptor tyrosine kinase because it can function both as a receptor and a catalytic unit. The atrial natriuretic peptides and nitric oxide are examples of hormones that bind directly to the guanyl cyclase molecules in the target cell membranes and use cGMP as their second messengers.

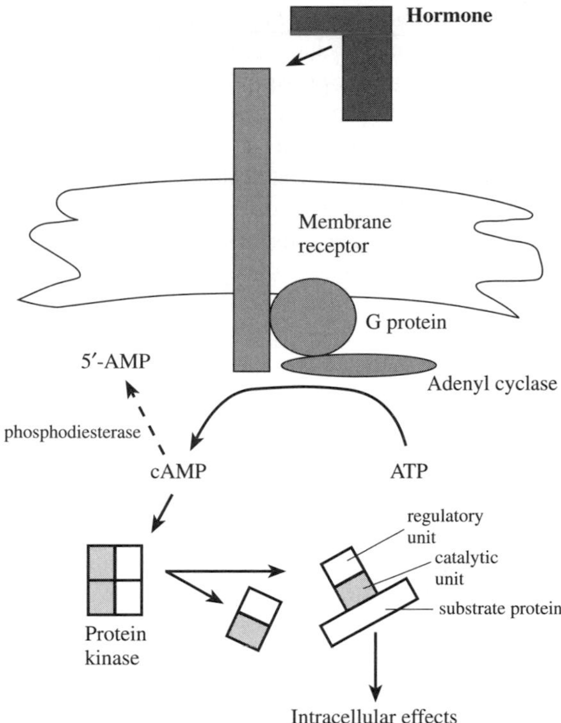

Fig. 2.5. Hormone binding to its membrane receptor can result in catalytic unit (in this case adenyl cyclase) activation. The second messenger cyclic AMP (cAMP) can then activate specific intracellular protein kinases (see text).

Table 2.1. Some hormones whose actions on specific target tissues involve the second messenger cAMP

Hormone	Target tissue
Thyrotrophin-releasing hormone (TRH)	Adenohypophysis
Gonadotrophin-releasing hormone (GnRH)	Adenohypophysis
Thyrotrophin	Thyroid
Luteinizing hormone (LH)	Ovary, testis
Adrenaline	Liver, adipose tissue
Vasopressin	Kidney
Glucagon	Liver, adipose tissue
Parathormone (PTH)	Kidney, bone

The phosphoinositides

Another important second messenger system involves the formation of active molecules from membrane phospholipids, following binding of the hormone to a membrane receptor. When the hormone interacts with its receptor (generally linked to a G protein complex) a membrane-bound enzyme, phospholipase C, is activated. This enzyme then acts on membrane phospholipids, specifically phosphatidylinositol 4, 5-bisphosphate (PIP_2), to produce inositol triphosphate (IP_3) and diacylglycerol (DAG). These molecules then act as second messengers which act to influence intracellular calcium levels. IP_3 stimulates the release of calcium ions from intracellular stores. This IP_3-sensitive calcium then appears to stimulate the release of further calcium from other, IP_3-insensitive, intracellular stores, so that a wave of calcium ions spreads rapidly across the cytoplasm. This release of calcium ions into the cytoplasm is, in essence, the formation of yet another intracellular second messenger. Calcium ions have many effects on metabolic processes (see below). Metabolism of IP_3 results in various other phosphorylated inositol forms most of which are inactive, although some may enhance the effects of IP_3 within the cell.

The other product formed from PIP_2 is diacylglycerol which activates the membrane-bound enzyme protein kinase C (PKC). This enzyme phosphorylates intracellular proteins which can then act on a variety of metabolic pathways within the cell, in cytoplasm and nucleus, to produce the actions associated with the initiator hormone. DAG activation of PKC may also result in stimulation of a calcium pump in the cell membrane as part of the recovery mechanism, restoring the cytoplasmic calcium ion level back to normal (see Fig. 2.6).

Calcium ions (Ca^{2+})

The mobilization of calcium ions is important in regulating various metabolic processes within cells. Therefore, calcium ions can be considered quite legitimately as being second messengers in their own right. The cytoplasmic Ca^{2+} concentration is approximately 10^{-7}M, compared with an extracellular concentration of the order of 10^{-3}M. The calcium gradient is maintained by a number of calcium channels, pumps, and transporters which in some cases are linked to the transport processes of other ions (e.g. sodium ions). There are two sources available to provide an increase in the cytoplasmic Ca^{2+} concentration: an extracellular source, which can be regulated through the availability of channels or the stimulation/inhibition of pumps, and an intracellular source, which consists of various intracellular organelles such as the endoplasmic reticulum, the mitochondria and the microsomes. These sources can be utilized following appropriate stimulation. As seen above, the binding of some hormones to their membrane receptors can result in stimulation of phospholipase C and the resulting formation of IP_3 from its precursor phospholipid. IP_3 then induces the release of Ca^{2+} from the intracellular stores of calcium ions. It is likely that extracellular Ca^{2+} can also participate in raising the cytoplasmic concentration of this ion.

One important effect of Ca^{2+} is to regulate the activity of various protein kinases, but in some cases it is first necessary for calcium to bind to intracellular binding proteins. The major calcium-binding proteins are the troponins in muscle cells and the calmodulins in non-muscle cells. The active calcium–calmodulin complex is then capable of interacting with a number of proteins including various

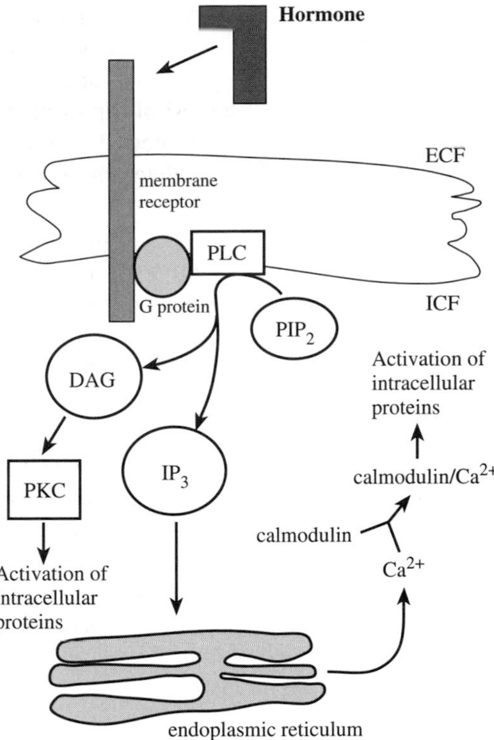

Fig. 2.6. Hormone binding to its membrane receptor can result in the activation of membrane-bound phospholipase C (PLC) which, in turn, can initiate the formation of inositol triphosphate (IP_3) and diacylglycerol (DAG) from precursor phosphatidylinositol diphosphate (PIP_2). IP_3 can increase the movement of calcium ions from intracellular stores into the cytoplasm while DAG activates protein kinase C (PKC).

protein kinases which may, or may not, be cAMP-dependent. Ca^{2+}-calmodulin can also stimulate calcium pump activity, thus leading to increased uptake of calcium by intracellular stores for example, resulting in a return of cytoplasmic Ca^{2+} concentration to basal levels (see Fig. 2.6).

The complex interactions and feedback loops which almost certainly exist within cells can best be exemplified by the inverse relationship which is believed to exist between the intracellular calcium ion concentration and cAMP. Thus, an increase in cAMP activity can lead to an increase in the cytoplasmic Ca^{2+} concentration which can then regulate the cAMP concentration by exerting an inhibitory feedback effect on the nucleotide.

Eicosanoids

Phospholipase enzymes in cell membranes, when stimulated by hormones, can act on phospholipid precursors to produce dihomo-γ-linolenic and arachidonic acids.

These molecules then act as substrates for the synthesis of various related molecules belonging to a family called the eicosanoids. Probably the best-known derivatives are the prostaglandins, which are variants of a 20-carbon unsaturated fatty acid, each containing a cyclopentane (5-carbon) ring. The first of these molecules to be discovered were found in an extract of human semen. Although it is now appreciated that the prostate gland is not a major source, the active substance was called prostaglandin. They are now known to exist in all cells, and since they are synthesized in response to hormones and can stimulate cyclic nucleotide formation (e.g. cAMP) they can be considered as intracellular 'second messengers'. Various prostaglandins have been isolated and each one is identified by a letter (e.g. A, B, C, D, E, and F) denoting the type of ring structure, a subscript numeral (e.g. 1 or 2) denoting the number of double bonds present, and finally by either α or β subscripts identifying the stereoisomeric form of the molecule.

The synthesis of prostaglandins (PG) involves the initial formation of extremely labile intermediates called endoperoxides which are precursors for other biologically active, although equally labile, molecules called thromboxanes. These, in turn, are rapidly metabolized to stable thromboxane B derivatives. The endoperoxides act as precursors for another active molecule called prostacyclin (PGI_2) following a different synthesis pathway. Arachidonic acid is the substrate for another group of active molecules called leucotrienes which are synthesized by leucocytes in the blood. Unlike the prostaglandins and thromboxanes, which appear to act chiefly as intracellular mediators, the leucotrienes and prostacyclin are released by the cells which synthesize them and can be considered to be hormones (Fig. 2.7).

Intracellular effects of hormones on protein synthesis

The various metabolic processes that regulate the functions of a cell are controlled by enzymes. These proteins consist of genetically determined arrangements of amino acids, the codes for which reside in the genes of nuclear chromosomes. Other proteins are synthesized for transport out of the cell. As mentioned previously some hormones, in particular steroids, are capable of penetrating the plasma membranes of cells to combine with their specific intracellular receptors. Some of the complexes thus formed appear to be able to influence protein synthesis at the nuclear level which suggests that they activate particular gene sequences.

Some peptide hormones which bind to membrane receptors on their target cell surface can influence nuclear gene transcription processes. It is quite possible that some may do so directly, following an internalization process. However, they can certainly do so indirectly, by activating specific intracellular protein kinases which themselves contain specific nuclear recognition elements, or which activate other intracellular transcription factors such as the STATs (signal transducers and activators of transcription) (see Fig. 2.2).

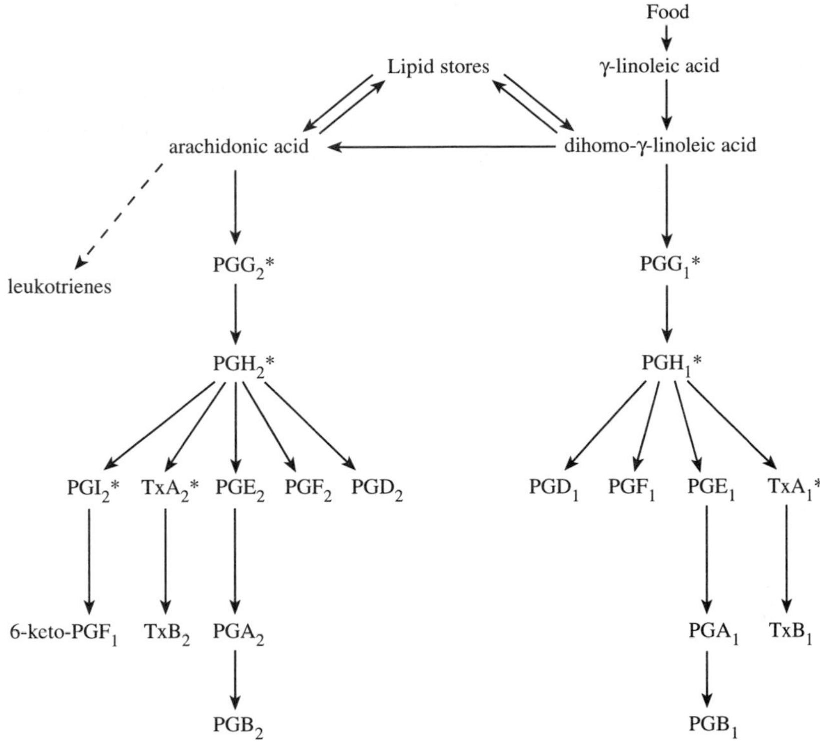

Fig. 2.7. The synthesis pathways for the various prostaglandins (PG) and thromboxanes (Tx) derived from precursors arachidonic and dihomo-γ-linoleic acids. Those intermediate molecules identified by an asterisk (*) are extremely unstable and short-lived.

Gene transcription

Much work on hormone-stimulated gene transcription has been done, particularly with respect to steroids. Most hormone-regulated genes share a common structural feature which is the presence of sequences of nucleotides that act as hormone-response (or hormone-binding) elements (HRE). These are similar to DNA sequences known as enhancers, and they bind specific transcription factors such as hormone-receptor complexes. Steroid hormones are an important group of transcription factors. They bind to the hormone-binding domains (D) of their receptors which have separate DNA-binding domains (C) and domains with transcription activation functions. The DNA-binding domains contain the two 'zinc fingers' which are necessary for the successful recognition and binding of the steroid hormone-response elements on the DNA. The purpose of the hormone-receptor complex linkage to the HRE on the target DNA is to modulate the transcription process for the ultimate synthesis of a protein molecule. Various mechanisms to explain transcription repression have been proposed, and these include binding of repressor sequences to DNA directly or binding to the transcription activator prior to DNA binding.

There are, in fact, two stages in the synthesis of protein that can be influenced by hormones: (1) the transcription of the code from DNA to RNA; and (2) the translation of the mRNA code to the synthesis of the protein on the ribosomes. Steroid hormones, such as cortisol and oestrogen, stimulate protein synthesis mainly at the transcription stage since their effects can be blocked by actinomycin D which irreversibly combines with the DNA. The effects of other hormones which stimulate cellular protein synthesis may be blocked by puromycin which inhibits the translation stage. Such hormones are therefore assumed to stimulate the translation stage possibly by increasing the rate at which tRNA takes up amino acids.

FURTHER READING

Carson-Jurica, M.A., Schrader, W.T., and O'Malley, B.W. (1990). Steroid receptor family: structure and function. *Endocrine Reviews*, **11**, 201–20.

Fantyl, W.J., Johnson, D.E., and Williams, L.T. (1993). Signalling by receptor tyrosine kinases. *Annual Review of Biochemistry*, **62**, 453–82.

Gordeladze, J.O., Johansen, P.W., Paulssen, R.H., Paulssen, E.J., and Gautvik, K.M. (1994). G-proteins: implications for pathophysiology and disease. *European Journal of Endocrinology*, **131**, 555–74.

Kolb, A., Busby, S., Buc, H., Garges, S., and Adhya, S. (1993). Transcriptional regulation by cAMP and its receptor protein. *Annual Review of Biochemistry*, **62**, 749–96.

Majerus, P.W. (1992). Inositol phosphate biochemistry. *Annual Review of Biochemistry*, **61**, 225–50.

Tsai, M-J. and O'Malley, B.W. (1994). Molecular mechanisms of action of steroid/thyroid receptor superfamily members. *Annual Review of Biochemistry*, **63**, 451–86.

Wilson, J.D. and Foster, D.W. (1992). *Williams textbook of endocrinology*. Eighth edition. See Chapters 3 and 4. W.B. Saunders Co.

3

Control of the endocrine system

INTRODUCTION

When there is an increased demand for a particular hormone the relevant endocrine gland is stimulated to produce it in increased quantities. Once the specific effect of the hormone on its target cells has satisfied that demand, then there is no further need for the hormone to be produced at the increased rate. Indeed, it is important that having done its job: (a) the biologically active hormone is removed from the circulation; and (b) the endocrine gland gets the message so that it can go back to its normal basal state. The latter process is concerned with feedback control and will be considered later in the chapter. First, we shall consider how the hormone is removed from the circulation.

HORMONE-RECEPTOR ENDOCYTOSIS

Some of the protein/peptide hormones bind to their cell membrane receptors, exert their specific effects, and then the hormone-receptor complexes are taken into the cells by receptor-mediated endocytosis. This process is unlike other forms of internalization, such as pinocytosis, because it involves the selective concentration of absorbed ligands (molecules that are recognized by a particular receptor), receptors, and other membrane proteins into clathrin-coated pits. Clathrin is a long protein which, associated with other proteins, forms the pits which 'trap' particular proteins such as receptors or receptor-hormone complexes. Some receptors appear to be captured readily by coated pits whereas others only become internalized once they have bound to their hormones (e.g. insulin receptors). Some hormone-receptor complexes are clustered together before becoming captured by coated pits. Once internalized, the hormone-receptor complexes rapidly appear in non-coated vesicles called endosomes in which the hormones can be separated from their receptors and be directed either to lysosomes for degradation, or back to the cell membrane as part of a recycling pathway (Fig. 3.1).

It is likely that receptor-mediated endocytosis plays an important role in removing a hormone from its receptor and directing it to a degradation pathway. It would also influence target tissue sensitivity by regulating the number of cell-surface receptors available for further hormone binding.

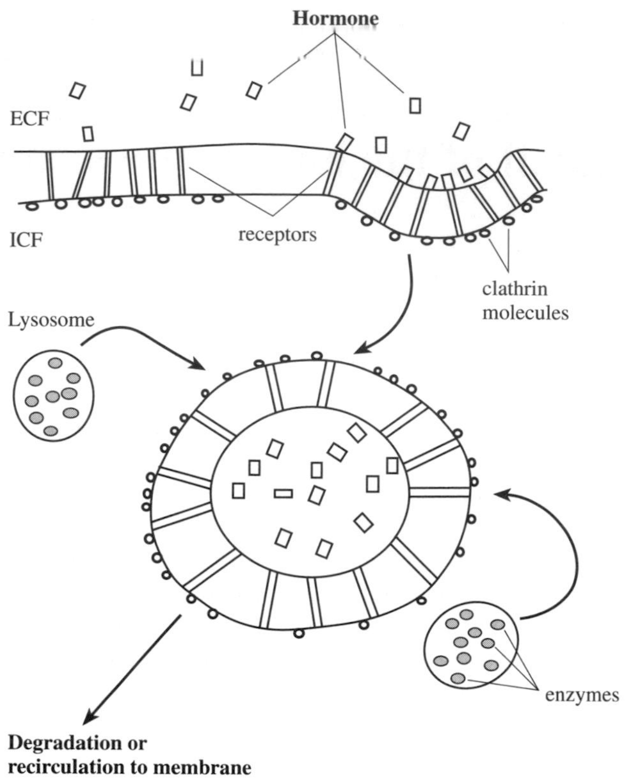

Fig. 3.1. Hormone receptor endocytosis. Once internalized, the hormone molecules can be degraded by lysosomal enzymes while the receptors can either be degraded or recirculated back to the membrane.

HORMONE INACTIVATION AND EXCRETION

The removal of a hormone from the bloodstream is a process which often takes place in two stages: (1) the inactivation (or degradation) of the hormone molecule; and (2) the excretion of the inactive metabolites.

Protein and polypeptide hormones are inactivated by the action of protease enzymes which cleave the large molecules into smaller components by acting at specific peptide bonds. For example, carboxypeptidases and aminopeptidases split molecules at the *C*- or *N*-terminal amino acids, respectively. Other enzymes work on specific components of the hormone molecule. For example, deiodinase enzymes split off iodine atoms from the iodothyronine hormones. Steroid hormones can be metabolized to inactive molecules by a process called conjugation which also renders them water-soluble and hence easier to excrete.

One site of inactivation for many hormones is the target tissue itself (see receptor-mediated endocytosis, p. 29). The lactating mammary gland has been implicated as an inactivation site and excretory organ for oxytocin, this hormone being detected in the milk of some mammals such as the goat and the cow. In addition, oxytocin is actually inactivated by a circulating enzyme called oxytocinase, found in the blood of pregnant women.

However, the two principal organs involved in the inactivation and excretion of hormones and their metabolites are the liver and the kidneys. Probably the most important is the liver which metabolizes many hormones, conjugating them with glucuronide or sulphate, for instance. Such water-soluble conjugates can then be secreted into the bile and excreted in the faeces (or reabsorbed via the enterohepatic circulation), or they can enter the bloodsteam to be excreted by the kidneys. It is important to remember that the liver and the kidneys not only convert certain hormones to inactive forms which can then be removed from the body, but also convert some inactive molecules (precursor prohormones) to biologically active molecules (hormones). Examples include the formation of the growth factors called somatomedins (insulin-like growth factors, IGFs) in the liver, and the potent dihydroxyvitamin D metabolite 1,25-dihydroxycholecalciferol from the (relatively) inactive hepatic precursor 25-hydroxycholecalciferol molecule in the kidneys.

Although some hormones are inactivated and excreted by different tissues, others may be degraded and excreted by the same organ. Some hormones are also excreted directly, as active molecules. Thus, on the one hand the kidneys inactivate some hormones and excrete the inactivated metabolites, and on the other, some low-molecular weight hormones are excreted directly into the urine. One example of such a hormone is vasopressin which appears in the urine in direct proportion to its concentration in the plasma (Fig. 3.2).

Hormone inactivation particularly in the liver is dependent on critical enzyme activity, predominantly the P-450 microsomal system. These enzymes can be induced by a wide variety of drugs in chemical usage, and this may account for many of the unwanted side-effects produced by chemicals used for the treatment of particular disorders.

The assay of hormones or metabolites in the urine is of value because it can be used to estimate the daily excretion of hormones, thus indicating (with certain limitations) the daily secretion rate of the hormones by their endocrine glands. For instance, the urinary excretion of pregnanediol, an inactive metabolite of progesterone, can be of (limited) value in determining the hormonal status of the fetoplacental unit during pregnancy.

FEEDBACK MECHANISMS

The basic function of a hormone is to regulate the activity of its target cells in a specific manner. To maintain this function it is essential that the endocrine gland cells receive constant, rapid information about the state of the systems being regulated. Release of the hormone can then be finely adjusted to the requirement of the target tissues by such feedback mechanisms. Usually, an endocrine gland continually receives signals from a variety of sources and the actual rate of hormone synthesis and secretion from the gland is therefore determined by the integration of

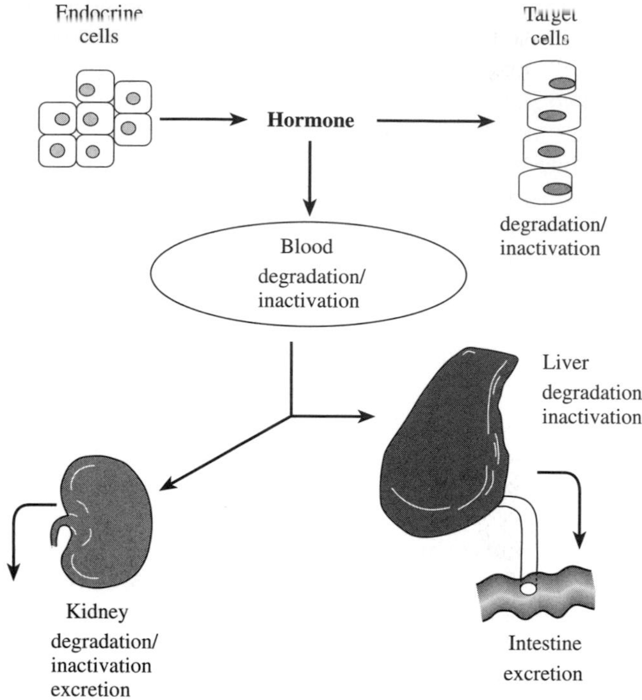

Fig. 3.2. The removal of hormone from the blood can be accomplished by enzyme degradation and/or inactivation in the blood itself, the target cells, the liver or the kidneys. Some hormone can be excreted (e.g. by the kidneys) unchanged.

these different signals. Various feedback loops have been shown to operate in endocrine systems, and these are briefly considered in the following sections.

Direct negative feedback

Probably the most straightforward feedback to an endocrine gland is the negative feedback system which relates the rate of production of the hormone to the blood concentration of that chemical substance which it controls, or to a chemical product of the metabolic process which it regulates, so that the response to the hormone opposes the generation of its stimulus. An example of this type of 'metabolite' feedback mechanism is the relationship between the hormone insulin and the principal variable which it controls, the blood glucose concentration. Insulin acts upon its target cells ultimately to decrease blood glucose levels; a change in these levels in turn alters the rate of secretion of insulin. Thus, a rise in blood glucose concentration (the stimulus) increases the rate of secretion of the hormone which then acts on its target cells to restore the blood glucose back to normal levels thereby reducing the stimulus for further insulin secretion (direct negative 'metabolite' feedback; see Fig. 3.3).

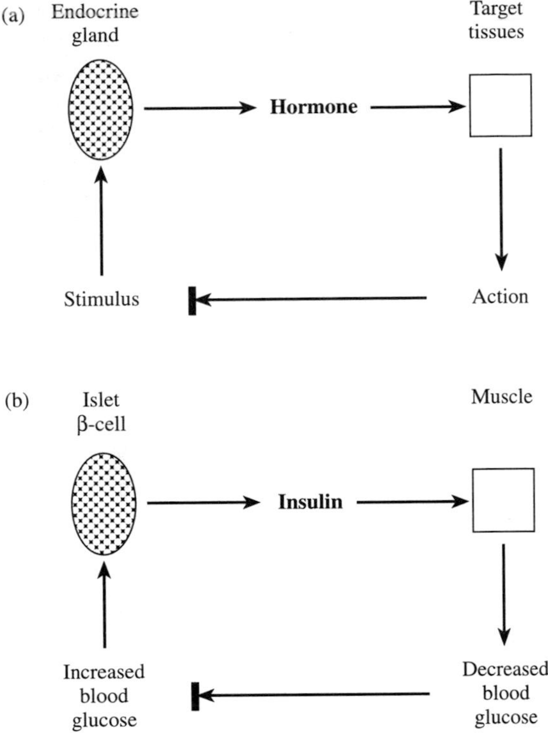

Fig. 3.3. Direct negative feedback: (a) the basic negative feedback loop principle; and (b) an example of a direct negative feedback loop using insulin and its effect on blood glucose concentration.

Some hormones from the adenohypophysis (anterior lobe of the pituitary gland) act primarily to regulate the secretions of other endocrine glands. For example, an endocrine gland (e.g. the thyroid) produces hormone A (in this case thyroxine, T_4 and/or triiodothyronine, T_3) when stimulated by hormone B (e.g. thyrotrophin) from the adenohypophysis. As the plasma level of hormone A increases it influences its own release by direct negative feedback on the adenohypophysial hormone B. Thus, an important action of hormone A is to act upon the cells which secrete the endocrine stimulus for its own release, inhibiting the secretion of hormone B (Fig. 3.4). The blood level of hormone A is regulated by its negative feedback influence on the stimulus for its own release (i.e. hormone B). If one considers the production of hormone A as the response to stimulus hormone B, then like any other direct negative feedback system, the response opposes the generation of its stimulus.

Indirect negative feedback

This term is used when the central nervous system, in particular the hypothalamus, is indirectly involved in the regulation of hormone secretion from an endocrine gland by influencing the release of the appropriate adenohypophysial hormone. Using the adenohypophysial–thyroidal axis described above, hormone A (tri-iodothyronine) from the target endocrine gland (the thyroid) has a direct negative feedback on the release of the adenohypophysial hormone B (thyrotrophin, see previous section), and an indirect negative feedback on the release of the hypothalamic hormone C (thyrotrophin-releasing hormone, TRH). This indirect involvement of the hypothalamus is particularly important in the control not only of thyroidal hormones (Fig. 3.4) but also adrenocortical and gonadal hormone secretions (see relevant chapters).

Auto (short-loop) negative feedback

As mentioned above, the hypothalamus controls the release of adenohypophysial hormones by the production of its releasing, or in some instances release-inhibiting, hormones. Some adenohypophysial hormones can influence their own release by having a feedback influence on the secretion of their release-stimulating or release-inhibiting hypothalamic hormones. This form of feedback control from

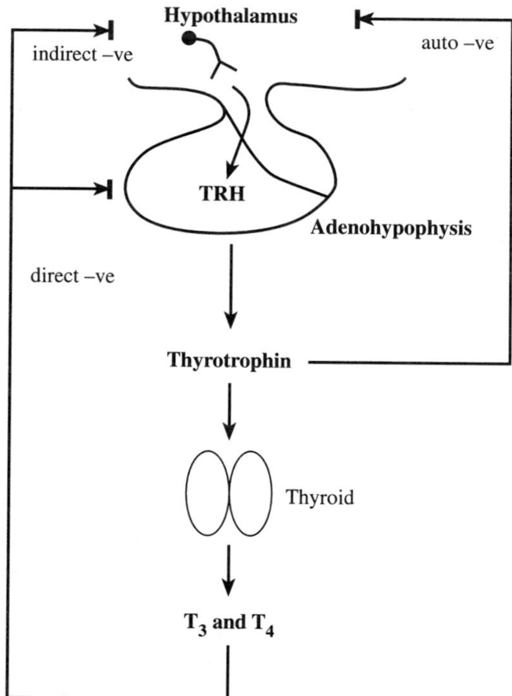

Fig. 3.4. The auto-, direct, and indirect negative feedback control loops linking target endocrine gland, adenohypophysis, and hypothalamus. The thyroid and its iodothyronine hormones (T_3 and T_4) is used as the example. (TRH, thyrotrophin-releasing hormone.) (See also Chapter 9.)

pituitary back to hypothalamus is called auto-feedback or short-loop feedback. One example of such a loop is the negative feedback exerted by somatotrophin (growth hormone) on its own release by a stimulatory effect on the production of somatostatin, a hypothalamic somatotrophin-inhibiting hormone (Fig. 3.4).

Indirect 'metabolite' negative feedback

In some endocrine systems, another negative feedback loop can operate, involving a metabolite acting on the hypothalamus to influence the release of a hypothalamic hormone, and therefore the release of the relevant adenohypophysial hormone under its control. An example of such a feedback is provided by the relationship between blood glucose concentration and the release of somatotrophin from the adenohypophysis. A decrease in blood glucose stimulates the release of somatotrophin, probably by inhibiting the release of hypothalamic inhibitory hormone somatostatin. Somatotrophin then participates in raising the blood glucose concentration, which in turn reduces the secretion of somatotrophin by the indirect 'metabolite' negative feedback at the hypothalamus.

Positive feedback mechanisms

Perhaps surprisingly, a hormone can, in particular circumstances, stimulate its own secretion. Thus, this kind of control, called positive feedback, involves the hormone acting as a stimulus of its own production. The principal positive feedback loops so far identified are the ones which exist between the ovarian hormone 17ß-oestradiol and certain hormones of the hypothalamo–hypophysial axis. A positive feedback loop can occur, under certain specific circumstances only (described in detail in Chapter 8), between high plasma concentrations of oestrogen and the adenohypophysial hormones follicle-stimulating hormone (FSH) and luteinizing hormone (LH), and the hypothalamic gonadotrophin-releasing hormone (GnRH). The positive feedback loop to the adenohypophysis is direct, whereas the loop to the hypothalamus is indirect (Fig. 3.5).

It is important to remember that any positive feedback loop is intrinsically unstable and consequently is a rarity. The reason why such instability does not usually get out of hand is that other feedback mechanisms are also operating to keep it under control. For instance, although positive feedback can occur at one particular level of the hormone, once the concentration has reached another, critical, level it can trigger a negative feedback mechanism which will then oppose the further rise in the hormone concentration.

Furthermore, it appears that 17ß-oestradiol produced by a developing ovarian follicle stimulates the growth of that follicle directly, thereby producing more of the hormone. This positive feedback effect by oestrogen is believed to act by stimulating the synthesis of receptors specific for circulating gonadotrophins. The follicle becomes increasingly sensitive to gonadotrophin by this action of oestrogen, and consequently produces increased quantities of this sex hormone.

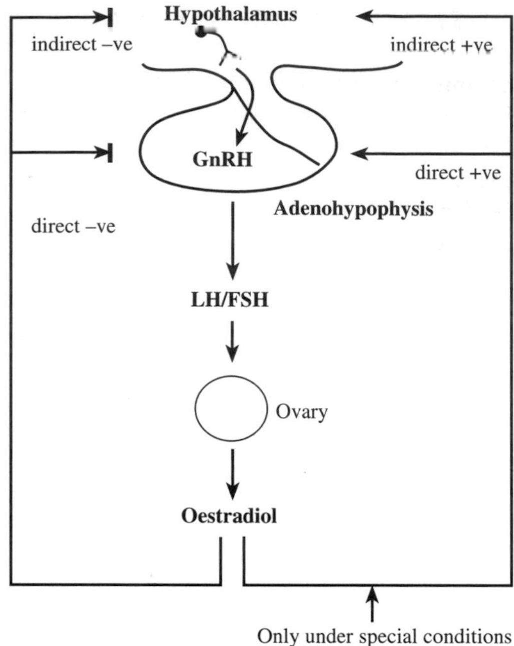

Fig. 3.5. The positive feedback loops (direct and indirect) which operate between the ovarian steroids (particularly oestradiol) and the hypothalamo–adenohypophysial axis under certain very specific conditions. (GnRH, gonadotrophin-releasing hormone; LH, luteinizing hormone, FSH, follicle-stimulating hormone.) (See also Chapter 8.)

The local production of growth factors is another way that the ovarian follicle can stimulate its own growth and development. In addition, growth factors such as the insulin-like growth factors, IGF-I and IGF-II, which are produced by the ovary probably exert an important influence on this increased sensitivity to gonadotrophins.

Intracellular feedback mechanisms

In addition to the 'extrinsic' feedback loops described in the previous sections, there are additional feedback mechanisms operating within the endocrine gland cells ('intrinsic' loops). Examples of such systems include the inhibition by organic iodide of iodothyronine hormone synthesis in the thyroid gland, the inhibition of 25-hydroxylation of cholecalciferol by previously formed 25-hydroxycholecalciferol in the liver, and the negative feedback loop which can exist between cAMP and the intracellular calcium ion concentration. There are probably many different intracellular feedback loops, and these are likely to be increasingly investigated as experimental techniques improve.

ENDOCRINE DISORDERS

Any endocrine system must include the source of hormone (the endocrine gland), the bloodstream which carries the hormone to its sites of action (the target tissues), the sites of inactivation and excretion, and finally the feedback loops linking the response to the hormone with the endocrine gland (Fig. 3.6). In such a system, there are many possibilities for disruption producing disorders which can be generally classified into two groups: (1) disorders which are associated with a decrease or absence of specific hormonal activity; and (2) those which are associated with increased hormonal activity. In either situation, the resulting disorder can be due to disruption at various levels in the system. For example (see also Fig. 3.6):

(a) The endocrine cells may fail to produce a hormone because of lack or absence of an enzyme crucial to the synthesis of that hormone (e.g. congenital adrenal hyperplasia).

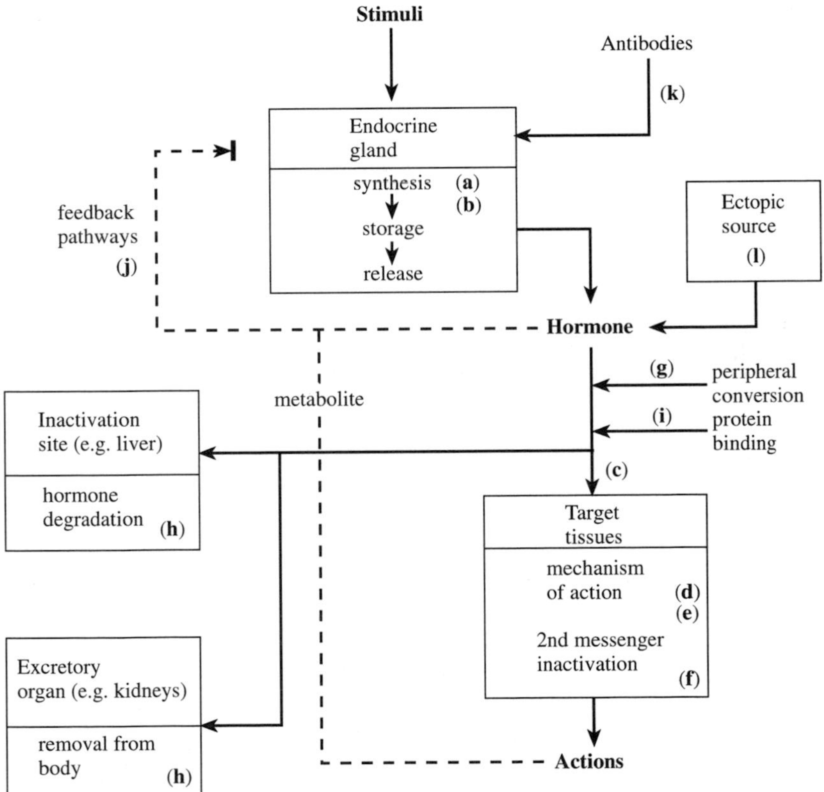

Fig. 3.6. Diagram showing some of the main disruption points in a typical endocrine system which can result in a clinical disorder.

(b) Synthesis failure may result from a genetic defect which results in the transcription of an abnormal, biologically inactive protein.

(c) The endocrine gland may function quite normally and secrete the hormone into the blood, but that hormone may be unable to stimulate its target cells because of an absence or deficiency of specific receptors (e.g. some forms of dwarfism).

(d) There may be a failure in some component of the mechanism of action initiated by the hormone within the target cell (e.g. perhaps the generation of the second messenger itself does not occur, even though the hormone has successfully bound to its receptor).

(e) It is possible that the second messenger is successfully generated but the defect lies at a later stage of the intracellular process.

(f) The excessive (uncontrolled) breakdown of the intracellular messenger may occur before it can initiate subsequent metabolic processes (one example of such a defect, the excessively rapid inactivation of the second messenger cAMP by phosphodiesterase enzyme, is a form of nephrogenic diabetes insipidus in mice).

(g) The lack or absence of a peripheral converting enzyme can be an important cause of endocrine abnormality. One particularly striking example is the absence of 5α-reductase enzyme in genetic males in whom the inability to convert testosterone to the more potent dihydrotestosterone during the early years of growth is manifest by their apparent outwardly female appearance. Interestingly, at puberty, such is the tremendous production of the weaker androgen testosterone that it can induce sufficient masculinization to alter the physical appearance from female to male.

(h) Abnormal inactivation mechanisms can also cause endocrine disorders: the syndrome of inappropriate antidiuretic hormone/vasopressin (ADH) can result from decreased inactivation by the liver in cirrhosis, for instance. Not surprisingly, hepatic and renal disease are often associated with secondary changes in endocrine function.

(i) Abnormal changes in plasma protein synthesis can be associated with liver disease. Since many of these proteins (e.g. specific globulins, growth factors, and precursor molecules) are associated with various endocrine systems, secondary endocrine disorders can develop.

(j) Impaired feedback mechanisms can also lead to endocrine disorders, the defect occurring at the endocrine cell itself. Modulation of receptors could be responsible in some cases; for instance, oestrogens increase the sensitivity of the thyrotrophin response to hypothalamic thyrotrophin-releasing hormone, with no alteration in the adenohypophysial thyrotrophin content.

(k) Autoimmune diseases can also cause endocrine malfunction. Graves' disease is one example of an autoimmune process in which antibodies to thyroid cell components are produced by the body, causing excessive thyroid hormone production. On the other hand, auto-immune diseases can be associated with decreased hormone production such as in autoimmune thyroiditis and adrenalitis.

(l) Finally, endocrine disorders can also occur as a result of excessive production of hormones, not from the endocrine gland but from another non-glandular source such as a tumour. This is called ectopic secretion. One example is the production of corticotrophin from a carcinoma of the lung.

FURTHER READING

Lutz, W., Salisbury, J.L., and Kumar, R. (1991). Vasopressin receptor-mediated endocytosis: current view. *American Journal of Physiology*, **261**, F1–13.

4

The hypothalamo–hypophysial axis

PHYSIOLOGY

The hypothalamus and its neurosecretions

The fundamental importance of the hypothalamus within the endocrine system was only truly appreciated following the classical experiments of Harris in the 1950s. This region of the brain is now considered as an 'endocrine gland', in addition to its previously accepted neural functions which include the regulation of autonomic nervous reflexes and temperature control. Its endocrine function is closely associated with that of the hypophysis (pituitary gland) and results from the various secretions by hypothalamic neurones which are released either into a special portal blood system linking hypothalamus to adenohypophysis (anterior pituitary), or into a capillary network in the neurohypophysis (posterior pituitary).

Anatomy

The hypothalamus consists of nervous tissue below the thalamus. It virtually surrounds part of the third ventricle, with afferent and efferent fibres connecting it to the rest of the central nervous system. There are numerous groups of nerve cells (hypothalamic nuclei) but it is not yet possible to designate specific functions to many of them. Some of the nuclei associated with endocrine function are shown in Fig. 4.1. The lower part of the hypothalamus, the median eminence, connects with the pituitary gland.

The hypothalamus is supplied with blood from the circle of Willis and most of the venous blood drains into the vein of Galen. Blood from the superior hypophysial arteries, which arise from the internal carotids, flows through a capillary plexus in the median eminence to enter a sinusoidal network in the pituitary stalk (the infundibulum). Blood passes from the sinusoids into a second capillary plexus in the anterior pituitary gland (the adenohypophysis). This is an example of a venous portal system linking two capillary networks, and is called the hypothalamo–hypophysial portal system (Fig. 4.2).

The hypothalamic neurosecretions

Certain hypothalamic nuclei contain nerve cell bodies which send their axons down to the median eminence where they terminate in close proximity to the capillaries of the primary network, or straight through the pituitary stalk to the posterior lobe of the pituitary gland (neurohypophysis). Many substances released by hypothalamic neurones have now been identified as peptides. The network of

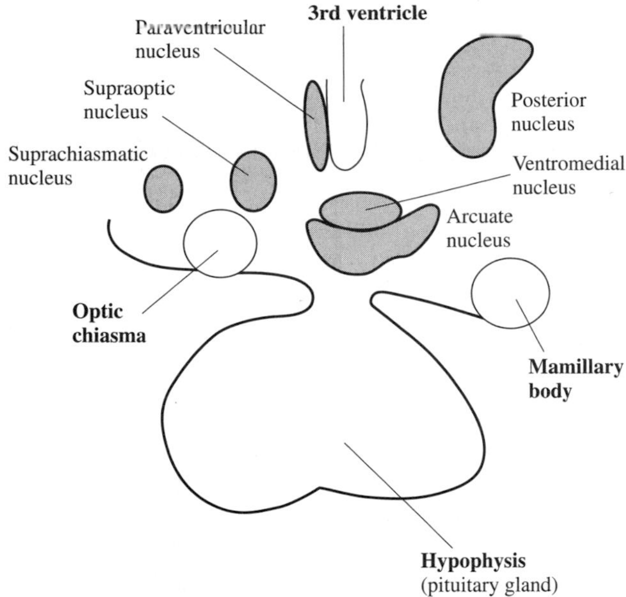

Fig. 4.1. Diagram showing some of the important hypothalamic nuclei associated with hormone production. These nuclei are composed of numerous neurone cell bodies which synthesize specific hormones; these may be released from nerve terminals in the median eminence or the posterior lobe of the pituitary (neurohypophysis).

neurones associated with the synthesis, storage, and release of these neuropeptides has therefore been called the peptidergic neuronal system. Many of these neurosecretions function as hormones: they are released from nerve terminals which are in close association with capillaries, and they then enter the bloodstream which carries them to their target cells in the adenohypophysis. The release of these peptides from nerve terminals into the blood is called neurosecretion. The peptides are initially synthesized as much larger pre-prohormones according to specific gene sequences. Following transcription, and translation on the endoplasmic reticulum, they are transferred to the Golgi complex where the final products of enzyme action are packaged into granules. The granules migrate down the axons and their contents are released to the exterior by exocytosis following depolarization of the nerve terminals. Thus, these peptidergic neurones have similar characteristics to other neurones.

The neurosecretory cells in the various hypothalamic nuclei have numerous connections with terminals from neurones originating in other parts of the central nervous system. Therefore, their overall activity is greatly influenced by signals received from other parts of the brain, these being either stimulatory or inhibitory. Neurotransmitters which have been shown to influence the activity of the different hypothalamic neurosecretory cells include noradrenaline, dopamine, acetycholine, serotonin, opioids, and GABA (γ-aminobutyric acid). Thus, the central nervous system can exert an important regulatory influence over many metabolic and other

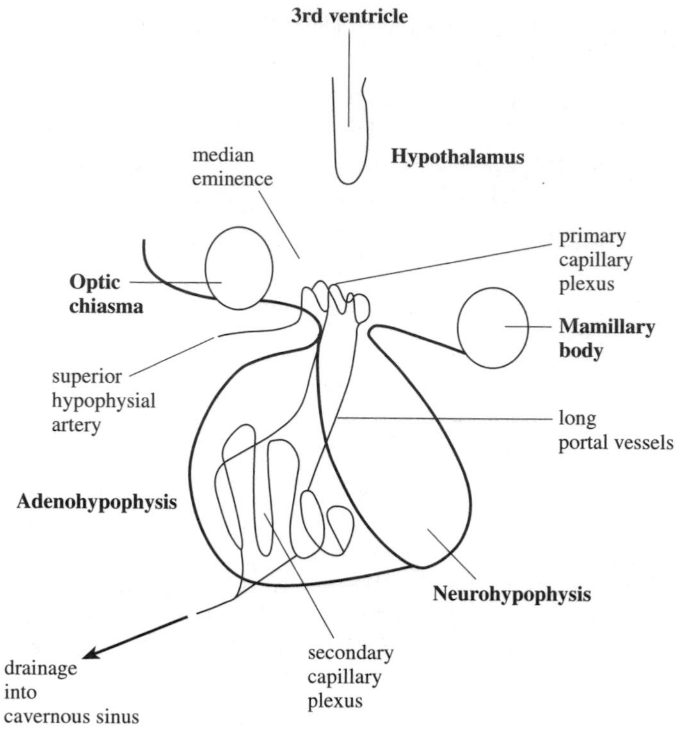

Fig. 4.2. Diagram showing the primary capillary plexus in the hypothalamic median eminence, the descending long portal vessels, and the second capillary plexus in the adenohypophysis (anterior pituitary). This system is called the hypothalamo–hypophysial portal system.

functions in the body by altering the synthesis and/or release of hypothalamic neuropeptides (hypothalamic hormones). These in turn act on their specific target cells in the adenohypophysis, controlling the release of the adenohypophysial hormones. This probably accounts for the important influence of external stimuli, such as environmental changes, emotions and stress on adenohypophysial function.

The hypothalamo–adenohypophysial system

Many hypothalamic neurosecretions are released into a primary capillary network in the median eminence, and thus enter the hypothalamo–hypophysial portal blood. These hormones are transported to their target cells in the adenohypophysis which they can then either stimulate or inhibit. The adenohypophysial cells also produce hormones and therefore the release of these adenohypophysial hormones is itself under hormonal control from the hypothalamus. Various hypothalamic hormones have so far been isolated and identified, and they are called releasing — or inhibiting — hormones depending on their primary action. They include:

(1) thyrotrophin-releasing hormone (TRH), a tripeptide which stimulates thyrotrophin and prolactin release;
(2) gonadotrophin-releasing hormone (GnRH), a decapeptide which stimulates the release of follicle-stimulating hormone (FSH) and luteinizing hormone (LH);
(3) corticotrophin-releasing hormone (CRH), also known as corticoliberin, a 41-amino acid polypeptide which stimulates corticotrophin release;
(4) the 44-amino acid polypeptide somatotrophin-releasing hormone (SRH), also known as somatoliberin and by the more cumbersome name growth hormone-releasing hormone (GHRH) which stimulates the release of somatotrophin (i.e. growth hormone); and
(5) somatostatin (SS), a tetradecapeptide which inhibits the release of somatotrophin (somatotrophin-inhibitory hormone).

When there is evidence for a hypothalamic hormonal influence on the release of an anterior pituitary hormone but the substance has not been chemically identified, it is generally called a releasing — or inhibiting — factor (see Table 4.1).

Not all the hormonal neurosecretions from the hypothalamus are peptides. For example, dopamine is clearly a hypothalamic hormone which inhibits the release of prolactin from the adenohypophysis. Other substances are also known to be

Table 4.1. The principal known hypothalamic releasing and inhibiting hormones and some of the adenohypophysial hormones which they influence

Hypothalamic hormones	Chemical structure	Adenohypophysial hormones
Thyrotrophin-releasing hormone (TRH)	3 aa	Thyrotrophin + Prolactin +
Gonadotrophin-releasing hormone (GnRH)	10 aa	Luteinizing hormone (LH) + Follicle-stimulating hormone (FSH) +
Corticotrophin-releasing hormone (CRH) (also known as corticoliberin)	41 aa	Corticotrophin +
Somatotrophin-releasing hormone (SRH) (also know as somatoliberin)	44 aa	Somatotrophin +
Somatostatin (SS)	14 aa	Somatotrophin – Thyrotrophin –
Antidiuretic hormone (ADH)/ Vasopressin	9aa	Corticotrophin +
Dopamine	1aa derivative	prolactin –

aa, amino acid; +, stimulation; –, inhibition.

released by neurones into the primary capillary plexus of the median eminence, and many of these are better known as molecules associated with other regions of the body. Natriuretic peptides and angiotensin II are such examples which probably have a modulatory influence on specific adenohypophysial hormone release. In addition, opioids, such as the enkephalins, may be released into the portal circulation and their role in adenohypophysial hormone regulation also requires elucidation.

One interesting, and important, finding is the coexistence of different biologically active molecules in the same nerve terminals in the median eminence. One example is the presence of corticotroprin-releasing hormone (CRH) and vasopressin in the same neurones; since both these molecules act together to stimulate the release of corticotrophin from the adenohypophysis it is likely that these particular neurones come into play under particular circumstances only. Probably pertinent is the recent finding that a volume depletion stress is associated with increased CRH mRNA, but not vasopressin mRNA, in these neurones.

Another point to appreciate is that some of the hypothalamic peptides are found in other parts of the body. One particularly ubiquitous molecule is somatostatin. Not only is it an important hormonal influence on somatotrophin release from the pituitary, but it is also found in other parts of the brain where it presumably acts as a neurotransmitter or neuromodulator, the gastrointestinal tract where it exerts various inhibitory effects (for instance on gut motility), and the endocrine pancreas where it can inhibit the release of insulin and glucagon.

As we have seen, the various identified hypothalamic hormones have been clearly related to stimulatory — or inhibitory — effects on specific adenohypophysial hormones (hence their names). However, it is important to appreciate that any one hypothalamic hormone can actually influence the release of more than one adenohypophysial hormone. As one example, consider thyrotrophin-releasing hormone (TRH), which is the dominant stimulator of thyrotrophin release from the thyrotrophe cells (see later). An additional action of TRH is to stimulate the lactotrophe cells of the adenohypophysis to produce prolactin. Thus, administration of TRH can be used to test pituitary function not only with respect to thyrotrophin release but also that of prolactin.

Finally, until recently it was believed that the hypothalamic innervation of the adenohypophysis was scarce and of little importance. Indeed, most nerve fibres are autonomic and terminate close to the blood vessels, hence the general assumption that any direct neural involvement with adenohypophysial function is purely concerned with regulation of blood flow (with a possible indirect influence over pituitary function). Now, there is increasing evidence of a direct hypothalamic innervation, with terminals actually on secretory cells of the adenohypophysis. Thus, it is likely that an additional, direct, control over adenohypophysial function is exerted by the hypothalamus.

Patterns of release

One characteristic of adenohypophysial hormones is that they are released in discrete pulses. These are associated with the pulsatile release patterns of the various regulatory neurosecretions from the hypothalamic neurones. Hence, this pulsatile release is related to the influence of the central nervous system, specifically the hypothalamus, over pituitary hormone release. The pulsatility of the release of these hormones may be vital for their normal function, and this is exemplified by the gonadotrophins luteinizing hormone (LH) and follicle-stimulating hormone (FSH). Normally, the pulses of LH and FSH follow the pulses of the gonadotrophin-releasing hormone (GnRH), with peaks approximately once each hour (circhoral) in primates. The GnRH 'pulse generator' is located in the arcuate nucleus of the medial basal hypothalamus. If the pulsatile release of GnRH is disrupted and replacement is given by continuous infusion, then after an initial increase the release of LH and FSH is inhibited. Administration of GnRH in regular pulses restores the normal release of LH and FSH, demonstrating how important the nature of hypothalamic hormone release can be, particularly with respect to the gonadotrophins. An interesting relationship between gonadal function and the light–dark sequence to which animals are exposed (in particular seasonal breeders) has pointed to a link between the hypothalamic GnRH neurones and the pineal gland (see below).

In addition to pulsatile release, some adenohypophysial hormones are secreted following diurnal rhythms. Again, this temporal relationship is associated with the hypothalamus and the secretion of releasing or inhibiting hormones. Interestingly, some diurnal patterns of release can be related to different stages in life. For example, a diurnal secretory pattern of LH and FSH is initiated during puberty, when large pulses are produced during the night, while in the adult this is much less marked.

The hypothalamus–pineal link: its influence on circadian and seasonal rhythms

The pineal gland is a small gland attached to the posterior wall of the third ventricle by a thin stalk. It consists of parenchymal cells called pinealocytes which contain features of typical secretory cells such as an extensive microtubular network, a prominent rough endoplasmic reticulum, a large Golgi complex, and numerous vesicles. Various roles have been ascribed to this gland in the past; it was once thought to be 'the seat of the soul' or the development of the rudimentary 'third eye' in invertebrates, and more recently simply to be a calcified vestigial organ. The principal innervation of the gland is by noradrenergic postganglionic sympathetic fibres arising from the superior cervical ganglia. This innervation is unusual because it forms the last link in a pathway relating responsiveness to light by the eye, through the suprachiasmatic nuclei in the hypothalamus (the 'biological clock' region) to the pineal (see Fig. 4.3). There is also some innervation directly from various nuclei in the brain, with different peptides (e.g. vasoactive intestinal peptide, somatostatin, neuropeptide Y, thyrotrophin-releasing hormone, and vasopressin) and acetylcholine the neurotransmitters so far identified. The pineal becomes increasingly calcified with age, although this is not necessarily related to decreased function of the pinealocytes. After puberty the principal pineal secretion, melatonin, does diminish but this is believed to be related more to the loss of catecholamine receptors or to other factors. Melatonin is a 5-methoxyindole synthesized from a precursor, serotonin (also known as 5-hydroxytryptamine)

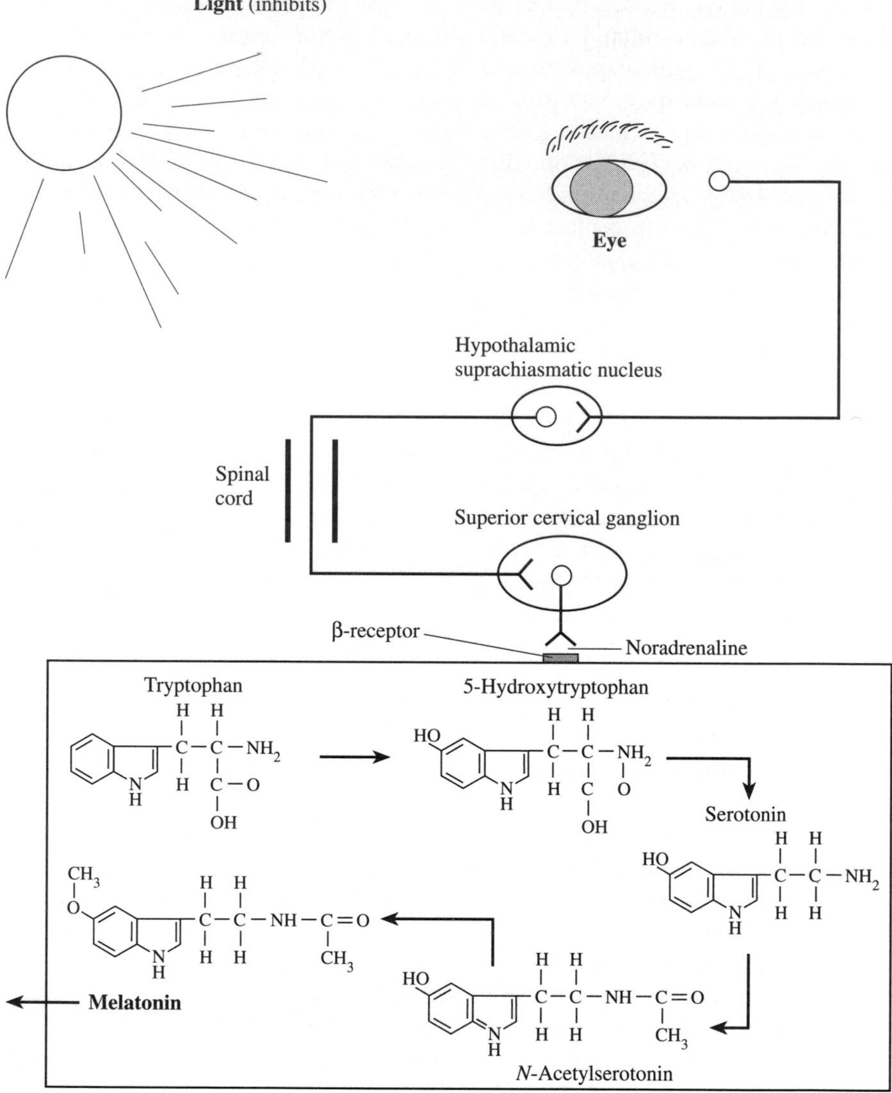

Fig. 4.3. The nerve pathway connecting the eye to the pineal gland, and (below) the synthesis of the principal pineal hormone, melatonin.

which is itself derived from tryptophan. Melatonin is metabolized in the liver to 6-hydroxymelatonin, which is excreted as either a glucuronide or a sulphate. The urinary excretory product 6-sulphatoxy-melatonin correlates well with circulating melatonin levels and can be used as a measure of 24-hour production. A circadian pattern of release normally occurs such that melatonin is released predominantly at night (i.e. during exposure to the dark) with exposure to bright light being associated with inhibition of release.

One function that has been associated with the pineal gland and melatonin is the regulation of circadian rhythms. Melatonin appears to be related to the setting of our 'biological clock', and its secretion is itself more firmly linked to this clock than to the night–day cycle. Thus, it may be relevant to aspects of our lives such as night-shift work and travel across time zones. It is interesting to note that melatonin receptors have now been located in the suprachiasmatic nucleus (SCN) which is believed to be important in setting our circadian rhythms (see above). Thus, the sensory pathway linking the eyes (i.e. light–dark cycle) to the pineal involves the SCN, and the pineal through melatonin may have a direct influence on the SCN.

A second function of the pineal is that it may exert an important influence on the hypothalamo–hypophysial–gonadal axis, and seasonal breeding in particular. Melatonin appears to switch off the GnRH neurones under specific conditions. For example, various stressors are associated with raised melatonin levels and reduced circulating gonadotrophins (LH and FSH). Interestingly, the gonadal steroids appear to modulate melatonin production, suggesting a degree of 'cross-talk' between the the reproductive axis and the pineal gland. The pineal may also be associated with the onset of puberty; circulating levels fall after puberty, pineal parenchyme tumours producing increased quantities of melatonin are associated with delayed puberty, while teratomas or other non-parenchymal tumours are associated with precocious puberty.

The neurohypophysial system

Some hypothalamic neurones have their cell bodies located in two pairs of relatively discrete nuclei called the supraoptic and paraventricular nuclei (SON and PVN, respectively). The majority of axons from these nuclei extend down through the median eminence to terminate on capillaries in the posterior lobe (pars nervosa) of the pituitary gland. These neurosecretory cells are much larger than other neurones in the central nervous system and are therefore called magnocellular neurones. Swellings along the magnocellular neurone axons are called Hering bodies. The term 'neurohypophysis' is used to describe the pars nervosa since it differentiates the posterior lobe of the pituitary from the anterior lobe (the adenohypophysis) by its different histological appearance (see below). Functionally, however, the term 'neurohypophysis' should also include the hypothalamic nuclei (SON and PVN) and the nerve tract (the hypothalamo–hypophysial nerve tract). A preferred alternative is therefore to refer to the neurohypophysial system when considering the nuclei, the nerve tract, and the pars nervosa of the pituitary.

Some axons terminate on the capillaries of the primary plexus in the median eminance (mentioned earlier) while another axonal component has been observed to terminate on the walls of the third ventricle (see Fig. 4.4). Yet other fibres have been detected terminating in other parts of the brain, such as the hippocampus and areas of the brain stem which are associated with cardiovascular control such as the nucleus tractus solitarius and the dorsal nucleus of the vagus. The cells which sends their axons down to the median eminence are smaller than the magnocellular neurones, so they are called parvocellular neurones.

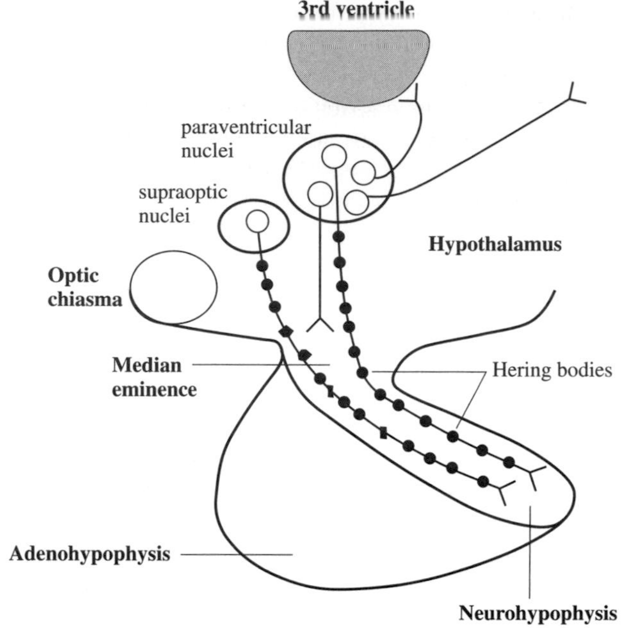

Fig. 4.4. The neurohypophysial system which includes the magnocellular neurones originating in the hypothalamic supraoptic and paraventricular nuclei, and the nerve tract passing through the pituitary stalk with fibres terminating in the neurohypohysis (posterior pituitary). Note that some nerve fibres from the hypothalamic nuclei terminate in other parts of the central nervous system, including the parvocellular fibres terminating in the median eminence.

There are two neurohypophysial hormones (both nonapeptides), called vasopressin (or antidiuretic hormone, ADH) and oxytocin.

Regulation of hypothalamic hormone secretion

The hypothalamic peptidergic neurones are subject to regulation by other nerves. These nerves may release neurotransmitters, such as the catecholamines, serotonin, vasoactive intestinal peptide (VIP), and acetylcholine which act on postsynaptic membranes, or neuromodulators such as the opioid enkephalins which may modulate the release of the neuropeptide hormones by acting on pre- and postsynaptic membranes. It is, of course, possible for any one hypothalamic neurosecretion to have more than one kind of action. For instance, TRH has been suggested to have three different roles: (1) as a hormone; (2) as a neurotransmitter; and (3) as a neuromodulator–depending on the site of action and the presence of specific receptors.

These neural control mechanisms, which influence the release of hypothalamic hormones (or factors), are one fundamental component of adenohypophysial hormone regulation. However, it must be emphasized that feedback mechanisms are also intimately involved in this regulation, and can act not only at the adeno-hypophysial level but also on the hypothalamus (see Chapter 3), and even on other ('higher') centres in the brain.

Certain feedback loops can have specific features. For example, the steroid hormone cortisol from the adrenal cortex can influence its own release by feedback on hypothalamus and adenohypophysis in two different time-frames, thus operating both fast and slow feedback mechanisms.

THE HYPOPHYSIS (PITUITARY GLAND)

The hypophysis, or pituitary, is an endocrine gland which lies in a bony cavity called the sella turcica. It is located at the base of the brain to which it is attached by an infundibular stem, or pituitary stalk. This link with the hypothalamus is crucial for the normal function of the hypophysis. As described earlier, hypothalamic neurones either have axons projecting to the median eminence where their secretions are released to influence anterior pituitary function, or send their axons down through the stalk to terminate in the posterior lobe of the pituitary.

The gland develops embryologically as a fusion between an up-growth of ectodermal cells from the roof of the primitive pharynx (buccal cavity), which forms the anterior lobe (the adenohypophysis), and a down-growth of neural tissue from the hypothalamus which forms the posterior lobe (the neurohypophysis). These two parts of the hypophysis are histologically different, and as a consequence of their development they function as two different endocrine glands. Between the two is a third lobe called the pars intermedia, or intermediate lobe. This is usually almost non-existent and vestigial in adult humans, although it is quite well developed in the fetus. It may increase in size during pregnancy or after pituitary stalk section.

The adenohypophysis (anterior pituitary)

The principal, and by far the largest, part of the adenohypophysis is the pars distalis. The upper part of the adenohypophysis which is 'wrapped' around the infundibulum is called the pars tuberalis. The pars distalis receives most of its blood supply from the paired superior hypophysial arteries in the hypothalamus. Arterial blood enters a network of capillary loops (primary plexus) in the ventral hypothalamus (the median eminence) drains into sinusoidal long portal vessels which descend through the pituitary stalk, and then flows into a second capillary network (secondary plexus) in the pars distalis. This blood system, involving two capillary networks linked by the portal vessels, is called the hypothalamo–hypophysial portal system (see Fig. 4.2). Approximately 15 per cent of the arterial blood reaching the pars distalis comes directly from the superior hypophysial arteries without going through the portal system. It is possible that some blood can flow to the anterior lobe via short portal vessels which originate in the posterior lobe of the pituitary. Although it is generally believed that blood flow through the hypothalamo–hypophysial portal system is unidirectional from median eminence to adenohypophysis, it is possible that blood flow can be reversed under certain circumstances. This would certinly tally with the evidence for short negative feedback loops which appear to operate between certain adenohypophysial hormones and their hypothalamic-releasing or -inhibiting hormones.

The pars distalis is innervated with sympathetic nerve fibres which probably have a vasomotor function in the region. Some of these fibres are not noradrenergic but contain other peptides such as vasoactive intestinal peptide. These neurosecretions may have an influence directly on specific adenohypophysial cell activity, or indirectly by influencing blood flow to the region. In contrast, although nervous connections with the hypothalamus are scarce, recent evidence suggests that this innervation is direct, with terminals seen on specific cells in the adenohypophysis. Thus, it is likely that some direct neural influence from the hypothalamus on adenohypophysial function may modulate the effects of releasing or inhibiting hormones released into the hypothalamo–hypophysial portal system.

Originally, histological staining techniques could identify only three types of cell: (1) acidophils (or eosinophils); (2) basophils; and (3) chromophobes. More specific immunohistochemical stains and electron microscopy now allow precise identification of the cells responsible for secreting the different hormones. The cell types are named after the hormones they produce; thus thyrotrophes, somatotrophes, and corticotrophes synthesize thyrotrophin, somatotrophin, and corticotrophin, respectively. The gonadotrophes are somewhat unusual because they synthesize two different gonadotrophins, luteinizing hormones (LH) and follicle-stimulating hormone (FSH). The fifth differentiated cell type is called the lactotrophe because it produces the lactogenic hormone, prolactin. Distribution of these cell types is not uniform within the adenohypophysis. This provides an explanation for the comparatively distinctive sites of tumour formation responsible for clinical endocrine states characterized by over-production of specific pituitary hormones. For example, somatotrophes, which form approximately 50 per cent of all endocrine cells in the adenohypophysis, are found mainly in the lateral wings. The exception is the wide, although not completely random, distribution of the lactotrophes throughout the anterior pituitary lobe.

The adenohypophysial hormones

The principal hormones from the adenohypophysis can be considered, somewhat arbitrarily, in two groups: (1) those which have their primary effect on target tissues directly; and (2) those whose primary effect is to stimulate other endocrine glands to secrete their hormones. Interestingly, the two hormones which act on more generalized target tissues, somatotrophin and prolactin, are both proteins with a high degree of homology in their structures. The other hormones are the glycoproteins thyrotrophin, LH and FSH, which also have certain similarities in structure, and the polypeptide hormone corticotrophin. Each of the adenohypophysial hormones (like other hormones) is released in quantities determined by the integration of the various signals, stimulatory and inhibitory, reaching the cell sites of synthesis.

Somatotrophin (growth hormone, GH)

The principal form of somatotrophin is a single-chain protein which, in humans, consists of 191 amino acids. It is synthesized mainly in the form of a molecule of approximately 22 kilodaltons, but other forms exist (e.g. a 20 kDa molecule). Initially, pre-prosomatotrophin is spliced to the precursor 27 kDa pro-somatotrophin molecule in the somatotrophe cells, and this is cleaved to the final secretory forms which are stored in cytoplasmic granules. Granule contents are released into the blood by exocytosis. In adults, the rate of secretion is variable during each 24 hours with a normal daily output of around 1.4 mg. In the plasma, various forms of somatotrophin have been identified, some of which are fragments.

Somatotrophin is closely related to prolactin (as well as placental lactogen, see Chapter 8) and shares many amino acid sequences. Not surprisingly, the genes for these three hormones are structurally similar, each one having four introns and five exons which code for the protein. The somatotrophin gene is located on chromosome 17 and is considerably smaller than the prolactin gene.

In the plasma, somatotrophin molecules bind to various binding proteins such that approximately 70 per cent is transported bound. The main binding protein (GHBP) has been found to have an amino acid sequence that is almost identical to the extracellular part of the somatotrophin target cell membrane receptor.

Actions of somatotrophin

The main physiological effect of somatotrophin is the promotion of linear growth and the maintenance of tissues which it induces most noticeably during adolescence. This is considered in more detail in Chapter 13. Its growth-promoting effect results partly from the stimulation of protein synthesis which is induced at the nuclear level and partly by an enhancement of amino acid transport through cell membranes. Many of its effects on linear growth are mediated by substances synthesized in many tissues, but mainly in the liver, under the influence of somatotrophin. These hormone mediators are polypeptides called somatomedins which stimulate cell proliferation (i.e. they are mitogenic) and/or cell differentiation depending on the tissue involved (see below).

It is important to appreciate that the growth and maintenance of tissues and the replacement of many cells are generally continuous processes under multifactorial regulation. There are numerous growth factors, many of them tissue-specific. These include epidermal growth factor, nerve growth factor, and the transforming growth factors. Many of the classical hormones also influence the growth and maintenance of tissues and these include the iodothyronines, insulin, the androgens, and the oestrogens (see relevant chapters), in addition to somatotrophin and the somatomedins.

The somatomedins

There are two somatomedins synthesized following stimulation of the hepatocytes by somatotrophin. These molecules both have considerable homology with each other, and with the proinsulin molecule. Because they have insulin-like effects in addition to their powerful growth-promoting action they are better known as insulin-like growth factors IGF-I and IGF-II, the latter having the greater insulin-like activity, while IGF-I has the greater growth-promoting effect. Many other tissues are now known to synthesize IGF-I, and this molecule has a wide range of activities in these different tissues, often of an autocrine regulatory nature. IGF-I is a 70-amino acid single-chain polypeptide, while IGF-II has 67 amino acids. Of the two hepatic molecules, IGF-I is the somatomedin more under the control of somatotrophin. Approximately 95 per cent of the somatomedins is transported in the blood bound to a variety of binding proteins (IGFBPs). Six such binding proteins have been identified, the principal one being IGFBP3 which is synthesized in the liver following stimulation by somatotrophin.

The IGF receptors are of two types, type 1 and type 2. The IGF type 1 and the insulin receptors are structurally similar. The IGF type 1 receptors have an extremely high affinity for IGF-I, a high affinity for IGF-II and a lesser affinity for insulin, and almost certainly mediate the main growth-promoting effects of IGF-I. The IGF type 2 receptor, on the other hand, has a high binding affinity for IGF-II, a lower affinity for IGF-I, and does not bind insulin at all. Many of the effects of IGF-II are probably mediated by the insulin and the IGF type 1 receptors although some are undoubtedly associated with the IGF type 2 receptors. The IGF type 1 receptors contain a tyrosine kinase domain which is activated once a ligand binds to the receptor. Not only can this result in the phosphorylation of tyrosyl units in intracellular proteins leading to induction of intracellular actions, but autophosphorylation of the receptor or adjacent receptors can occur leading to amplification of the initial signal.

Metabolic actions of somatotrophin

The increase in the growth of soft and skeletal tissues, induced by somatotrophin mainly through the mediation of IGF-I (and to a lesser extent IGF-II), is accompanied by changes in electrolyte metabolism. Indeed, nutritional factors (particularly dietary protein and energy) are an important regulatory influence on IGF-I production through hormones such as somatotrophin, insulin and iodothyronines on IGF and IGFBP synthesis. The somatotrophin–somatomedin-induced increase in protein synthesis results in a positive nitrogen and phosphorus balance, while blood urea levels fall. The intestinal absorption of calcium is increased and the urinary excretion of sodium and potassium fall probably as a consequence of the increased uptake of these ions by the growing tissues. Somatotrophin stimulates the uptake of non-esterified fatty acids (NEFA) by muscle and causes a significant but delayed increase in the mobilization of NEFA from adipose tissue. The hormone influences lipolysis through the mediation of cAMP. Somatotrophin also stimulates hepatic glycogenolysis and antagonizes the effect of insulin on glucose uptake by peripheral cells (see Chapter 11), so that the blood glucose concentration can increase. The roles of somatotrophin and insulin are complementary in inducing growth since they have protein anabolic effects and stimulate the transport of amino acids into peripheral cells, while their respective effects on the blood glucose level will tend to oppose each other. The picture is complicated by the insulin-like actions of IGF-I and IGF-II, which promote the uptake of glucose

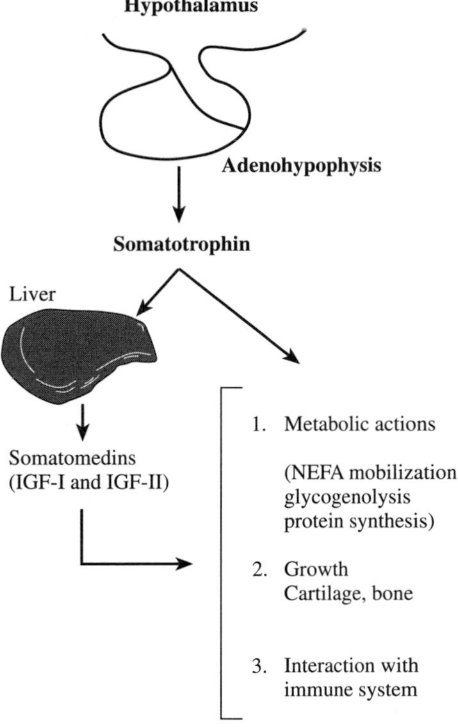

Fig. 4.5. The principal actions of somatotrophin (growth hormone), including the production of the intermediary somatomedins (insulin-like growth factors IGF-I and IGF-II).

(hence reducing the blood glucose concentration), probably via the insulin receptors. If excess somatotrophin is released due to an adenoma, the chronic overall effect is one of increasing insulin resistance and a hyperglycaemia which can become permanent (diabetes mellitus). An interaction between somatotrophin and the immune system is suggested by the enhanced T cell proliferation which is induced by this hormone (see Fig. 4.5).

Mechanism of action of somatotrophin

The hormone binds to two adjacent receptor molecules in the target cell membrane, forming a dimeric unit. The receptor is associated with a tyrosine kinase called JAK2 (a kinase belonging to the Janus family of proteins) which is activated by the hormone-receptor complex. Subsequent protein phosphorylation within the cytoplasm, for instance of the mitogen-activated protein kinase (MAPK), ultimately results in the intracellular mediation and expression of somatotrophin actions. An additional pathway induced by somatotrophin-receptor binding is the activation of membrane-bound phospholipase C mediated by a G protein. Subsequently, the increase in phosphoinositide metabolism and diacyl-

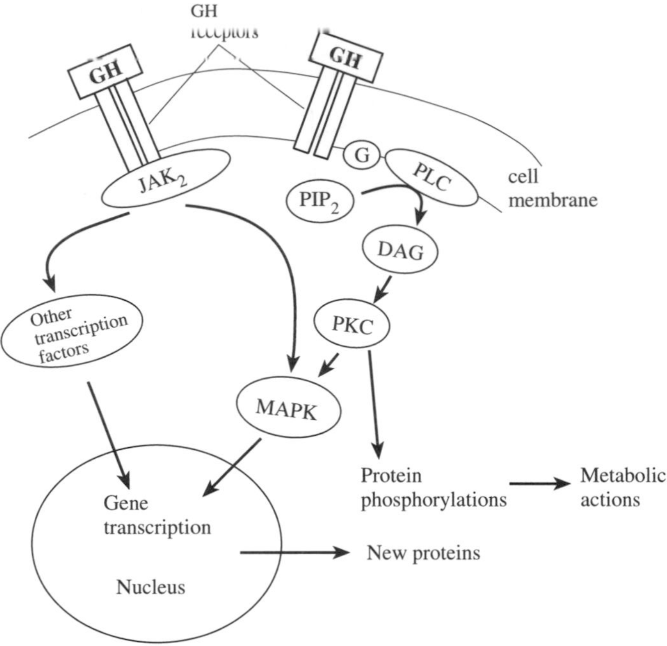

Fig. 4.6. The intracellular mechanisms of action of somatotrophin (growth hormone, GH) induced after the hormone binds to its membrane receptor and its associated G protein and kinase (JAK). (PLC, phospholipase C; PIP_2, phosphoinositol diphosphate; PKC, protein kinase C; DAG, diacylglycerol; MAPK, mitogen-activated protein kinase.) (See text and Chapter 2.)

glycerol formation results in increased cytoplasmic Ca^{2+} mobilization, and activation of protein kinase C which, in turn, activates other intracellular proteins such as transcription factors (Fig. 4.6).

Control of somatotrophin release

Somatotrophin is released in discrete pulses (as are all adenohypophysial hormones primarily controlled from the hypothalamus) and shows a diurnal variation with greater pulses occurring during stage IV sleep. Its release from the adenohypophysis is primarily under the control of two hypothalamic substances released into the portal blood system from terminals in the median eminence. The most important influence is exerted by somatotrophin-releasing hormone (SRH), sometimes called somatoliberin (also called growth hormone-releasing hormone, GHRH) which stimulates the release of somatotrophin. In fact, three forms exist in humans, but the two most biologically active are the larger two, one with 40- and the other with 44-amino acid sequences. The other, lesser, influence on somatotrophin release is the 14-amino acid polypeptide somatotrophin-inhibiting hormone, better known as somatostatin. Again, other forms of somatostatin exist and can be biologically active.

Somatostatin in its various forms has a wide distribution in the body. For instance, it is found not only in the hypothalamus but also in other parts of the brain, the gastrointestinal tract, and in the delta (δ) cells of the pancreatic islets of Langerhans. It binds to a variety of membrane receptor subtypes, two of which are found in the pituitary and mediate the inhibitory effect on somatotrophin release. Two G proteins are known to mediate intracellular effects of somatostatin (Gi_1 and Go). The Gi_1 protein is associated with the inhibition of cAMP formation which, via protein kinase A, inhibits calcium channels in the cell membrane. These channels are also inhibited directly by somatostatin through an interaction with the Go protein. These two actions lower the cytoplasmic calcium ion concentration in the somatotrophic cells of the adenohypophysis and this results in the inhibition of somatotrophin production. Interestingly, somatostatin's actions appear to be generally inhibitory. It not only inhibits somatotrophin release but also inhibits the release of thyrotrophin and, under certain conditions, corticotrophin and prolactin secretion. In the pancreas, it inhibits islet cell insulin and glucagon hormone production (see Chapter 11), as well as the exocrine secretions into the pancreatic duct. It can also inhibit the release of hormones from a variety of adenomas including insulinomas and glucagonomas.

Control of the release of the two hypothalamic neurosecretions is mediated by monoaminergic and serotoninergic pathways so that α-adrenergic, dopaminergic, and serotoninergic agonists, as well as β-adrenergic antagonists, all stimulate somatotrophin release in man. The serotoninergic pathway is involved in the increased production of somatotrophin which accompanies the onset of deep sleep. In addition, enkephalins and endorphins apparently stimulate somatotrophin release, an effect which is blocked by the drug naloxone. Other stimuli, such as emotional, febrile, and surgical stress act through these various nerve pathways in the hypothalamus.

Physiological stimuli such as changes in the levels of energy substrates in the blood including hypoglycaemia, increased amino acid concentrations and decreased free fatty acid concentrations all increase somatotrophin secretion. In addition, the blood level of circulating somatotrophin is thought to exert an influence on the release of the hypothalamic neurosecretions (e.g. somatostatin) through a short feedback loop. Somatomedins may also influence somatotrophin release by means of negative feedback loops at hypothalamic and/or adenohypophysial levels. Oestrogens stimulate somatotrophin production, possibly by altering the number of receptor sites for hypothalamic hormones on the somatotrophes (Fig. 4.7).

Prolactin

Prolactin is a protein whose chemical structure has some similarity to that of somatotrophin, with approximately 16 per cent of the amino acids being homologous. It has 199 amino acids and its molecular weight is approximately 25 kDa. The prolactin gene is located on chromosome 6. The hormone is synthesized initially as a precursor prohormone in acidophilic cells in the adenohypophysis. Various dimeric forms (e.g. 46 kDa) are present in the circulation, in addition to the main monomeric form.

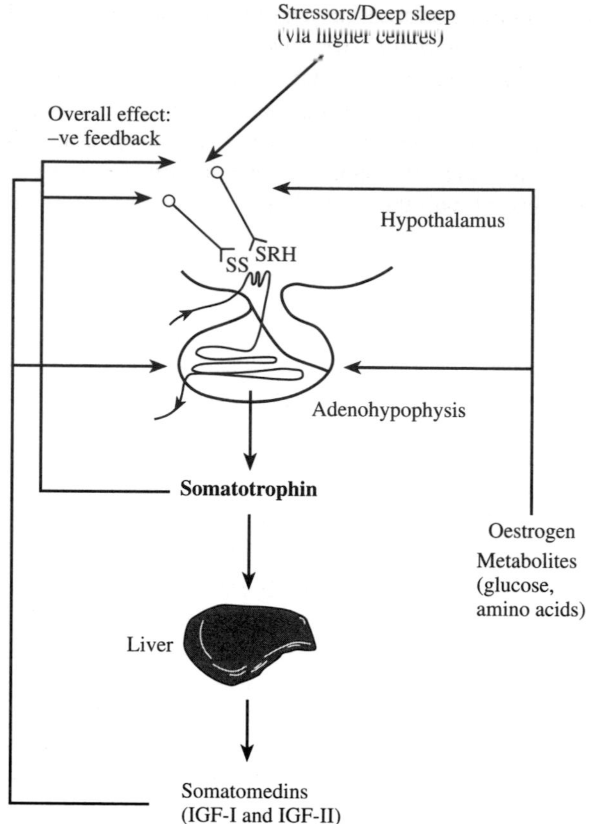

Fig. 4.7. Control of somatotrophin production. The two hypothalamic hormones are somatostatin (SS) and somatrophin-releasing hormone (SRH).

Actions of prolactin

The principal established functions for prolactin are the growth and development of the breasts and the initiation and maintenance of lactation in postpartum women. These actions require the influence of various other hormones such as oestrogens, corticosteroids, and insulin. Prolactin is also involved in the regulation of gonadal function. For example, it stimulates the generation of LH receptors in the gonads of both sexes. In the male, LH receptor synthesis in the Leydig cells is stimulated by prolactin while in the female this effect occurs in the ovarian corpus luteum (see Chapter 8). Interestingly, and on the face of it paradoxically, hyperprolactinaemia is associated with a loss of reproductive function. It is probable that this inhibition of the reproductive axis results at least partly from the increased production of dopamine, the hypothalamic prolactin-inhibiting hormone, consequent upon the short-loop feedback effect of the raised plasma prolactin level. Therefore, men commonly become impotent, lose their libido, and can become infertile; and women often develop amenorrhoea or oligomenorrhoea (the complete or partial loss of regular menstrual cycles). General metabolic functions similar to those of somatotrophin have also been observed, but the importance of prolactin for these is unclear. A natriuretic action has been proposed for prolactin, and such an effect has been observed in some other species. Prolactin also interacts with the immune system since it can stimulate lymphocyte proliferation; such an interaction may prove to be an important function of this hormone.

Mechanism of action of prolactin

As for somatotrophin, prolactin binds to its membrane receptor which is associated with a tyrosine kinase (JAK) molecule. As a result of hormone binding to its receptor, the tyrosine kinase is activated and subsequent phosphorylation of intracellular proteins induces the intracellular actions of the hormone.

Control of release of prolactin

Prolactin release is primarily under the control of the hypothalamus which receives afferent impulses initiated from sensory receptors, particularly those round the nipples in lactating women. Two hypothalamic neurosecretions have been implicated in prolactin regulation. The dominant hypothalamic influence is inhibitory and the predominant inhibitory hormone is dopamine. Thus, bromocriptine and other dopamine agonists are often successful in the treatment of hyperprolactinaemia. Various other monoamines have also been shown to be involved in the control of prolactin secretion. In addition to dopamine, noradrenaline, histamine, and serotonin all influence the release of prolactin, acting at either the hypothalamic or pituitary level. The tripeptide thyrotrophin-releasing hormone (TRH), in addition to being the principal releasing hormone for thyrotrophin, also stimulates prolactin release from the lactotrophe cells. Prolactin is released in pulses and has a diurnal variation with the greatest pulses occurring during the night.

The most important physiological stimulus for its release occurs when the infant suckles at the breast. Tactile receptors round the nipple are stimulated and increased afferent nerve activity reaches the hypothalamus culminating in increased prolactin release. This neuroendocrine reflex arc involves the inhibition of dopamine release and, probably, the stimulation of TRH release from hypothalamic neurones into the hypothalamo–hypophysial portal system. Various stressors stimulate the release of prolactin, the central pathway possibly involving histamine as a neurotransmitter (Fig. 4.8). Vasoactive intestinal peptide (VIP), which is found within the adenohypophysis as well as in the hypothalamus, may have a paracrine stimulatory effect on prolactin secretion. Thyroidal iodothyronine hormones and oestrogens also affect prolactin secretion. Thyroxine and oestrogens may modulate the number of TRH receptors in lactotrophes, thereby influencing prolactin release indirectly. Thyroxine, by negative feedback, decreases the number of TRH receptor sites while oestrogens increase their availability. Oestrogens also stimulate prolactin gene expression; consequently, premenopausal women usually have higher serum prolactin concentrations than men or postmenopausal women.

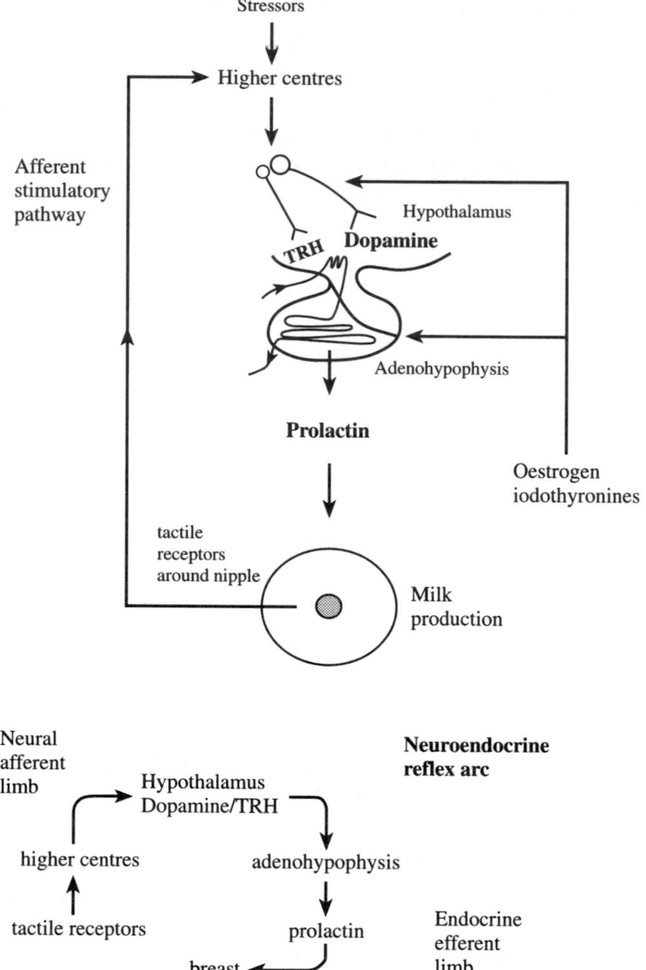

Fig. 4.8. Diagram showing the neuroendocrine reflex are relating tactile (stretch) receptors around the nipple and the release of prolactin. The dominant hypothalamic influence is inhibitory via dopamine. Various stimulatory (releasing) hormones are likely, an important one being thyrotrophin-releasing hormone (TRH).

Thyrotrophin (thyroid-stimulating hormone, TSH)

Thyrotrophin is a glycoprotein hormone comprising two non-covalently bound chains of amino acids (α and β) which is synthesized and stored in the thyrotrophes of the adenohypophysis. The 92-amino acid α-chain is identical to that found in the other adenohypophysial glycoprotein hormones FSH and LH, the biological activity of each hormone residing in the specificity of the β-chains. This chain for thyrotrophin is 110 amino acids long. Thyrotrophin is released in low-amplitude pulses following a diurnal rhythm, with higher levels attained during the night and decreasing in the early hours of the morning.

Actions of thyrotrophin

The primary action of thyrotrophin is to stimulate the thyroid gland to secrete two of its own hormones, the iodothyronines triiodothyronine (T_3) and thyroxine (T_4) into the bloodstream. This action of thyrotrophin on the thyroid gland is the result of several different effects on the intracellular mechanisms involved in the synthesis and release of the thyroidal metabolic hormones. These effects include:

(1) stimulation of the iodide pump in the cell membrane which transports iodide from the blood into the cells against an electrochemical gradient;

(2) stimulation of the synthesis of the thyroidal storage protein thyroglobulin;

(3) stimulation of T_3 and T_4 synthesis; and

(4) stimulation of the release of T_3 and T_4 from the thyroglobulin complexes.

In addition, the vascularity of the gland increases, and the follicular cells increase in size and number, an effect which can result in an enlarged thyroid (goitre). Thyrotrophin may also have extrathyroidal effects, such as the lipolysis induced in isolated (e.g. adipocyte) tissues, but the physiological importance of such actions is unclear.

Mechanism of action of thyrotrophin

Thyrotrophin binds to its membrane receptor on the follicular cells of the thyroid. The receptor has seven transmembrane domains, four intracellular domains, and a long extracellular sequence which contains six potential glycosylation sites. In the cell membrane, it is linked to a Gs protein and consequently the associated catalytic unit adenyl cyclase is activated with the subsequent generation of cAMP. The activation of protein kinase A then follows, and this results in the phosphorylation of various intracellular proteins involved in follicular cell regulation. Auto-antibodies formed against the thyrotrophin receptor are an important cause of thyroid clinical disease.

Control of release of thyrotrophin

Like all other adenohypophysial hormones, thyrotrophin release is pulsatile. Furthermore, there is a circadian rhythm with plasma levels raised during the night. Thyrotrophin release is controlled mainly by the hypothalamic thyrotrophin releasing hormone, TRH, with small inhibitory effects exerted by somatostatin and dopamine. The other major controlling influence is from circulating factors, such as the thyroid iodothyronine hormones (thyroxine and triiodothyronine), which exert direct and indirect negative feedback effects at pituitary and hypothalamic levels, respectively. It is likely that T_3 is the intracellular regulator of thyrotrophin production in the adenohypophysis. Oestrogens increase the number of TRH receptors on thyrotrophe cells in the adenohypophysis. Consequently, thyrotrophin release in response to TRH is greater in women than in men. Certainly, some relationship between the gonadal steroids and the adenohypophysial–thyroidal axis is suggested by the far greater occurrence of thyroidal disorders in women. Modulation of TRH release probably occurs in the hypothalamus since serotonin consistently decreases, and noradrenalin increases, its secretion from incubated hypothalamic tissue. A decrease in the ambient temperature is a potent stimulus for thyrotrophin release. However, in general, stressors inhibit thyrotrophin release and this is at least partly due to a reduced TRH release from the hypothalamus.

Corticotrophin (adrenocorticotrophic hormone, ACTH)

This hormone is a polypeptide of 39 amino acids, which is synthesized and stored in corticotrophe cells of the adenohypophysis. Its biological half-life is estimated to be approximately 8 minutes. The initial precursor prohormone is a large 241-amino acid protein called pro-opiomelanocortin (POMC). The POMC gene is found on chromosome 2 in humans. Post-translational processing of POMC is species- and tissue-specific; in the human adenohypophysis it is cleaved into corticotrophin, β-lipotrophin (β-LPH), a joining peptide, and an *N*-terminal peptide (Fig. 1.3). In the intermediate lobe in humans, which is almost non-existent except in the fetus and during pregnancy, β-LPH is further processed to β-endorphin while corticotrophin is cleaved to form α-melanocyte-stimulating hormone (α-MSH) and corticotrophin-like intermediate lobe peptide (CLIP). The pigmentation associated with hypersecretion of corticotrophin is actually due to the direct stimulation of melanocytes by excess corticotrophin and β-LPH rather than to intermediate lobe processing and subsequent α-MSH production. On the other hand, α-MSH has been found in the hypothalamus, for instance, in neurones originating in the arcuate nucleus, and may have a role as a neurotransmitter or neuromodulator.

The endorphins

Endorphins comprise a group of *endo*genous substances which have mo*rphine*-like activity; that is, they interact with opiate receptors to produce opioid-like effects. The discovery of such specific receptors in the brain certainly explained why drugs such as morphine could exert their profound analgesic ('pain-killer') effects. The likely explanation for the presence of such receptors came subsequently, with the discovery of the 31-amino acid polypeptide β-endorphin and the pentapeptide enkephalins. Pituitary β-endorphin has not yet been shown to have any specific effects, but it is found in other parts of the body together with methionine enkephalin (met-enkephalin) and the related molecule leucine-enkephalin (leu-enkephalin). They are located in various parts of the brain (in particular the hypothalamus) and in the adeno- and neurohypophysial systems. Dynorphin, for example, is an endorphin located in magnocellular neurones originating in the hypothalamic paraventricular nucleus, coexisting with vasopressin. The brain endorphins have been implicated in the control of pain (the important analgesic action), the regulation of adaptive behaviour, the response to stressors, the modulation of hypothalamic hormone release, and possibly the regulation of neurohypophysial hormone secretion. These opioid peptides probably function as neurotransmitters, neuromodulators, and possibly as hormones. Opioid receptors have also been identified in axon terminals in the adrenal medulla and sympathetic ganglia. Various endorphins have been located in cells of the gastrointestinal tract (e.g. the stomach) in addition to being present in the myenteric plexus

Actions of corticotrophin

The primary function of corticotrophin is to stimulate the two innermost zones of the cortex of the adrenal gland, the zonae fasciculata and reticularis, which secrete the glucocorticoid hormones (primarily cortisol in man) and small quantities of sex hormones (androgens and oestrogens). It is also believed to sensitize the outermost zone of the adrenal cortex, the zona glomerulosa, to other stimuli which induce the release of the mineralocorticoid hormone, aldosterone ('permissive' role, see Chapter 5).

Mechanism of action of corticotrophin

Corticotrophin binds to specific membrane receptors on its target cells, and consequently adenyl cyclase is activated. Generation of intracellular cAMP results in increased protein kinase A activity and subsequent phosphorylation of intracellular proteins mediating the actions of the hormone. Acutely, enzyme stimulation results in rapid (within minutes) synthesis and release of cortisol followed over a more prolonged time course by a more profound production rate. This includes synthesis of the enzymes involved in steroid hormone production (see Chapter 5).

Control of release of corticotrophin

Corticotrophin is released in spontaneous pulses but nevertheless normally follows a distinct circadian rhthym, with peak plasma levels measured in the early hours of the morning and lowest levels in the late evening. Consequently, plasma cortisol concentrations also show an early morning (around the time of waking up, between 7 a.m. and 8 a.m.) peak and a nadir around midnight. This normal circadian rhthym can be disrupted by prolonged night-shift work or by a major time shift, such as on intercontinental flights. The release of corticotrophin is controlled principally from the hypothalamus. Various corticotrophin-releasing factors have been isolated, but the most potent is the 41-amino acid polypeptide called corticotrophin-releasing hormone (CRH, also known as corticoliberin). Some CRH coexists with vasopressin (antidiuretic hormone) in parvocellular neurones originating in the paraventricular nuclei. These hormones can be released together from these parvocellular nerve terminals in the median eminence into the hypothalamo–hypophysial portal system. Vasopressin (VP) acts synergistically with CRH to stimulate corticotrophin release from the corticotrophe cells of the adenohypophysis. Various neurotransmitters, including acetylcholine and noradrenaline, are involved in the regulation of CRH and VP. All stressors, almost by definition, cause the release of corticotrophin from the adenohypophysis and consequently cortisol from the adrenal glands. Stressors act on the paraventricular neuronal pathway involving the CRH/VP neurones. There is an additional extensive network of CRH neurones elsewhere in the brain, particularly around the hypothalamus.

Another important controlling influence on corticotrophin release is the negative feedback exerted by the glucocorticoids. Cortisol is a potent inhibitor of corticotrophin release by a direct action on the adenohypophysis and by an indirect action through the inhibition of CRH release. A negative feedback effect by corticotrophin itself (short-, or auto-loop, feedback) has also been identified.

Gonadotrophins

The two gonadotrophins produced in the adenohypophysis are luteinizing hormone (LH) and follicle-stimulating hormone (FSH). They are both glycoproteins composed of two subunits (α and β). The 92-amino acid, 2 carbohydrate side-chain, α-subunits are identical to the thyrotrophin α-subunit. The gene for the α-subunit is located on chromosome 6. The specific biological activity of each hormone resides in its β-subunit. A double staining technique has identified the gonadotrophe cells as being the sites of synthesis of both LH and FSH.

Luteinizing hormone (LH)

The human LH β-subunit gene is located on chromosome 19. The LH β-subunit consists of 115 amino acids and has two carbohydrate side-chains. The β-subunit of human chorionic gonadotrophin (HCG), a placental glycoprotein hormone which has comparable biological activity to LH (see Chapter 8), is similar to that of LH but has an additional 32 amino acids. LH is secreted in pulses in males and females, and this pulsatile release pattern is vital for the normal regulation of gonadal function. Its biological half-life is approximately 30 minutes. In contrast to other adenohypophysial hormones there is no clear indication of a diurnal variation in LH production in adults. However, in pubertal adolescents the first indicator of maturation of the hypothalamo–hypophysial–gonadal axis is the increased nocturnal release pattern of LH. A sexual dimorphism becomes readily apparent once maturity of this axis is attained. The establishment of regular menstrual cycles in women is then associated with a small rise in plasma LH during the follicular phase, an LH surge mid-cycle, and a decrease during the luteal phase (see Chapter 8).

Actions of LH

In females, it acts on the ovaries to stimulate ovarian steroid hormone production (see Chapter 8). Thus, during the follicular phase of the cycle it acts on follicular thecal cells to stimulate the production of androgens, particularly androstenedione. Just prior to the pre-ovulatory surge in gonadotrophin production the outer layers of granulosa cells begin to synthesize LH receptors as a result of FSH and oestradiol action on these cells. The effect of the LH surge is to stimulate: (1) the final maturation of the oocyte (even though there are no LH receptors on the ovum itself); (2) progestogen synthesis by the outer granulosa cells; and (3) the process of ovum release itself — ovulation. At this stage of the cycle, LH stimulates the conversion of the follicle to a corpus luteum, and then stimulates the corpus luteal cells to synthesize large quantities of progesterone. This latter action continues during much of the luteal phase. The effects of LH on the ovaries are generally the result of its collaborative actions with FSH.

In males, the hormone acts primarily by stimulating the interstitial Leydig cells in the testes which secrete testosterone. Since testosterone is involved in the regulation of spermatogenesis, it is clear that in both sexes LH functions as a stimulator of steroidogenesis and gametogenesis. Interestingly, it is FSH which appears to be necessary to initiate spermatogenesis, while testosterone is necessary for the subsequent maintenance of the process (see Chapter 7).

Mechanism of action of LH

Luteinizing hormone binds to membrane receptors in their ovarian and testicular target cells, the associated G protein complex is activated and consequently adenyl cyclase is stimulated. Subsequent cAMP generation results in protein kinase activation which in turn leads to phosphorylation of specific intracellular proteins.

Control of release of LH

The release of LH is primarily under hypothalamic control through the mediation of gonadotrophin-releasing hormone GnRH (also known as LHRH). However, modulation of this mechanism occurs at both the hypothalamic and adenohypophysial levels. Dopamine, for example, appears to have excitatory and inhibitory actions with respect to GnRH release; this modulating influence of dopamine appears to be dose-dependent. Indeed, prolactin, when present in the circulation in very high concentrations, probably exerts at least part of its inhibitory influence on LH secretion through the stimulation of dopamine release. The pulsatile nature of LH secretion is vital for normal gonadal function, and it is dependent on the pulsatile release of GnRH. If GnRH is administered as a continuous infusion, LH production is suppressed and gonadal function impaired. In women oestrogens and progesterone influence LH release through feedback mechanisms at both hypothalamic and adenohypophysial levels. One oestrogen influence on LH release may be the alteration in the number of GnRH receptors on the gonadotrophe cells in the adenohypophysis. The usual feedback influence by oestrogens and progesterone is negative, acting through a direct loop on the pituitary and an indirect loop on GnRH release from the hypothalamus. However, if plasma oestrogen levels are maintained sufficiently high for a period of approximately 36 hours in the absence of raised plasma progesterone concentrations, then a positive feedback influence is exerted and an LH surge occurs. After the menopause, when ovarian function is greatly reduced and circulating oestrogen levels are relatively low, the negative feedback influence is removed and plasma LH (and FSH) concentrations rise. In men, testosterone has a direct and an indirect negative feedback influence on LH release (see Chapters 7 and 8).

Follicle-stimulating hormone (FSH)

Follicle-stimulating hormone is a glycoprotein consisting of two subunits, the α-subunit being identical to the α-subunits of LH and thyrotrophin. The β-subunit, which confers its specific biological activity, consists of 115 amino acids and two carbohydrate side-chains, as in luteinizing hormone. The β-subunit gene is located on chromosome 11. The biological half-life of FSH is estimated to be approximately 150 minutes.

Actions of FSH

This glycoprotein hormone stimulates follicular development in the ovary in females, and it is important in stimulating aromatase enzyme activity in the granulosa cells particularly during the early (pre-antral) follicular phase of the menstrual cycle. Thus, androgens reaching the granulosa cells are aromatized to oestrogens as a consequence of the stimulatory action of FSH. During the late antral phase (pre-ovulatory) phase FSH stimulates the outer layer of granulosa cells to synthesize LH receptors; consequently, these cells respond to LH and begin to secrete progestogens. Although FSH is present throughout the cycle, relatively little is known about its physiological role during the later phases. For instance, an FSH surge accompanies the LH surge just prior to ovulation; although smaller than the LH surge it is likely that FSH influences the final maturation of the ovum and may participate in the process of ovulation by acting in conjunction with LH. During the luteal phase the same situation prevails, and FSH may have some corpus luteal-stimulating activity along with LH.

In males, FSH acts on Sertoli cells and initiates the process of spermatogenesis. Thus, following hypophysectomy (removal of the pituitary) spermatogenesis stops, and can be restarted only by the administration of FSH.

Mechanism of action of FSH

Follicle-stimulating hormone binds to its receptors on the membranes of its target cells in the ovaries and testes and the process activates the generation of intracellular cAMP through the signal transducer (the G protein complex). Intracellular protein kinase activation by cAMP-induced phosphorylation results in increased enzyme activity which is associated with the effects of FSH.

Control of release of FSH

Release of FSH from the adenohypophysis is similar in some ways to the regulation of LH discussed above. However, since the adenohypophysial gonadotrophe cells are capable of synthesizing both LH and FSH there must be some discrimination between control systems, allowing for the varying pattern of release of the two hormones which can occur. For example, although the release of FSH is also stimulated by GnRH the possibility that a specific FSH-releasing factor might exist cannot be discounted at present. Another difference is related to the production by FSH target cells of the protein inhibin. This molecule is produced by follicular granulosa cells in the female and Sertoli cells in the male, and it inhibits FSH, but not LH, secretion by the gonadotrophe cells. In addition, the gonadal steroid hormones are of particular importance in modulating the gonadotrophic cell response to GnRH. Experiments on pituitary cell cultures indicated that oestrogens stimulate GnRH-induced LH and FSH release, whereas androgens inhibit LH, but stimulate FSH, release. In the presence of oestrogens the effect of progesterone is stimulatory for FSH release but is only excitatory initially for LH, this being followed by a marked inhibition. *In vitro* experiments strongly support feedback effects by the various gonadal hormones on the adenohypophysis, as well as on the hypothalamus. It is also likely that separate populations of FSH- and LH-producing gonadotrophes exist in the adenohypophysia.

The neurohypophysis (posterior pituitary)

Anatomy, histology, and development

The neurohypophysis functionally consists of the supraoptic and paraventricular nuclei in the hypothalamus, the hypothalamo–hypophysial nerve tract and the pars nervosa (the posterior or neural lobe) of the hypophysis. However, the term 'neurohypophysis' is often used to describe the posterior pituitary as a separate unit, to differentiate this lobe from the adenohypophysis (the anterior lobe of the pituitary). The cells associated with the neurohypophysis are neurones which have their cell bodies grouped together in the supraoptic and paraventricular nuclei in the hypothalamus. The unmyelinated axons of most of these neurosecretory cells pass down through the pituitary stalk to terminate on the walls of capillaries in the neural lobe. The cells are larger than other hypothalamic neurosecretory cells and are called magnocellular neurones. They have another characteristic: they have small swellings (varicosities) all along the length of the axons, called Hering bodies. In addition, the dendrites from these cell bodies are particularly profuse and contain numerous peptide (e.g. vasopressin) containing granules. Other, smaller, cells are called parvocellular neurones; they release their neurosecretions into the primary capillary plexus in the median eminence region of the hypothalamus. Yet other paraventricular neurones send their axons to other parts of the brain (Fig. 4.4). Interspersed between the nerve fibres in the posterior pituitary are numerous glial cells called pituicytes, thought at one time to be the sites of synthesis and release of the neurohypophysial hormones and controlled by the neurones; their actual function is at present undetermined but while they may be simply structural, it is also possible that they have a direct regulatory effect on neurohypophysial hormone release.

The neurohypophysis receives most of its arterial blood supply from branches of the inferior hypophysial artery in the lower part of the pars nervosa. An extensive capillary network is fairly regularly distributed throughout the posterior lobe; the blood ultimately drains into the jugular veins. Some of the arterial blood may reach another capillary plexus which is linked to the adenohypophysis by short portal vessels. A vascular link between the two lobes of the pituitary may have a functional purpose, but details are lacking.

The neurohypophysial hormones

The cells bodies of the supraoptic and paraventricular neurones synthesize various molecules which can be secreted from the nerve terminals in the neural lobe. The two principal secretory products of the magnocellular neurones are the hormones vasopressin and oxytocin. Each cell body synthesizes either vasopressin or oxytocin, hence the neurones are called either vasopressinergic or oxytocinergic. Other peptides are synthesized by the magnocellular neurones and can be released with these hormones; the opioid peptide dynorphin, for example, is released from vasopressinergic neurones, whereas corticotrophin-releasing hormone (CRH) is colocalized in oxytocinergic neurones. Vasopressin and oxytocin are nonapeptides with similar chemical structures, consisting of six amino acids linked together by a disulphide bond and a short chain of three amino acids. Two forms of vasopressin have been identified in mammals. One contains the amino acid arginine, and is called arginine vasopressin (AVP); it is found in most mammals including humans. The other contains lysine, instead of arginine, and is called lysine vasopressin (LVP); it is present in the pig and the hippopotamus. The structures of both vasopressins are otherwise identical and include the amino acid phenylalanine. Oxytocin differs from the vasopressins by having the amino acid leucine instead of arginine or lysine, and isoleucine instead of phenylalanine.

Both vasopressin and oxytocin are intially synthesized as larger prohormones (pro-vasopressin and pro-oxytocin). The genes for both prohormones consist of exons separated from each other by introns (Fig. 4.9). The exon 1 regions contain the vasopressin or oxytocin sequences while the exon 2 regions contain the sequences for specific proteins called neurophysins which are released in equimolar amounts with their respective hormones. Exon 3 of the vasopressin gene

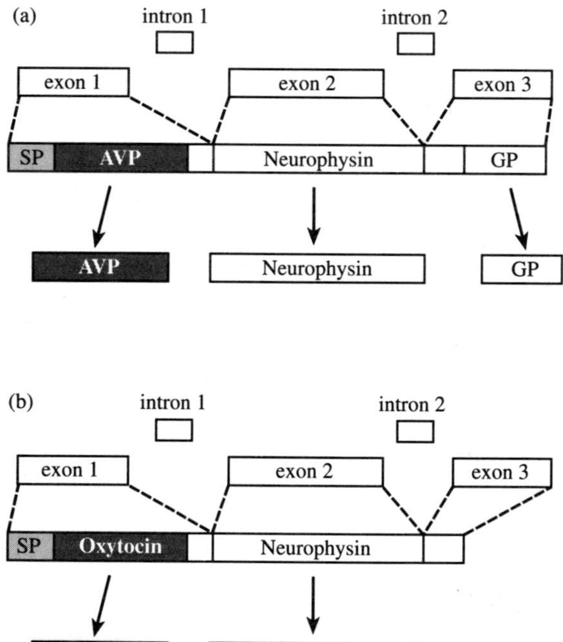

Fig. 4.9. The genes for (a) arginine vasopressin (AVP) and (b) oxytocin, showing the three coding regions (exons) and two non-coding regions (introns) in each case. (SP, signal peptide; GP, glycopeptide.)

contains the sequence for a glycopeptide (GP) of unknown function also released with the hormone. No such glycopeptide is transcribed from the oxytocin gene.

These molecular complexes become incorporated into granules which then migrate down the nerve axons as a result of axoplasmic flow (axonal transport). The rate at which the hormone complexes travel down the nerve fibres has been estimated by using labelled molecules, and two components have thus been identified: (1) a fast component which migrates down the axons at a rate of 1–3 mm/h; and (2) a more controversial slow component travelling at a rate of 1 mm/24 h. The latter could represent a non-granular component, but its existence is disputed. The granules collect at the nerve terminals and in the Hering bodies along the nerve axons, which may act as storage sites. The nerve endings lie close to the capillaries in the posterior lobe of the pituitary. Release of the neurohypophysial hormones is associated with the arrival of action potentials at the nerve endings which depolarize the terminal membranes. The granule contents are believed to be released into the bloodstream by exocytosis. An influx of calcium ions, occurring when the membrane is depolarized, is necessary for the excitation–secretion coupling process. Dissociation between neurohypophysial hormone and neurophysin protein is believed to occur prior to the releasing process. The neurophysins are released with the neurohypophysial hormones although they are not bound to them in the bloodstream.

Vasopressin (VP)

Most vasopressin is synthesized in cell bodies located in the supraoptic and paraventricular nuclei. It is released from nerve terminals of magnocellular neurones in the pituitary neural lobe, and also from parvocellular neurones in the median eminence. This vasopressin enters the systemic circulation or the hypothalamo–hypophysial portal system, respectively. The vasopressin released from at least some of the fibres with terminals in the median eminence coexists with corticotrophin-releasing hormone (CRH). Other vasopressinergic neurones have their cell bodies located in the suprachiasmatic nucleus. Some of the paraventricular (and suprachiasmatic) vasopressinergic neurones project to various parts of the central nervous system where the peptide acts as a neurotransmitter. Areas of the brain which receive these projections include the nucleus tractus solitarius (involved in cardiovascular regulation) and regions associated with behavioural processes including memory. Vasopressin has also been identified in other parts of the body including the adrenal glands, the gonads, sympathetic ganglia, and even in pancreatic islet tissue. In the circulation, most vasopressin is found within the platelets in humans.

Vasopressin receptors

Two vasopressin receptors have been identified and sequenced, and they are called v1 and v2 receptors. They are both members of a receptor superfamily, each one having seven transmembrane domains, with four extracellular regions and three intracellular regions. The v2 receptors are found in the renal collecting ducts and mediate in the principal physiological action of the hormone. The v1 receptors are located in many other target cells for vasopressin, and are associated with various other effects of the hormone (see below). An additional receptor which is similar to the v1 receptor but has certain different characteristics is located in the adenohypophysis. It has been called the v1b receptor, to differentiate it from the other more common receptor which is therefore called the v1a receptor.

Actions of VP

Antidiuretic action of VP

The principal physiological action of vasopressin is to stimulate the reabsorption of water from the tubular fluid in the cortical and (mainly) the medullary collecting ducts of the renal nephrons in the presence of a net absorption (osmotic) pressure gradient. The blood level of the hormone therefore directly determines the water balance of the body, and indirectly regulates the concentration of osmotically active solutes in the extracellular fluid, the most important solute being sodium. As the main action of vasopressin is to increase the volume of water reabsorbed from the nephrons, the urinary concentration rises. In the presence of vasopressin the urine excreted by the kidneys is small in volume and highly concentrated (antidiuresis). For this reason, the hormone is sometimes called the 'antidiuretic hormone' (ADH). The increase in water reabsorption is initiated when vasopressin binds to its v2 receptors on the basolateral membranes of the collecting duct cells.

Cardiovascular action of VP

The name 'vasopressin' denotes a vascular (vaso) effect on the blood pressure (pressor) and this was the first action of a pituitary extract observed by Oliver and Schafer in 1895, later to be ascribed to the hormone. The increase in blood pressure produced by vasopressin is normally only observed when relatively large quantities are present in the circulation, and is not usually considered to be a physiological effect. However, this is somewhat surprising because vasopressin is an extremely potent naturally occurring vasoconstrictor molecule, being particularly effective on arteriolar smooth muscle in the skin and splanchnic bed. This vasoconstrictor action is associated with the v1 receptors, which are found on vascular smooth muscle cells. The explanation for this paradox is at least partly because vasopressin produces a simultaneous bradycardia and a decrease in cardiac output, which normally compensate for the increase in total peripheral resistance produced by the arteriolar vasoconstriction. Indeed, vasopressin may potentiate the baroreceptor reflex which mediates the decrease in cardiac output. The vasoconstrictor action of vasopressin may be of physiological importance in volume depletion states, such as severe haemorrhage or dehydration, when very high plasma concentrations of the hormone are present. A v2 receptor-mediated vasodilatory effect has been indicated by recent research. Also worth noting are the various interactions which probably occur between vasopressin and other hormones, such as angiotensin II, the catecholamines, the atrial natriuretic peptides, and steroids such as the adrenal and gonadal hormones.

Other actions of VP

1. *Renal effects.* Vasopressin can increase renal sodium chloride reabsorption in the thick ascending limb of the loop of Henle through a direct effect on either sodium or chloride transport. In the cortical collecting duct also, vasopressin appears to stimulate sodium reabsorption, and urea transport from lumen to interstitial fluid is increased, particularly in the inner medullary collecting duct. These effects of vasopressin on solute transport are important in maintaining the osmotic gradient from the cortex down to the papilla, which is a necessary prerequisite for the concentrating ability of the kidneys.

2. *Corticotrophin-releasing activity.* Vasopressin stimulates corticotrophin release from the adenohypophysis, which it reaches mainly via the hypothalamo–hypophysial portal system. Depending on the species, it either mainly acts directly on the corticotrophe cells as a corticotrophin-releasing factor (CRF) or it mainly potentiates the effect of the separate hypothalamic CRH. Thus, it is involved in the control of cortocotrophin release, and may be important in the activation of the adrenocortical stress response. It is worth noting that vasopressin may also influence the stress-related inhibition of LH release, so that in the absence of vasopressin the normal inhibition of LH is attenuated.

3. *Central effects.* Vasopressin has been implicated in various behavioural studies on memory consolidation and learning. However, the precise nature of the memory improvement induced by this neuropeptide is unclear and still controversial. A central involvement of vasopressin is also possible with regard to the control of drinking behaviour.

4. *Other effects.* Various other effects have been described for vasopressin. These include the stimulation of hepatic glycogenolysis and a possible stimulatory effect on insulin release from pancreatic islets. Vasopressin also appears to stimulate the hepatic synthesis of factor VIII and the production of Von Willbrandt factor from an undetermined site, and thus influences the blood coagulation process.

Mechanism of action of VP

The principal physiological action of vasopressin is to stimulate water reabsorption in the renal collecting ducts. Here, vasopressin binds to its v2 receptor on the basolateral surface of the epithelial principal cells and via a G protein the catalytic unit (adenyl cyclase) is stimulated. The subsequent increase in intracellular cAMP concentration is associated with protein kinase (probably protein kinase A, PKA) activation. Although the subsequent sequence of events is still unclear, the movement of water channels (proteins called aquaporins) to the luminal membrane occurs in clathrin-coated vesicles called aggrephores (see Fig. 4.10). The precise function of the clathrin proteins is unknown but they may act as recognition molecules. The insertion of water channels into the luminal membrane in the presence of vasopressin (specifically aquaporin-2 proteins) is associated with the presence of

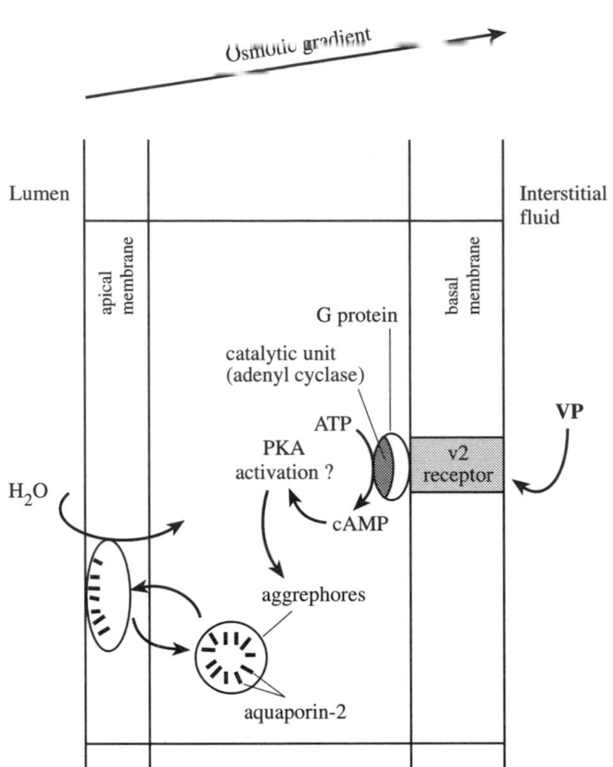

Fig. 4.10. The proposed mechanism of action for vasopressin (VP) on water reabsorption in the renal collecting duct. It involves the v2 receptor in the basal membrane, and its associated G protein and catalytic unit (adenyl cyclase), the second messenger cAMP, protein kinase A (PKA) activation, the synthesis/mobilization of water channels (aquaporin-2 molecules), and the transport of the vesicles (aggrephores) to and from the apical membrane.

intramembraneous particles which can be seen with the electron microscope. Recirculation of the water channels also may be influenced by vasopressin. Disruption of microtubules (polymers of the protein tubulin having a diameter of approximately 25 nm) and microfilaments (which have similar biochemical properties to actin found in muscle, and have a diameter of approximately 5 nm) impairs the water transport response to vasopressin in some preparations, so these intracellular structures have also been implicated. However, the relevance of such observations to the mechanism of action of vasopressin in humans is still speculative. Some prostaglandins appear to stimulate the release of vasopressin, while in the kidneys, PGE_2 is capable of inhibiting the antidiuretic action of the hormone. Since vasopressin can itself stimulate PGE_2 production in renal cells it would appear that the peptide can induce a self-regulatory process in these target cells.

The actions of vasopressin which are mediated by the v1 receptors do not involve stimulation of adenyl cyclase and cAMP formation. Instead, the mechanism of action induced through these receptors involves the inositol triphosphate and diacylglycerol pathways which are both concerned with an increase in intracellular (cytoplasmic) calcium ion concentration.

Control of release of VP

The most important physiological mechanism involved in the control of vasopressin synthesis and release is a variation of the plasma osmolality. As a change of hydration commonly leads to an alteration in the concentration of osmotically active solutes in the extracellular fluid, this mechanism ensures the regulation of water balance and the maintenance of the plasma solute concentration. For example, an increase in plasma osmolality results in an increased release of vasopressin from the neurohypophysis. The change in plasma osmolality is detected by specialized cells called osmoreceptors believed to send axons to the cell bodies of the supraoptic and paraventricular nuclei in the hypothalamus. It is generally accepted that the osmoreceptors must lie outside the blood–brain barrier, in one (or more) of the circumventricular organs. One such site that has been implicated in the osmotic control of vasopressin is the subfornical organ. The magnocellular neurones may respond directly to osmotic changes in their immediate environment but it is unclear how physiologically relevant this would be. Not all solutes appear to stimulate the osmoreceptors, however, despite increasing the plasma osmolality. Sodium ions and mannitol, which cross the blood–brain barrier relatively slowly, are potent stimulators of vasopressin release while urea, which is a very permeant molecule, has no effect. Glucose, on the other hand, crosses the barrier with relative ease mostly by means of a glucose transporter molecule; it appears to inhibit the release of vasopressin despite a raised plasma osmolality. Other observations suggest that some osmoreceptors are in contact with the cerebrospinal fluid in the brain.

Thus, increased osmoreceptor activity stimulates the vasopressinergic neurones which then release increased quantities of vasopressin from their nerve endings into the general circulation. Consequently, more water is reabsorbed from the collecting ducts as a result of vasopressin's action on the kidneys and the plasma osmolality falls. Interestingly, the pattern of discharge of electrical activity in vasopressinergic neurones appears to be quite characteristic, occurring in short, phasic but asynchronized bursts of activity. This is in contrast to the discharge pattern seen in oxytocinergic neurones which occurs in synchronized bursts during milk ejection — at least in the rat.

A second mechanism involved in the control of vasopressin release concerns changes in blood volume. The stimulus for the release of vasopressin during a haemorrhage, for example, is a decrease in the stretch of certain mechanoreceptors, called volume receptors. These are situated mainly in the left atrium of the heart but are also present in the walls of the main veins, for instance, and they function as low-pressure receptors. In addition, the baroreceptors (high-pressure receptors) in the carotid sinus and aortic arch are also an important influence on vasopressin release. A reduced blood volume results in a decreased frequency of action potentials from these various stretch receptors. This fall in frequency stimulates the release of vasopressin by decreasing the tonic inhibitory effect normally operated by this baroreceptor reflex pathway. Normally, an increased stimulation of these receptors, following volume expansion for example, increases the inhibition on the paraventricular and supraoptic cell bodies; consequently the release of vasopressin from the neurohypophysis is then reduced.

The higher centres of the brain also exert a profound influence over neurohypophysial hormone release through nerve pathways to the hypothalamus. Stimuli such as emotional or surgical stress may cause the massive release of vasopressin through such pathways (Fig. 4.11).

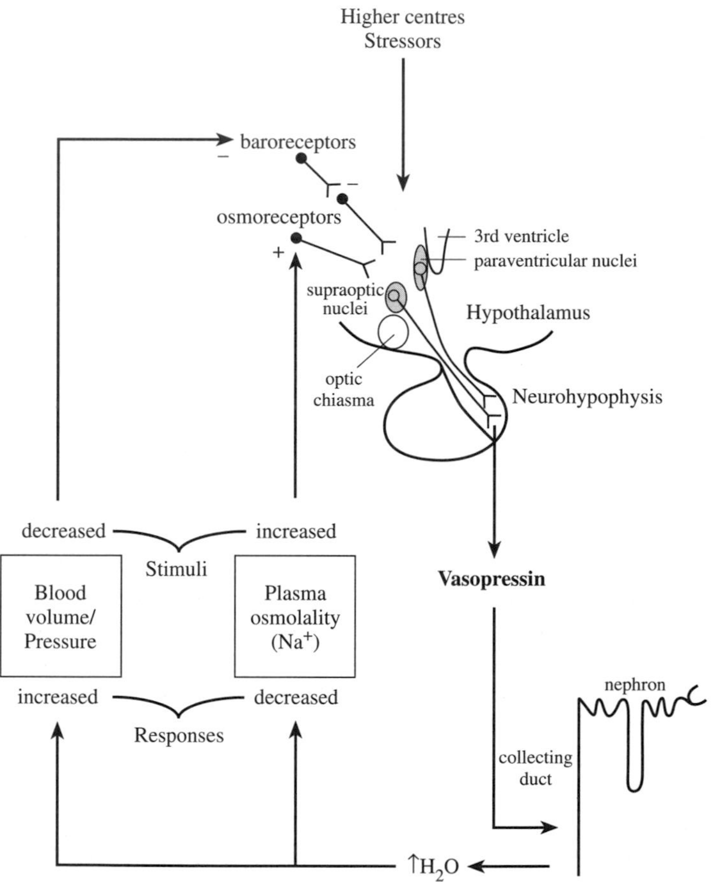

Fig. 4.11. The control of vasopressin production by changes in plasma osmolality and/or blood volume. Note that the final pathways linking hypothalamic osmoreceptors and the peripheral baroreceptors and volume receptors to the paraventricular and supraoptic vasopressinergic neurones are still unclear.

Other controlling influences on vasopressin release involve the renin–angiotensin system and atrial natriuretic peptides. Angiotensin II injected into the third ventricles of experimental animals stimulates vasopressin release. The existence of such a control system is supported by the observation that vasopressin inhibits renin release from the nephron, thus exhibiting a neat negative feedback loop between the two systems. It is worth appreciating that all the components of the renin–angiotensin system are present in the brain. Atrial natriuretic peptide (ANP) appears to decrease vasopressin release, and again a related molecule called brain natriuretic peptide has been isolated and characterized.

The presence of opiate receptors and enkephalin-secreting neurones in the neurohypophysis have led to experiments which suggest a dose-dependent stimulatory effect by the endogenous opiates on vasopressin release. Various nerve pathways originating from other parts of the brain terminate on the cell bodies of the paraventricular and supraoptic neurones and their neurosecretions, which include acetylcholine and noradrenaline, influence vasopressin release.

Oxytocin

Oxytocin is the other neuropeptide released from magnocellular neurones which terminate in the neural lobe of the pituitary. Oxytocin is synthesized in a similar manner to vasopressin in cell bodies in the supraoptic and paraventricular nuclei. As for vasopressin, some oxytocinergic neurones send axons to other parts of the brain.

Actions

Oxytocin is synthesized in both sexes but its principal, well-recognized, physiological effects occur only in females. Oxytocin stimulates the contraction of the smooth muscle of the oestrogen-primed uterus (the myometrium) and the myoepithelial cells surrounding the ducts of the lactating mammary glands. Contraction of the myometrium in response to oxytocin is only observed during the late stages of pregnancy when oestrogens may be secreted in increasing quantities relative to the concentration of circulating (or local) progestagens. The oxytocin receptor resembles the vasopressin receptors, consisting of seven transmembrane domains separating four extracellular and three intracellular regions. Oxytocin increases the movement of calcium ions into the myometrial cells probably by opening calcium channels in the membrane. Oxytocin also increases prostaglandin synthesis, PGE_2 being particularly effective in mobilizing calcium ions from intracellular stores. Oestrogens and progesterone stimulate and inhibit the synthesis of oxytocin receptors, respectively. While it is clear that oxytocin plays a part in parturition, its physiological importance in this process is debatable. Nevertheless, oxytocin can be an effective and useful therapeutic agent in inducing labour.

Oxytocin is necessary for the contraction of the myoepithelial cells of the milk ducts in the lactating mammary glands. Consequently, milk is ejected from the breasts when an appropriate stimulus (e.g. suckling) is applied and this is known as the milk-ejection reflex.

Oxytocin may have central effects, and an involvement in memory and learning behaviours (oxytocin impairing these processes) has been suggested. Oxytocin is also present in the male but its physiological functions are undetermined. However, there is some evidence to suggest that it is released from the neurohypophysis on stimulation of the male genitalia, and is present in high con-

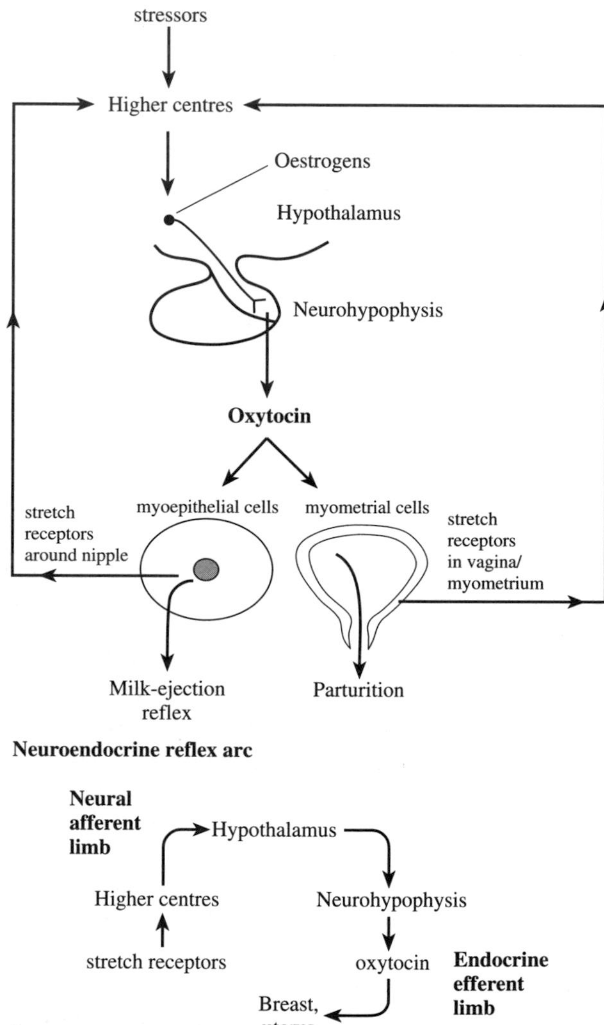

Fig. 4.12. Control of oxytocin production. The neuroendocrine reflex arcs linking stretch receptors around nipple and in vagina/myometrium to the release of oxytocin under appropriately steroid-primed conditions (see text) are also illustrated. The neuroendocrine reflex arc linking oxytocin to the breast, producing milk ejection from the nipple, is known as the milk-ejection reflex.

centrations in the blood during ejaculation. Behavioural effects may also be relevant in men.

Control of release

Oxytocin release is stimulated in the lactating mother by suckling. Tactile receptors in the breasts, especially round the nipples, when stimulated initiate action potentials which propagate along afferent nerve fibres through the spinal cord and midbrain to the hypothalamus. The oxytocinergic cell bodies in the paraventricular and supraoptic nuclei are then stimulated, resulting in the release of oxytocin. It is also believed that receptors in the uterus, and possibly in the mucosal walls of the vagina respond to stretch and initiate action potentials in afferent nerve fibres which ultimately stimulate the release of oxytocin from the neurohypophysis. Both the milk-ejection reflex and the myometrial contraction are examples of neuroendocrine reflex arcs, involving afferent neural and efferent endocrine components (Fig. 4.12). The influence of the higher centres of the brain on the release of oxytocin-mediating effects, such as emotional stress inhibiting lactation, is well documented. Enkephalins have been shown to be capable of inhibiting the release of oxytocin, at least in certain situations. In general, vasopressin and oxytocin are released independently.

CLINICAL DISORDERS

The various endocrine disturbances will be considered as excess or deficiency syndromes for each individual hormone. Although increasingly documented, single adenohypophysial hormone deficiency is quite rare, and it is more common to find that the secretions of several hormones are affected together. Accordingly, at the end of this section, the causes, investigation, and management of the clinical syndromes of hypopituitarism will be discussed.

Early diagnosis of any pituitary disorder requires high clinical acumen and a continuous awareness of the subtlety of early presentation. Once suspected, comparatively simple and precise methods are available for confirming or rejecting a provisional diagnosis.

Systematic approach to investigating pituitary disorders

Evaluation of hormonal excess

(a) Measurement of basal values of relevant pituitary or target gland hormone (i.e. thyroxine, cortisol) in plasma or urine.

(b) Attempted suppression of an elevated basal hormone level using a known feedback mechanism (e.g. glucose suppression of elevated growth hormone in suspected acromegaly; synthetic corticosteroid suppression of elevated cortisol level in suspected Cushing's syndrome). Pathological hypersecretion is confirmed by non-suppressible (autonomous) hormone production. Such suppression tests are essential, since wide fluctuations of hormone levels, particularly cortisol and growth hormone occur commonly even under physiological conditions.

Evaluation of hormonal deficiency

1. Measurement of basal values of relevant pituitary or target gland hormones in plasma or urine.

2. Attempted stimulation of decreased basal value using known feedback or stimulatory pathways (e.g. induction of hypoglycaemia to stimulate an initially low basal growth hormone level in suspected pituitary dwarfism).

Evaluation of anatomical disruption of parapituitary structures

1. *Skull radiograph* — double contour or minor irregularity of the floor of the pituitary fossa, although sometimes a normal finding, may indicate the possibility of a space-occupying lesion. Larger tumours produce generalized enlargement of the fossa, posterior displacement and erosion of the posterior clinoid processes, or downward erosion into the sphenoidal sinuses. Some pituitary tumours are first identified as a result of skull X-ray for a totally unrelated condition (e.g. head trauma). Many pituitary tumours are either entirely intrasellar or do not affect the bony sella confines, and therefore cannot be identified with conventional skull radiology. (Figure 4.13.)

2. *Computed tomography or magnetic resonance imaging (CT or MRI scan)* provide information not only on bone configuration, but because they can resolve

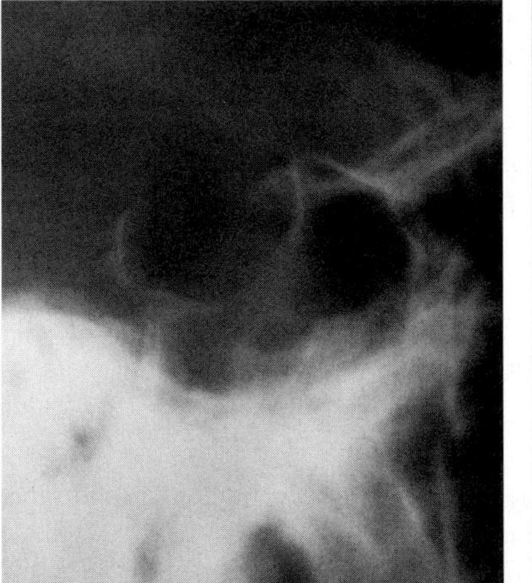

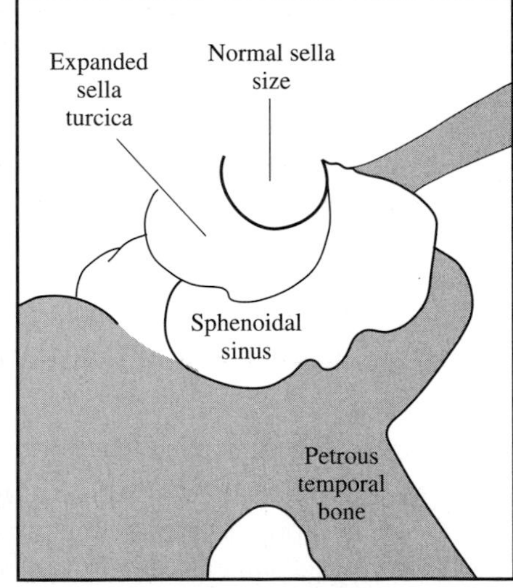

Fig. 4.13. Acromegaly: note enlargement of sella compared with normal pituitary dimensions.

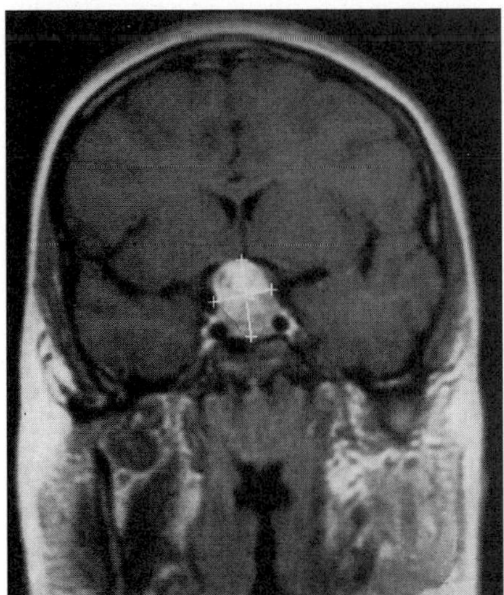

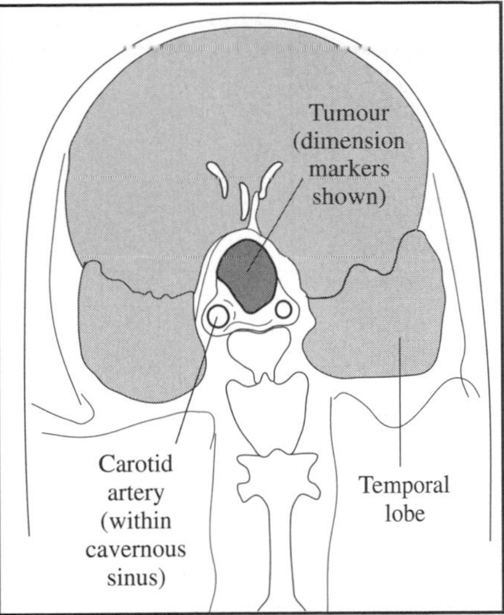

Fig. 4.14. MRI scan of non-functioning pituitary tumour. High density of tumour due to intravenous contrast medium (gadolinium).

soft tissue density, they enable size, position, and extent of any intrasellar mass to be identified, with accurate definition of any extrapituitary extension laterally, inferiorly, or superiorly. Contrast medium is used to enhance the density differences between vascular and relatively avascular tissue. (Figure 4.14.)

3. *Carotid angiography* is sometimes required to exclude carotid artery aneurysm, or to delineate the extent of superior extension of a large suprasellar tumour.

4. *Assessment of visual fields.* Superior and lateral extensions of tumour beyond the pituitary fossa may produce compression of the optic chiasm. In early stages, this produces a bitemporal upper quadrantanopia. In more advanced cases complete bitemporal hemianopia occurs. Larger tumours may result in complete blindness. Visual fields are assessed clinically by confrontation, and more precisely by a number of automated perimetry methods. (Figure 4.15.)

Indirect evidence of hormonal excess or deficiency

There may be indirect evidence of a long-standing hormone disturbance in some cases; for example, delayed skeletal growth in somatotrophin deficiency, demineralization of bone in Cushing's syndrome, increased heel pad thickness and mandibular enlargement in acromegaly.

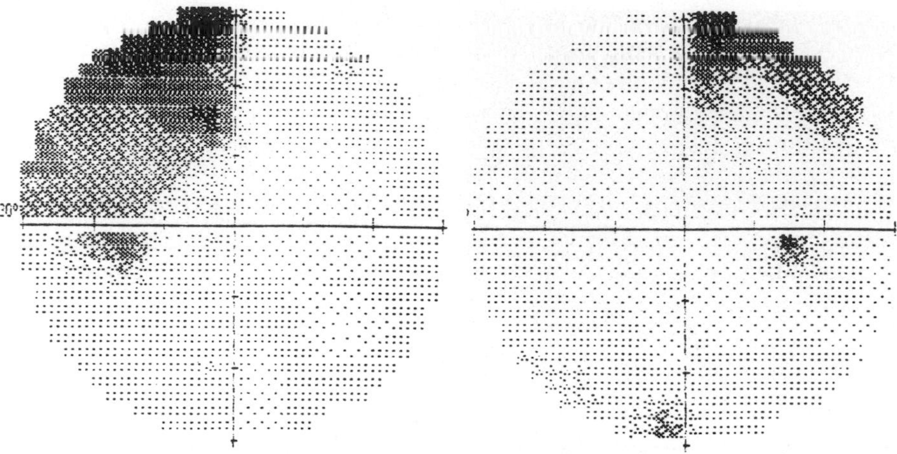

Fig. 4.15. Visual fields of patient in Fig. 4.14: note upper quadrantic bitemporal hemianopia due to chiasmal compression. Fields reverted to normal two weeks after tumour resection.

Individual hormone disturbances

Gonadotrophin

Excess

Sexual precocity associated with increased gonadotrophin secretion is usually induced by tumours in the region of the hypothalamus (occasionally aberrant pinealomata), in which case there are often changes associated with hypothalamic disturbances such as diabetes insipidus and appetite disorders (see also Chapter 13). Recently, LH- and FSH-producing pituitary adenomas have been reported in adults.

Deficiency

Gonadotrophins are often the earliest and occasionally the only trophic hormones to be affected by lesions of the adenohypophysis. In the young, accessory sex organs and secondary sex characteristics fail to develop. Subsequent delay in the maturation and fusion of the epiphyses of long bones results in continued longitudinal growth, and eventual tall stature if treatment is delayed into adult life.

Isolated gonadotrophin defects may be congenital and familial, sometimes occurring together with anosmia, and with other defects such as cleft palate, harelip, and facial asymmetry (Kallman's syndrome). The endocrine lesion is thought to be at the hypothalamic level, based on the usual responsiveness of gonadotrophins to repeated GnRH stimulation. There may be a congenital defect of LH alone in the male, a condition referred to as the 'fertile eunuch syndrome'. It is assumed that LH (and hence testosterone) is secreted in sufficient quantity to maintain spermatogenesis but insufficient to fully develop secondary sex characteristics.

If gonadotrophin deficiency develops in the adult, secondary sex characteristics show evidence of regression and there is scanty or absent pubic and axillary hair, infertility, and possible impotence and loss of libido. In the female, amenorrhoea and some atrophy of external genitalia and vagina occurs. In the male, facial hair growth diminishes, the testes become soft, but penile size usually remains unaltered.

Perhaps the most common cause of gonadotrophin deficiency is encountered in young females with amenorrhoea in response to stress — the so-called 'functional hypothalamic anovulation'. This is encountered in its more severe form in anorexia nervosa. In these clinical situations the abnormality is reversible by correction of the appropriate provocative situation, a procedure sometimes involving psychotherapy (see also Chapter 8).

Diagnosis

Both gonadotrophin and relevant gonadal hormone concentrations are low, in contrast to the hypogonadism of primary gonadal origin in which FSH and LH concentrations are elevated. Theoretically, the adenohypophysial response to GnRH should distinguish between hypothalamic and pituitary causes of hypogonadotrophic hypogonadism, but in practice this test is unreliable.

Treatment

Where infertility is not the primary problem, the clinical features are usually treated by administration of synthetic target hormones, rather than by therapy with gonadotrophins themselves, these being expensive and requiring parenteral administration. Testosterone oenanthate 250 mg every two to four weeks in the male, or ethinyloestradiol 20 to 50 μg daily (usually in combination with a progestogen) in the female are comparatively standard treatments, although there are a wide variety of alternative preparations. In pituitary dwarfism, gonadal replacement therapy is usually deferred until longitudinal growth has been achieved with growth hormone therapy.

Where correction of infertility is the objective, use of gonadotrophins is essential to induce either spermatogenesis or ovulation. In the male, combined LH/FSH therapy is usually employed with or without testosterone over a minimum period of four to six months. Non-response may be due to seminiferous atrophy consequent on prolonged understimulation. In the female, ovulation induction can often be achieved by LH/FSH injections. However where the lesion is at the hypothalamic level, pulsed GnRH, given via a subcutaneous infusion pump is now the principal approach used, with the aim of simulating a normal gonadotrophin secretory pattern, and with a significantly higher rate of ovulation. Such therapy needs to be carefully monitored to avoid ovarian hyperstimulation and consequent multiple pregnancy (see also Chapters 7 and 8).

Simple delayed puberty, a physiological 'functional' form of hypogonadotrophic hypogonadism is paradoxically associated with short stature, and occurs mainly in boys. This condition, its diagnosis and management is dealt with in Chapter 13.

Prolactin

Excess

Hyperprolactinaemia may be induced by a number of drugs and disorders (see Table 4.2), most of which act directly or indirectly on the hypothalamic dopaminergic system. The principal clinical manifestation is galactorrhoea, a milky and normally bilateral breast discharge in females (and rarely in the male). Galactorrhoea is not invariable, even with markedly raised levels. As indicated, serum prolactin is also very responsive to stress of different types. However, consistently elevated prolactin levels are most frequently due to pituitary microadenomata, which are benign and judging by longitudinal radiological studies, extremely slow growing. Disease of the hypothalamic–pituitary pathways, by interfering with dopamine-mediated prolactin inhibition, may also induce elevated prolactin levels; the so-called 'pituitary disconnection syndrome'.

Hyperprolactinaemia suppresses gonadal function by short-loop negative feedback inhibition of LH release. However, it has also been shown that gonadal responsiveness to gonadotrophin is partially inhibited in the presence of raised serum prolactin. Therefore, in addition to the galactorrhoea, infertility and amenorrhoea often occur. Hyperprolactinaemia in men is also occasionally a cause of hypogonadism and infertility, with a loss of libido which is thought to be a direct effect of hyperprolactinaemia, rather than being due to associated hypogonadism.

Hyperprolactinaemia has also been suggested as a cause of premenstrual tension, idiopathic oedema, migraine, the fluid retention seen in heart failure, and eclampsia. However, these claims have little support.

Diagnosis

Hyperprolactinaemia clearly needs to be considered in every patient with non-puerperal galactorrhea, as well as with the wide variety of other presenting

Table 4.2. Major causes of hyperprolactinaemia

Prolactinoma
Pregnancy and breast-feeding
Breast stimulation
Stress (psychological, physical, infection)
Pituitary disconnection
Drugs
Antipsychotics
Neuroleptics
Tricyclic antidepressants
Phenothiazines
Metoclopramide
Cimetidine/ranitidine
Hypothyroidism
Hypoadrenalism
Acromegaly

symptoms listed above. Basal serum prolactin levels more than three times the upper limit of the normal range are usually pathological: lower levels may be due to stress and need reconfirmation before embarking on detailed studies. Microadenomata have values from 1500 mU/l upwards, with macroadenomas (defined as tumours greater than 1 cm diameter and occasionally as large as 4 cm diameter) occasionally producing prolactin levels as high as 500 000 mU/l. Such tumours may behave invasively, extending inferiorly into the sphenoidal sinus, laterally into the cavernous sinus, and even into the middle cranial fossa. Suprasellar extensions are often responsible for various visual field abnormalities (classically bitemporal hemianopia) and even blindness. By compressing or interfering with the circulation to remaining normal pituitary tissue, these larger tumours may also induce varying degrees of hypopituitarism which needs independent investigation.

As with all other pituitary adenomas, prolactinomas may form part of the multiple endocrine neoplasia syndrome (MEN I) and is discussed more fully in Chapter 16. Although systematic screening of all cases for additional endocrinopathy is not justified, routine serum calcium (for hyperparathyroidism) is cheap and has quite high specificity in this setting. In due course, gene probes for MEN genes may prove to be a valid assessment.

Imaging of a possible tumour is essential with prolactin levels above 1500 mU/l: either high resolution CT scanning or (ideally) MRI can be used, both for diagnosis as well as a baseline to assess the effect of any therapeutic approaches.

Treatment

Hyperprolactinaemia requires therapy only under specified circumstances. When due to the dopamine antagonist action of psychotropic drug therapy, values as high as 5000 mU/l are commonly seen, simply noted, and are not themselves an indication for altering drug treatment. The use of dopamine agonists in this situation reverses any beneficial psychopharmacological effects.

In macroadenomas, treatment involves the use of one of the many ergot-related dopamine agonist drugs, of which bromocryptine has had the biggest clinical exposure. All may have the side-effects of nausea and dizziness, unless commenced in low dosage (1.25 mg of bromocryptine or equivalent dose in alternative drugs), taken at night with a snack, and titrating with fortnightly increments against prolactin levels. Newer non-ergot drugs, such as quinagolide, tend to be better tolerated, and longer-acting pharmacological formulations, such as cabergoline also probably diminish side-effects. All these drugs are capable of normalizing or markedly reducing prolactin levels, with a co-incident major reduction in tumour mass, sometimes down to 10 per cent of its initial volume. Lowering of prolactin level by drugs is not necessarily matched by proportional reductions in tumour mass. Only rare cases of tumours becoming refractory to dopamine agonists have been reported, so that long-term and even life-long treatment is often used. Surgery, with its attendant risks of induction of hypopituitarism can therefore be largely avoided.

Some centres advocate radiotherapy to the tumour, once its mass has been reduced in size, but irradiation can result in brain necrosis, optic nerve damage, and late development of hypopituitarism, largely due to co-incident hypothalamic irradiation: accordingly, radiotherapy is often restricted to those patients with a significant demonstrable post-operative residual tumour. Finally, it is now known that between 5 and 10 per cent of tumours appear to spontaneously regress, possibly due to infarction and perhaps due to a direct effect of the dopamine agonist. Accordingly, drug therapy may be discontinued on a trial basis every few years, to avoid needless ongoing therapy.

The approach to microadenomas has evolved from a common surgical approach to a more selective treatment philosophy, particularly in the United States, where dopamine agonists have only recently become available due to licensing formalities: under those circumstances, many women with microadenomas previously required surgical treatment and both residual hyperprolactinaemia and hypopituitarism occurred with significant frequency. Dopamine agonists are now widely available. Women presenting with infertility or galactorrhea can usually be effectively treated with quite small doses. Amenorrhoeic, but otherwise asymptomatic women may not require therapy at all unless circulating oestrogen levels are low. However, in the presence of low oestrogen secretion, it has been shown that age-related loss of bone is accelerated, increasing the risk of later osteoporosis. Accordingly, dopamine agonist therapy in this subgroup is mandatory.

The natural history of microadenomata, as currently perceived from sequential CT and MRI imaging, is for little if any growth over a period of years. Accordingly, frequent re-scanning is not called for in this group of patients. In the rare instance of drug intolerance, transnasal, transsphenoidal removal of a microadenoma in specialized hands can produce acceptable results in terms of treatment of galactorrhoea and infertility, and minimal interference with remaining pituitary function.

Particular care is required when pregnancy arises from successful dopamine agonist treatment of a woman with a prolactinoma. There is a general tendency for prolactinomas to increase in size during pregnancy, partly due to increased pituitary blood flow, but mainly associated with the direct growth-promoting effect of high oestrogen levels. Microadenomata are unlikely to increase significantly in size: accordingly, dopamine agonists are discontinued as soon as conception is confirmed to avoid unnecessary fetal exposure. Macroadenomata, especially those which prior to treatment had significant extrasellar extension, justify continuation of medical treatment throughout pregnancy: previously, cases in which this had not been done have sometimes required urgent neurosurgery. Initial (preconception) surgery or pituitary irradiation have also occasionally been recommended in such high risk cases.

Deficiency

The only known clinical effect of prolactin hyposecretion is the inhibition of lactation in puerperal women. Of the causes of failure of lactation, psychogenic factors and normal physiological variation are the major factors. However, hypopituitarism, especially due to postpartum pituitary necrosis (Sheehan's syndrome) needs to be considered particularly if clinical evidence of other pituitary deficiencies is present.

Somatotrophin (growth hormone)

Excess: acromegaly

Circulating growth hormone levels are particularly labile, rising to high levels in response to any form of stress, as well as to exercise, deep (stage 4) sleep, fasting, uncontrolled diabetes mellitus, and several drugs including propranolol, clonidine, and other drugs with beta-adrenergic blocking activity.

Autonomous hypersecretion of growth hormone, however, is virtually restricted to patients with growth hormone-producing pituitary tumours. The cause of such tumours is unknown. However, the multiplicity of stimulating or inhibiting hypothalamic–pituitary pathways for growth hormone secretion has been referred to earlier in this chapter. Prolonged stimulation of pituitary somatotrophes by disordered hypothalamic mechanisms and receptor status could be envisaged in a number of ways. In fact, a variety of pituitary tumours have been induced experimentally in animals by ablating the relevant target organ (e.g. pituitary thyrotrophe tumours following thyroidectomy and gonadotrophe tumours following gonadectomy). These so-called feedback tumours may provide a clue to a variety of mechanisms which could underlie somatotrophe (and other pituitary) tumours in the human.

Autonomous growth hormone hypersecretion is almost invariably associated with elevations of somatomedin-C (IGF-I), representing the action of integrated growth hormone levels on liver receptors responsible for initiating somatomedin synthesis. The clinical effects in acromegaly can be best seen as due to a combination of growth hormone and somatomedin effects.

Excessive secretion of growth hormone in a child produces the rare syndrome of gigantism: growth is accelerated and heights in excess of 1.5 metres (8 feet) may be reached. Initially, muscular strength is increased but this is replaced by weakness (myopathy) in longstanding cases. If the condition continues untreated after skeletal maturity is reached, the more common changes of acromegaly are seen.

Acromegaly is the name given to the characteristic clinical appearance of adult patients who have growth hormone-producing pituitary adenomas (see Plate 4.3). Such patients have a characteristic clinical appearance manifest by coarsening of facial features due to an increase of connective tissue. Increased cartilaginous growth results in an enlargement of the ears and nose, and growth of the mandible leads to a jutting jaw (prognathism), while alveolar bone growth causes the teeth to separate. The enlargement of the frontal and maxillary sinuses results in a prominent brow and a long face. In addition there is a well-recognized broadening and enlargement of the hands and feet due both to increased periosteal growth as well as thickening of skin and subcutaneous tissue (see Plate 4.4). The facial appearance may superficially resemble that of hypothyroidism, partly because in the latter condition there is also facial swelling and enlargement of the tongue. A husky voice is also a feature of both disorders.

There is also generalized visceral enlargement involving the spleen, liver, kidneys, and almost invariably the heart. Hypertension is common, and is at least partly related to the sodium and water retention consequent upon renal actions of growth hormone. Additional clinical features result from anatomical effects of the pituitary tumour on neighbouring structures, such as the optic chiasm and the cavernous sinuses, and from interference with function of other pituitary cells induced: accordingly, hypopituitarism of varying degrees is quite often seen in acromegaly.

In the florid case described above, the diagnosis is obvious, but the disease normally has a subtle presentation and follows a slow and insidious course with clinical features which have (usually in retrospect) evolved over a period of years or decades. Normally, there are warning symptoms such as joint pains (due to associated synovial hypertrophy and degenerative arthritis), excessive sweating (a direct growth hormone effect), and paraesthesiae of the hands and feet (due to nerve entrapment by thickened bone and subcutaneous tissue) some years before the typical physical changes appear. Headaches may occur: although superficially attributable to fossa expansion, they more frequently represent sensory nerve entrapment.

In some cases, the progress of the disease may appear to halt spontaneously. This 'burnt out' or inactive phase is usually more apparent than real: even in patients with stable clinical features, growth hormone levels are almost invariably raised. Nevertheless, in rare cases, spontaneous infarction of somatotrophe (as indeed other pituitary) tumours does occur. This may be a dramatic event, simulating meningitis with cardiovascular collapse, or a more subtle event which passes unnoticed. In all such cases, clinical features, especially those due to soft tissue changes, actually regress. Usually, the disease will gradually progress, with increasing deformity and disability due to arthropathy. Treatment is indicated not only for symptoms but also because mortality is increased due to accelerated atheromatous cerebro- and cardiovascular disease, cardiomyopathy and hypertension and rarely as a result of the tumour itself.

Associated endocrine disorders

Most patients have slightly elevated prolactin levels and women occasionally present with galactorrhoea, due to cosecretion of prolactin with somatotrophin. Approximately 25 per cent of patients have impaired glucose tolerance due to increased gluconeogenesis: only half of these develop overt diabetes mellitus. While basal metabolic rate may be increased and patients complain of feeling warm, hyperthyroidism is uncommon but a goitre is present in approximately 20 per cent of cases as part of the generalized visceral enlargement. Hypogonadism, hypothyroidism, and even hypoadrenalism may occur as a result of secondary hypopituitarism, with associated fatigue, reduced libido, impotence, and amenorrhoea together with all the other features referred to elsewhere in this chapter. Occasionally, diabetes insipidus may occur due to suprasellar tumour extension.

Multiple endocrine adenomatosis is a rare condition in which there are associated but physiologically unrelated parathyroid and pancreatic islet cell tumours (see Chapter 16).

Diagnosis

Because of large physiological variations, random growth hormone levels have no diagnostic value whatsoever. Serum growth hormone levels, measured at half-hourly intervals after a 75 g glucose load, are unsuppressable (to less than 3 mU/l) in acromegaly and in very few other situations such as severe anxiety, depression, or uncontrolled insulin-dependent diabetes. The same procedure can be used for following the progress of this disease in response to treatment. Administration of 200 μg intravenous TRH will produce a significant (doubling) growth hormone rise in acromegaly which is qualitatively unique and diagnostic. Serum IGF-I levels are also diagnostically useful, being almost invariably raised in acromegaly. However, because IGF-I is nutrition-dependent, any serious associated disorder may falsely lower IGF-I levels and thereby produce diagnostic confusion.

Only in about 70 per cent of cases will an enlarged pituitary fossa be seen using routine skull radiology because the tumour is often small. Computed tomography (CT) or magnetic resonance (MRI) scanning will always identify the tumour. An increase in subcutaneous tissue (as in the heel pad) or skin thickening is often measurable by radiological techniques, but these findings have no absolute diagnostic value. Visual field assessment, most conveniently by automated perimetry identifies those cases with anatomically significant suprasellar extension.

Treatment

Pharmacological Although tumours associated with acromegaly are relatively autonomous, growth hormone secretion can be modified and sometimes totally suppressed by drugs acting through pathways known to modify physiological growth hormone secretion. First employed were dopamine agonists, of which bromocryptine has had the greatest exposure. Increasing doses gradually to tolerance (up to 40 mg daily) reduces growth hormone levels in most patients, but only rarely to the target (normal) value of less than 3 mU/l. There are, however, little firm data upon which to base any target growth hormone value which could be confidently relied on to confer some level of improved prognosis. Alternative dopamine agonists can be used; other ergot derivatives (lysuride, pergolide, cabergoline) and non-ergot compounds (quinagolide). In general, it is rare to achieve a normal growth hormone profile with these compounds.

More recently, somatostatin analogues have been used: in subcutaneous doses of octreotide 100–200 μg 8-hourly, suppression of growth hormone to the consistently low values referred to above can be achieved in about 50 per cent of cases. Because of the inconvenience of such frequent parenteral dosage, longer-acting injectable and orally effective analogues are currently being evaluated. These newer compounds are likely to be of great therapeutic importance, since other destructive approaches to tumours associated with acromegaly are often functionally incomplete (see below).

Although there was an initial impression that tumour shrinkage was significant with the above pharmacological approaches (as is the case with prolactinoma), in acromegaly, such reduction of tumour size is statistical rather than clinically useful: accordingly, where there is anatomical expansion of clinical significance, surgery is the most appropriate initial step.

Surgical For definitive cure of acromegaly, small intrasellar tumours of less than 1 cm diameter can be resected by a transnasal, trans-sphenoidal approach.

This is a comparatively minor surgical procedure with a high success rate and low morbidity: other pituitary functions are often preserved. Therefore, it represents the treatment of choice with such small tumours. A striking post-operative diuresis and a remarkably rapid regression of soft tissue changes (including reversal of cardiomegaly) are often seen.

With increasing tumour size, the responses to surgery are progressively less satisfactory, due to tumour cell remnants often embedded in the lateral fossa walls. However, surgery also has a significant role as a debulking procedure particularly where there is chiasmal compression. Trans-sphenoidal surgery may not provide optimum access, and a formal craniotomy is then necessary. In all situations where incomplete tumour removal has been demonstrated by persistently raised growth hormone levels, either pharmacological or radiotherapy approaches are normally considered, depending on the age and life expectancy of the patient.

Irradiation This is usually performed over a four- to six-week period by conventional external irradiation using a cobalt source, or a linear accelerator, using a maximum dose which does not exceed 4500 rad (cGy) given through multiple intersecting fields in order to avoid irradiation damage to surrounding structures. More directional alpha-particle or proton-beam therapy is available in a few centres, allowing a larger dose to be delivered with even less risk of damage to parasellar structures. Conventional irradiation therapy alone is effective in no more than half of the cases treated, and the clinical benefits, even in responsive cases, may take up to 10 years to become apparent. Radiation therapy risks the development of other adenohypophyseal deficiencies by irradiation of normal (but more radioresistant) pituitary tissue. It is likely that both the beneficial and adverse effects of radiotherapy may be based at least in part on the incidental irradiation of more radiosensitive neighbouring hypothalamic centres. Whatever the mechanism, life-long follow up of endocrine function is mandatory: for example, 50 per cent of patients thus treated become thyroxine- or cortisol-requiring over a 10-year follow-up period.

Cases of brain necrosis and optic nerve damage due to irradiation have been noted, particularly in older patients, and spectral MRI analysis has shown minor but possible significant changes in the brains of treated patients. Accordingly, renewed concern is being directed at this form of treatment for what is fundamentally a non-malignant tumour.

Deficiency

As indicated earlier, growth hormone levels are very labile, and a value which is undetectable by routine growth hormone assay may be obtained even in normal subjects under appropriate conditions (e.g. post-prandially).

True deficiency is based on abnormal hypothalamic or pituitary function. Suprasellar tumours, such as craniopharyngioma (which may frequently calcify) in children, and chromophobe adenoma and parasellar tumours in adults, are the common causes. Growth hormone deficiency is also one of the most common adenohypophysial defects in generalized pituitary disease resulting from any cause. However, so-called 'idiopathic growth hormone deficiency' is a common subgroup occurring as an isolated defect in hormone release, and may reflect either a primary hypothalamic or pituitary disorder.

The manifestations of growth hormone deficiency are dominated by growth failure in childhood. In the adult, clinical manifestations may include impaired hair growth and proneness to fasting- and alcohol-induced hypoglycaemia, and a wide variety of less dramatic symptoms such as poor muscular tone, malaise, osteoporosis, and a variety of psychological changes.

Growth hormone does not appear to play a significant role in the growth of the fetus, and a deficiency of somatotrophin at this stage does not affect birth weight. It is, therefore, only after birth that there is impairment of growth, and hence the condition is not usually recognized before the first year of life.

Clinical features

Parents usually bring their affected child because of growth failure. The child has an immature face and is short and often overweight for his/her age; radiological skeletal immaturity may be marked, and there is progressive growth failure below expected percentiles. It is difficult to define normal growth rates without referring to standard growth charts (see Chapter 13).

Pituitary dwarfism must be distinguished from other causes of short stature, including malabsorption syndrome and a wide range of systemic and skeletal disorders, all of which need to be considered in the full differential diagnosis of short stature. These are dealt with in Chapter 13.

In growth hormone deficiency, other adenohypophysial deficiencies may be present at the onset, or may develop in the course of subsequent treatment. This is particularly so in regard to hypothyroidism due to TSH deficiency.

A clinically similar syndrome to growth hormone deficiency may occur due to defective hepatic growth hormone receptors, so that somatomedin (IGF-I) deficiency is then the cause of the growth failure (Laron syndrome).

Diagnosis

CT scans or MRI are used to exclude hypothalamic or pituitary tumours, infiltrates, and rarer developmental abnormalities such as aqueductal stenosis.

Because of the fluctuating serum levels of growth hormone, a random growth hormone sample is of little value. A screening test employing very strenuous exercise to the point of exhaustion (e.g. exercise bicycle or brisk stair climbing) usually causes an elevation of serum growth hormone beyond the normal diagnostic level of 20 mU/l. Non-responders can then be challenged by more complex, costly, and occasionally dangerous procedures such as stimulation by combined arginine infusion and insulin-induced hypoglycaemia (see Chapter 13).

In adults, the diagnosis of growth hormone deficiency has until recently been considered irrelevant. However, treatment of growth hormone-deficient adults with growth hormone has been shown to produce occasionally impressive correction of more or less minor but important symptoms, which were otherwise attributable to 'ageing'. Indeed, growth hormone deficiency itself is probably one of the accompaniments of normal ageing: accordingly, it may prove feasible and desirable to treat such deficiency, especially if it is pharmacologically possible to enhance endogenous growth hormone release.

Treatment

Prior to the occurrence of epiphysial fusion, the appropriate treatment is human growth hormone derived by recombinant DNA technology. This is expensive and must be given until longitudinal growth is complete. The normal dose range of subcutaneous growth hormone is between 0.5–1.0 unit/kg week in divided dosage, until completion of growth. This is normally supplemented by additional hormone replacement depending on associated deficiencies. Gonadal hormone replacement is usually deferred as long as possible to avoid premature epiphyseal fusion. Associated tumours require independent assessment and therapy.

The knowledge that some cases of growth hormone deficiency are based on defective hGH-releasing hormone release, has led to the use of parenteral hGH-RH analogues such as hexarelin in the management of some cases. At this stage, it is not known whether such an approach is more effective than growth hormone itself, but there may be considerable biological and financial advantages as well as the theoretical possibility of oral or at least less frequent parenteral administration. Somatomedin therapy is also under investigation, and its use will broaden the variety of disorders capable of being treated for growth delay, including the Laron syndrome.

Corticotrophin (ACTH)

Excess

Effects are mainly due to enhanced quantities of cortisol and androgens from the adrenals. The resulting clinical picture which this induces (Cushing's syndrome) is discussed in Chapter 5 . Excluding iatrogenic causes and ectopic secretion from non-endocrine tumours (see Chapter 15), Cushing's syndrome in some 75 per cent of cases is pituitary-dependent.

Deficiency

Typically, corticotrophin is one of the least frequent hormones to be involved when adenohypophysial function is impaired. The clinical picture is essentially similar to that seen in primary adrenocorticoid deficiency (see Chapter 4), with non-specific fatigue as the primary symptom. Because of ACTH deficiency the skin is not pigmented (in contrast to primary adrenocortical deficiency): similarly, since aldosterone secretion can be maintained in the absence of ACTH, dehydration is not a clinical feature.

Diagnosis

Current plasma ACTH assays do not have the sensitivity to invariably distinguish between normal and subnormal levels. Although basal cortisol levels are low, these too are not diagnostic. Because the unstimulated adrenals atrophy as a result of ACTH deficiency, even after a few weeks, the short tetracosactrin stimulation test referred to under primary adrenocortical deficiency, will be abnormal: serum cortisol will not stimulate to the normal minimum value of 550 nmol/l. Other tests have been used but are not often required. Metopirone (metyrapone), an 11-hydroxylase inhibitor, reduces cortisol secretion and in normal subjects produces a secondary increase in endogenous ACTH and cortisol precursors which can be measured. The stimulus of insulin-induced hypoglycaemia produces a stress-induced rise of ACTH in normal subjects: either ACTH or cortisol can be measured to identify this response.

Treatment

Standard glucocorticoid replacement consists of oral hydrocortisone (cortisol) 20–30 mg daily in divided dosage, incremented as indicated in Chapter 5, in response to stress situations. As discussed earlier, mineralocorticoid replacement is not required, since adrenal aldosterone production is almost entirely independent of ACTH control.

Thyrotrophin (TSH)

Excess

The hyperthyroidism of Graves' disease was initially believed to be due to an excess secretion of TSH. It is now clear that thyroid-stimulating immunoglobulins are the primary cause of that disorder, and pituitary TSH secretion is almost completely suppressed by negative feedback in almost all cases of hyperthyroidism. Only very rarely is thyroid hyperfunction due to oversecretion of TSH. This has been recorded in acromegaly and in rare TSH-producing pituitary tumours: treatment in these cases is directed at the underlying tumour.

Deficiency

Reduction of thyrotrophin induces a similar clinical picture to that of primary thyroid deficiency (see Chapter 9). However, there is often evidence of other trophic hormone deficiency which gives a clue to adenohypophysial aetiology.

Diagnosis

In contrast to the hypothyroidism of primary thyroidal origin, in which low total and free T_4 (and sometimes free T_3 levels) are accompanied by elevated TSH levels, the hypothyroidism of pituitary origin is associated with a low or normal TSH level. Therefore, evaluation of the biochemically hypothyroid patient always demands concurrent estimation of TSH for accurate identification of the primary cause. Serum TSH concentration may be expected to be diagnostically low on assay. However, even with the most sensitive assays, it is not possible to discriminate between low normal and hypopituitary levels. Administration of TRH might similarly be expected to provide additional evidence of the site of the lesion: in hypothalamic disease, a normal (or occasionally excessive) response of the serum TSH, while in pituitary disease an reduced response. There are exceptions to these expected patterns, and the test does not usually provide information which cannot be obtained more reliably by imaging techniques.

Treatment

Thyroxine is normally given as for primary hypothyroidism. However, if the patient has co-existent ACTH deficiency, as is frequently the case, steroid replacement must be commenced concurrently: otherwise, by increasing the relative cortisol requirement, thyroxine may precipitate a pituitary 'crisis' (see following section).

Clinical and aetiological characteristics of hypopituitarism

A number of pathological processes result in variable degrees of disturbance to pituitary function. Although the term 'pan-hypopituitarism' is used to describe the situation where all trophic hormones are involved, in practice, the clinical syndrome varies according to the dominant cell type involved.

The initial concept of a precise sequence of involvement of trophic hormones with increasing destruction/compression has now been shown to be fallacious. Nevertheless, somatotrophin and gonadotrophin production and release tend to be impaired in comparatively early disease affecting the pituitary, while thyrotrophin and corticotrophin deficiencies usually reflect a more severe involvement by the pathological process.

The clinical presentation may be quite subtle, with tiredness the first and only symptom, occasionally associated with a chronic normochromic anaemia. Indeed, the disorder may only be unmasked by a superimposed stress situation such as an accident, anaesthetic, or infection. These events can induce a pituitary 'crisis' with nausea, vomiting, dehydration, hypotension, and ultimately coma. Apart from the absence of gross dehydration, this clinical picture closely resembles an acute adrenal crisis. Hyponatraemia is common, but usually dilutional in origin and due to defective water excretion which is a direct consequence of adrenocortical and thyroid hormone deficiencies.

The appearance of the patient with early hypopituitarism may be normal, but the combination of severe hypogonadism, hypothyroidism, and hypoadrenalism produces a curious waxy pallor with fine, comparatively hairless skin in a slightly obese patient, an appearance which in its gross form can be quite characteristic (see Plate 4.3). Early concepts of pituitary 'cachexia' have now been shown to be incorrect: very thin patients were almost certainly examples of anorexia nervosa.

Aetiology (see table 4.3)

Intrasellar tumours

Of these, the microadenomata of pituitary-dependent Cushing's syndrome are least likely to be associated with interference with other pituitary functions, while those of acromegaly, the common non-functioning chromophobe tumours, and prolactinomas are more likely to induce trophic hormone deficiencies.

Table 4.3. Major causes of hypopituitarism

Intrasellar pituitary tumours
Prolactinoma
Acromegaly
Cushing's disease
Non-functioning pituitary adenoma
Metastasis
Secondary (extrasellar) tumours
Craniopharyngioma
Pinealoma
Meningioma
Glioma
Infiltration/inflammation
Idiopathic hypophysitis
Tuberculosis
Sarcoidosis
Haemochromatosis
Eosinophilic granuloma/histiocytosis
Amyloidosis
Meningitis
Other causes
Carotid artery aneurysm
Trauma
Postpartum pituitary infarction
Pituitary apoplexy
(Primary empty sella syndrome)

Primary extrasellar tumours

Sphenoidal ridge meningioma, optic nerve glioma, and various secondary (metastatic) tumours, as well as suprasellar tumours, such as craniopharyngioma and pinealoma, often produce significant hypopituitarism. In some cases, this is due more to interference with the hypothalamic–pituitary neurovascular connections, rather than direct involvement of specific groups of pituitary cells. In addition, these tumours are more likely to involve the supraoptico–hypophysial tract, thereby inducing diabetes insipidus as an additional hormone deficiency.

Carotid artery aneurysms

These may expand medially into the pituitary fossa, inducing multiple hormone deficiencies and simulating an intrasellar tumour.

Infiltration

A number of pathological processes, including sarcoidosis, haemochromatosis, tuberculous meningitis, and rarities, such as granulomas of Hand–Schüller–Christian disease, may all provide differing degrees of interference with adenohypophysial function.

The empty sella syndrome

This is an increasingly recognized phenomenon characterized by a radiologically normal or enlarged pituitary fossa and occupation of the sella by an extension of the subarachnoid space. An empty sella may occur either as a primary anatomical variant, or following the spontaneous infarction, surgery or radiotherapy of a tumour: a CSF-containing arachnoid extension evolves in order to occupy the space left by the tumour. If hypopituitarism is present, it is unlikely to be due to the empty sella itself, but rather the pathology which preceded it. However, visual field changes may occur due to prolapse of the optic chiasma into the sella. Many cases are incidentally diagnosed, when skull radiology or CT or MRI are performed for an unrelated reason, and the characteristic lucency of CSF identified within the sella.

Pituitary infarction or haemorrhage

Sheehan's syndrome. During pregnancy, blood flow through the pituitary is markedly increased. Although a less common problem than previously, major postpartum haemorrhage causes sufficient acute reduction in blood flow through the pituitary to result in infarction of this previously well-vascularized organ. Although this may produce quite acute postpartum symptoms, a more delayed presentation with amenorrhoea and vague symptomatology is more usual, even years later.

Pituitary apoplexy. A similar but more dramatic presentation is that in which a pre-existing pituitary adenoma undergoes infarction, usually together with some parapituitary haemorrhage. The cause of this is never easy to identify, but may represent a tumour outgrowing its blood supply. Patients present with a meningitic-type syndrome with or without acute collapse. Since routine skull radiology is often normal, the diagnosis can be overlooked until CT or MRI is performed. Pituitary apoplexy is followed by selective or multihormonal hypopituitarism, and with later appearance of an empty sella on high-resolution scanning.

Idiopathic hypopituitarism

As a 'cause' of hypopituitarism, this is second in frequency only to intrasellar tumours. It appears to be due either to an immunodestructive process in the pituitary (allied to the thyrogastric autoimmune group) or to primary hypothalamic disease, for which no structural defect has been shown to be responsible. Much clarification is required in the understanding of this important group of disorders which may also present as single hormone (monotrophic) deficiencies.

Severe head trauma

Although this is more likely to be associated with transient diabetes insipidus due to neurohypophysial damage, in rare cases severe injury will produce either transient or permanent adenohypophysial damage.

Irradiation

Megavoltage therapy of pituitary or other intracranial lesions, including tumours of the nasopharyngeal area, quite frequently leads to hypopituitarism. Whether this is based on primary hypothalamic or pituitary damage is not clear, although there is evidence that hypothalamic tissue is more radiosensitive.

Diagnosis

The confirmation of a diagnosis may not always be possible prior to the need for immediate treatment. This applies particularly to various forms of pituitary 'crisis' referred to above. In this latter situation, rehydration and administration of hydrocortisone 400 mg by continuous infusion over the first 24 hours is usually life-saving. Subsequently, more detailed evaluation can be performed to clarify the precise pathology and extent of endocrine involvement. In less acute cases, the characteristic abnormalities described in the separate sections earlier in this chapter should clarify the diagnosis.

Treatment

Treatment is precisely based on the demonstrated deficiencies, as indicated in the appropriate sections discussed above. While cortisol and thyroxine replacement are mandatory when these are demonstrated to be deficient, growth hormone replacement is normally only used where short stature is an additional problem in children. Nevertheless, as previously discussed, adult growth hormone deficiency is being increasingly viewed as a clinically important syndrome, justifying at least a consideration of replacement therapy. Similarly, androgen and oestrogen replacement is not always indicated, particularly in patients past middle age, although in women, an early menopause whatever its cause, is associated with a much higher risk of osteoporosis: accordingly, premenopausal loss of oestrogen is an indication for oestrogen replacement (see Chapter 8).

Clearly, treatment of the underlying pathology is also necessary, and endocrine evaluation needs to be repeated at intervals to ensure no change in the endocrine profile, particularly after pituitary surgery or radiotherapy. Education is of utmost importance, since replacement therapy is life-long, and appropriate instruction for increasing steroid replacement is essential to avoid risk of crisis with intercurrent infection or other form of stress.

Clinical disorders of the neurohypophysis

An excess of oxytocin has not been described, and the deficiency of oxytocin which complicates hypothalamic disease is probably not clinically significant. Accordingly, this section will be entirely devoted to arginine vasopressin (AVP) using the title antidiuretic hormone (ADH) which is the usual clinical term employed.

Excess

Inappropriate ADH secretion. As yet there has been no reported case of excess ADH secretion by a tumour of the pars nervosa. However, ADH secretion may

Table 4.4. Causes of inappropriate ADH secretion (SIADH)

CNS Disease
Meningitis
Head injury
Brain tumour/abscess
Subarachnoid/subdural haemorrhage
Cerebral thrombosis/haemorrhage
Guillain–Barré syndrome
Acute intermittent porphyria
Endocrine disease
Hypothyroidism
Hypoadrenalism
Hypopituitarism
Other causes
Pneumonia/lung abscess
Bronchogenic carcinoma
Tuberculosis/sarcoidosis
Aspergillosis
Postoperative
Hepatic cirrhosis
Drugs: chlorpropamide, clofibrate, phenytoin
Idiopathic

persist in a wide variety of clinical conditions in which it would be expected to be suppressed: this condition has been entitled the 'syndrome of "inappropriate" secretion of ADH' (SIADH). Its causes are summarized in Table 4.4. It is assumed that if the syndrome exists the following are present: hyponatraemia, hypo-osmolar serum, urine osmolality in excess of plasma, and normal renal and adrenal function. The syndrome has been redefined such that its occurrence is accepted when 'the amount of ADH released and the elevation of urine osmolality which it produces are considered to be inappropriate only in relationship to the plasma osmolality'. Since assay of ADH is one of the least readily available, the diagnosis is normally made indirectly, and the presence of the syndrome inferred by characteristic clinical features.

Clinical features

Even though hyponatraemia may be severe, symptoms are often absent. This is in strong contrast to the hyponatraemia associated with significant sodium depletion from a number of other causes. However, there may be generalized weakness, malaise, poor mental function, anorexia, and nausea. Serum sodium concentration may fall to less than 110 mmol/l, resulting in confusion, clouding of consciousness, epileptiform attacks, and ultimately coma if the condition remains unrecognized and untreated.

In the differential diagnosis, hyponatraemia is seen to occur in many other conditions, such as gastrointestinal sodium loss, sodium-losing nephritis, adrenocortical deficiency, and in chronic oedematous states, including congestive cardiac failure. True hyponatraemia must also be differentiated from the pseudohyponatraemia of hyperproteinaemia (e.g. myeloma) or of hyperlipidemia (where plasma space is occupied by excess lipid).

Diagnosis

This is usually confirmed by demonstrating hyponatraemia (serum sodium less than 130 mmol/l) together with plasma hypo-osmolality and inappropriately elevated urine osmolality. Where indicated, standard tests are employed to exclude adrenal and renal dysfunction.

Treatment

The underlying lesion should be treated when possible, or the causative drug discontinued. Water intake is restricted to 500–600 ml per 24 hours, or in severe cases withheld altogether. Fludrocortisone and other corticosteroids should not be administered, as this will cause retention of greater quantities of water without altering plasma sodium concentration. Similarly, intravenous saline will not significantly raise the plasma sodium and may be detrimental since such patients already suffer from excess body water and have a normal total body sodium. The antibiotic demeclocycline inhibits tubular receptors for ADH, and in doses of 900–1200 mg daily corrects the hyponatraemia by creating temporary nephrogenic diabetes insipidus. A number of other drugs have been used for a similar effect, but are less certain in their action and usually less well tolerated.

Deficiency

Diabetes insipidus

This disorder results from a relative or complete absence of ADH, and is sometimes referred to as cranial diabetes insipidus in order to avoid confusion with nephrogenic diabetes insipidus, which is due to insensitivity of the renal tubule to ADH.

The most common cause of diabetes insipidus is head injury or surgical procedure in the vicinity of the pituitary gland. Suprasellar tumours and other pathologies, such as granulomatous infiltration, sarcoidosis, and Hand–Schüller–Christian disease, give rise to diabetes insipidus only if the lesion involves the median eminence as well as the pars nervosa. This observation is based on the fact that sufficient secretion of ADH can occur directly into the circulation from the median eminence, even with complete trans-section of the pituitary stalk.

No causal factor can be detected in approximately one-third of patients presenting with diabetes insipidus, although some studies using MRI imaging have demonstrated minor hypothalamic abnormalities in a proportion of patients. Some cases are familial and may date from infancy. This observation, together with the concurrence of diabetes insipidus, diabetes mellitus, optic atrophy and deafness in the same individual (DIDMOAD or Wolfram syndrome) suggests a major genetic factor which has so far not been characterized. Another form of diabetes insipidus occurs only during pregnancy and resolves postpartum. There is evidence to suggest that such patients have borderline basal ADH secretion even in the non-pregnant state: the placenta enhances catabolism of ADH and thereby renders the deficiency clinically significant only during pregnancy.

Clinical features

There is insatiable thirst and intense polyuria (up to 20 litres daily). While the onset of these changes is usually gradual, it may sometimes be sudden and dramatic. The danger of dehydration in adverse environmental conditions is very real. The same danger occurs in the unconscious patient following head injury or intracranial surgery when adequate fluid replacement may not be maintained.

There are three major conditions which may be confused with diabetes insipidus: first, *compulsive water drinking* (psychogenic polydipsia), in which the polydipsia represents a unique response to stress and anxiety, somewhat akin to the rather more common stress-induced hyperphagia. In more severe cases, the polydipsia becomes surreptitious and manipulative, usually with more severe metabolic disturbance (dilutional hyponatraemia resulting in disordered brain function). Secondly, *nephrogenic diabetes insipidus*, where there is renal tubular resistance to ADH. This may be a consequence of chronic pyelonephritis, hypercalcaemia, or hypokalaemia. The drug lithium, which is commonly used in the treatment of bipolar depression, also induces ADH resistance by a direct tubular action, as does demeclocycline which is specifically used to induce ADH insensitivity in the treatment of inappropriate ADH referred to earlier in this chapter. Finally, patients with hypothalamic tumours may manifest *neurogenic polydipsia*, due to direct stimulation of hypothalamic thirst centres by tumour or surgical injury. Recognition of this disorder is important, since inappropriate administration of ADH may result in acute fluid overload, cerebral oedema, and death.

Diagnosis

Plasma urea and electrolyte concentrations demonstrate the effects of selective water deficit with hypernatraemia and elevated blood urea. In addition, urine osmolality shows an inadequate rise following dehydration, but unlike nephrogenic diabetes insipidus, responds normally to administration of a therapeutic dose of ADH. The compulsive water drinker, when subjected to an ADH bolus, often shows a greater increase in urine osmolality (800–1000 mOsm/kg compared with 600–800 mOsm/kg in diabetes insipidus), but is occasionally and inexplicably unable to optimally concentrate the urine in response to fluid deprivation.

Treatment

Desamino-D-arginine vasopressin (DDAVP), an analogue of AVP has greater antidiuretic potency and less vasopressor side-effects, and has simplified the treatment of diabetes insipidus. Therapy consists of administering 10–20 μg DDAVP intranasally once or twice daily. DDAVP is also available in parenteral form and an oral preparation of which doses vary from 300 to 600 μg daily.

Mild cases of diabetes insipidus were previously treated using chlorpropamide, which in addition to its hypoglycaemic effect, enhances the renal tubular action of suboptimal ADH concentrations. With the advent of oral desmopressin the use of this and other compounds, such as clofibrate, are of historic interest only.

Nephrogenic diabetes insipidus, occurring either as a primary disease entity, or secondary to a wide variety of renal disorders is clearly unresponsive to the usual measures but may be controlled using a thiazide diuretic which reduces free water clearance.

FURTHER READING

PHYSIOLOGY

Breyer, M.D. and Ando, Y. (1994). Hormonal signaling and regulation of salt and water transport in the collecting duct. *Annual Review of Physiology*, **56**, 711–39.

Crowley, W.R. and Armstrong, W.E. (1992). Neurochemical regulation of oxytocin secretion in lactation. *Endocrine Reviews*, **13**, 33–65.

Kalra, S.P. (1993). Mandatory neuropeptide-steroid signaling for the preovulatory luteinizing hormone-releasing hormone discharge. *Endocrine Reviews*, **14**, 507–38.

Stojilkovic, S.S., Reinhart, J., and Catt, K.J. (1994). Gonadotrophin-releasing hormone receptors: structure and signal transduction pathways. *Endocrine Reviews*, **15**, 462–99.

Thissen, J-P., Ketelslegers, J-M., and Underwood, L.E. (1994). Nutritional regulation of the insulin-like factors. *Endocrine Reviews*, **15**, 80–101.

Vamrakapoulos, N.C. and Chrousos, G.P. (1994). Hormonal regulation of human corticotrophin releasing hormone gene expression: implications for the stress response and immune/inflammatory reaction. *Endocrine Reviews*, **15**, 409–430.

Webb, S.M. and Puig-Domingo, M. (1995). Role of melatonin in health and disease. *Clinical Endocrinology*, **42**, 221–34.

CLINICAL

Bates, A.S., Van't Hoff, W., Jones, J.M., and Clayton, R.N. (1993). An audit of outcome of treatment in acromegaly. *Quarterly Journal of Medicine*, **86**, 293–9.

Beshyah, S.A., Freemantle, C., Shahi, M., *et al.* (1995). Replacement treatment with biosynthetic growth hormone in growth hormone deficient hypopituitary adults. *Clinical Endocrinology* **42**, 73–84.

Faglia, G., *et al.* (1993). Pituitary tumours: diagnosis and management (symposium). *Acta Endocrinol.* **129** (Suppl.1), 1–40.

Grua, J.R. and Nelson D.H. (1991). ACTH-producing pituitary tumours. *Endocrinology Metabolism Clinics North America*, **20**, 319–62.

Katznelson, L., Alexander, J.M., and Klibanski, A. (1993) Clinically non-functioning pituitary adenomas. *Journal of Clinical Endocrinology and Metabolism,* **76**, 1089–94.

Laws, E.R. (1987) Pituitary surgery, *Endocrinology Metabolism Clinics North America*, **16**, 647–65

Levy, A. and Lightman, S.L. (1993). The pathogenesis of pituitary adenomas. *Clinical Endocrinology*, **38**, 559–70.

Lightman, S.L. (1993) Molecular insights into diabetes insipidus. *New England Journal of Medicine*, **328**, 1562–3.

Mankin, H.J. (1994) Progress in the management of hyperprolactinaemia. *New England Journal of Medicine*, **331**, 942–3.

Molitch, M.E. (1992) Clinical manifestations of acromegaly. *Endocrinology Metabolism Clinics North America*, **21**, 597–614.

Reid, R.L., Quigley, M.E., and Yen, S.C.C. (1985) Pituitary apoplexy: a review. *Archives Neurology*, **42**, 712–8.

Soskin, A., *et al.* (1995). New developments in the treatment and diagnosis of acromegaly (symposium). *Clinical Endocrinology*, **44**, (Suppl.1), 1–33

Vance, M.L. (1994). Hypopituitarism, *New England Journal of Medicine*, **330**, 1651–62.

5

The adrenal cortex

PHYSIOLOGY

The adrenal cortex can be considered as an endocrine gland quite distinct from the adrenal medulla. Control of the adrenal cortical cells is principally by the action of other hormones and by variations in the plasma concentrations of certain chemical substances. It secretes steroid hormones (corticosteroids) which control either salt and water balance (mineralocorticoids), or regulate metabolic processes (glucocorticoids), although their actions are not sharply differentiated. In addition, small amounts of oestrogens and androgens, also steroid hormones, are normally secreted by the adrenal cortex. Extirpation of the adrenal cortices is rapidly fatal, so that, unlike the adrenal medullae, they play a vital role in the normal homeostatic regulation of many important physiological functions.

Anatomy, histology, and development

The bilateral adrenal glands are recognizable in the fetus at two months' gestation. Each gland is derived from mesenchymal cells forming the primitive outer layer, or cortex, which is invaded by neuroectodermal (chromaffin) cells forming the central medulla. In the fetus the glands become very vascular and large. A thin outer layer of cells forms, surrounding a much larger 'fetal zone' which disappears rapidly after birth. At this stage the thin outer layer already has two distinct regions, the zonae glomerulosa and fasciculata, while the innermost layer (the zona reticularis) develops soon after. Thus, the adult adrenal cortex consists of three relatively distinct bands of cells. The outermost layer, the zona glomerulosa, is relatively narrow and consists of small cells grouped together in poorly defined clusters. The wider middle zone, the zona fasciculata, consists of larger cells which are arranged in parallel chains running radially down towards the centre of the gland. The innermost zone, the zona reticularis, consists of cells which are similar to those of the zona fasciculata, but are arranged as an interconnecting network (Fig. 5.1). Some glomerulosa cells are innervated by axons containing catecholamines and vasoactive intestinal peptide which appear to originate mainly from the chromaffin cells of the medulla. While much of the autonomic innervation of the adrenal glands passes through the cortex to the medullary chromaffin cells, some sympathetic axons innervate the subcapsular arterial plexus and presumably exert a regulatory effect on adrenal arterial blood flow. Furthermore, there is evidence for some autonomic innervation of glomerulosa cells. In addition, various chromaffin cells are scattered throughout the cortex.

The arterial blood supply to the adrenal gland is provided by a number of small arteries branching mainly from the aorta and the inferior, phrenic, and renal

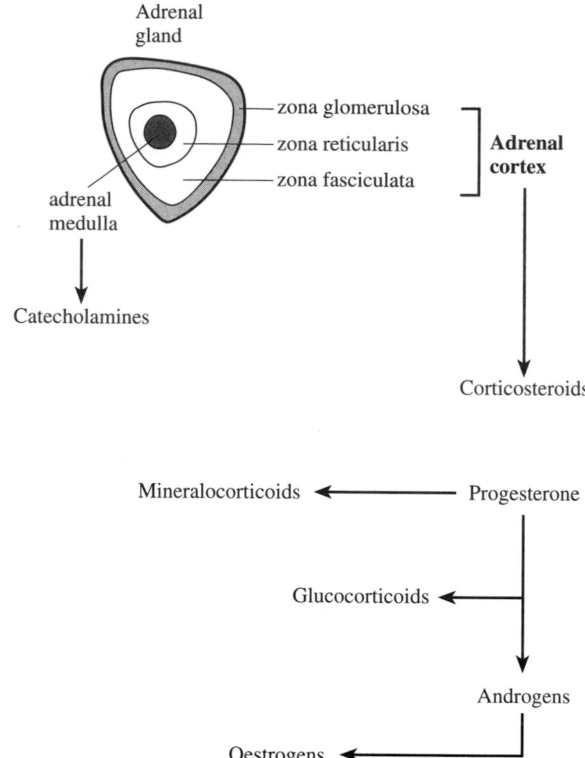

Fig. 5.1. The three regions of the adrenal cortex and the corticosteroid hormones they produce.

arteries. Many smaller branches form an arteriolar plexus below the capsule from which blood drains into a capillary network in the zona glomerulosa, many of them anastomosing as they penetrate into the zona fasciculata to form a sinusoidal plexus around the cells of the zona reticularis. Thus, the two innermost layers of the cortex receive a partly deoxygenated arterial blood supply draining down through the gland towards the medulla where it finally empties into the central vein. Most of the venous blood from the right gland enters the inferior vena cava while from the left gland it flows into the left renal vein directly or via the left inferior phrenic vein.

Corticosteroids

Synthesis, storage, and release

The hormones of the adrenal cortex are all derived from cholesterol which can itself be synthesized within the gland from acetate or, mostly, is taken up from the circulation as lipoprotein cholesterol. The adrenocortical hormones are therefore steroid hormones with a common structure, the cyclopentanoperhydrophenanthrene nucleus. Their synthesis involves four cytochrome P-450 enzymes located within the cell in different compartments, including the mitochondria, the microsomes, and the smooth endoplasmic reticulum. Early precursors formed from cholesterol are pregnenolone and progesterone, the latter at least being a hormone in its own right. The main final hormone products from the adrenal cortex, the adrenocortical hormones, may be conveniently considered according to their principal effects: mineralocorticoids, glucocorticoids, androgens, and oestrogens. The first two groups of hormones, like pregnenolone and progesterone, have 21 carbon atoms in their chemical structures and are sometimes called C21 steroids. The androgens from the adrenal cortex are normally synthesized in very small quantities relative to the gonadal secretions in the adult male, but can form a significant part of the total output in the adult female. Androgens contain 19 carbon atoms in their chemical structure and are sometimes called C19 steroids. Oestrogens derived from the androgens are C18 steroids; only very small amounts are normally released from the adult gland (see Fig. 5.1).

The main mineralocorticoid in humans is aldosterone. Its biosynthesis pathway is shown in Fig. 5.2. The final stage, from 18-hydroxycorticosterone to aldosterone, is catalysed by a mitochondrial P-450$_{c11}$ enzyme which also catalyses the

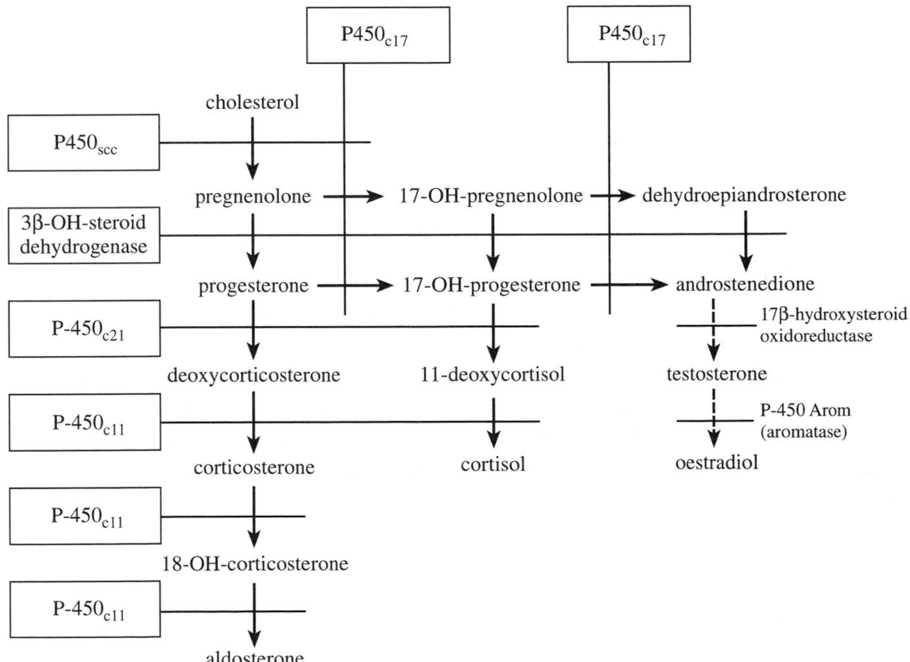

Fig. 5.2. The corticosteroid hormone biosynthesis pathways with the relevant enzymes involved in the various conversions. (P-450scc, the short-chain cholesterol cytochromal P-450 enzyme, also known as desmolase.)

earlier 11α-hydroxylation and the 18-hydroxylation steps. This enzyme is present in the zona glomerulosa, and aldosterone is only synthesized in this part of the adrenal cortex. Cortisol, which is the principal glucocorticoid in humans is also synthesized from the progesterone derived from cholesterol (Fig. 5.2). However, progesterone is then converted to 17α-hydroxyprogesterone in the presence of P-450_{c17} (17α-hydroxylase activity), an enzyme which is only found in the zonae fasciculata and reticularis. Subsequent conversions of progesterone and 17α-hydroxyprogesterone to deoxycorticosterone and 11-deoxycortisol respectively occur in the presence of the P-450_{c21} enzyme in the smooth endoplasmic reticulum. The final conversion of 11-deoxycortisol to cortisol is catalysed by another, different, mitochondrial P-450_{c11} enzyme. Of the androgens secreted by the adrenal cortex, dehydroepiandrosterone (DHEA) is the most important, being secreted in greatest (relative) quantities. Physiologically significant quantities of these hormones may only be produced if the adrenal cortex is hyperactive in disease in females, when the effects of excess androgens may be observed. In this chapter only the principal mineralocorticoid (aldosterone) and the principal glucocorticoid (cortisol) in humans will be considered. Androgens and oestrogens are discussed in Chapters 7 and 8.

Cholesterol, the original precursor molecule for steroid hormone synthesis, is stored mainly within cytoplasmic lipid droplets in the cells in the adrenal cortical cells. The various hormones are only stored in very small quantities. Stimulation of adrenal cells through various control mechanisms therefore induces new synthesis and release of hormone. The secretion rate for aldosterone normally ranges from between 0.1 and 0.4 μmol/24 h whereas cortisol is secreted in far greater quantities, usually varying between 30 and 80 μmol/24 h in humans.

Once in the blood, approximately 75 per cent of cortisol is tightly but reversibly bound to a plasma globulin called transcortin, which also has a high affinity for other corticosteroids, such as deoxycorticosterone and corticosterone, and transports significant quantities of progesterone. Only about 10 per cent of the cortisol in the blood is in the free and active state, the remainder being loosely bound to plasma albumin. If the total peak concentration (highest normal level) exceeds 850 nmol/l, the free cortisol rises disproportionately because the binding capacity of transcortin is saturated, and albumin only binds a small quantity of the hormone. Aldosterone has a lower affinity than cortisol for transcortin and, furthermore, since it is released in much smaller quantities, it does not seriously compete for binding sites on the carrier protein. The biggest proportion of the secreted aldosterone is bound to albumin. In the normal individual the secretion of cortisol follows a diurnal variation which closely follows the diurnal pattern of release of corticotrophin from the adenohypophysis, with a time lag of approximately 40 minutes. The plasma corticotrophin and cortisol levels rise during sleep to reach highest levels in the morning, just before or soon after waking up. The levels then decrease to reach lowest values in the evening (Fig. 5.3). This diurnal variation appears to depend on the central nervous system acting via the hypothalamus which controls corticotrophin release, which in turn controls cortisol secretion. The endogenous circadian 'pacemaker' is probably located in the suprachiasmatic nucleus in the hypothalamus.

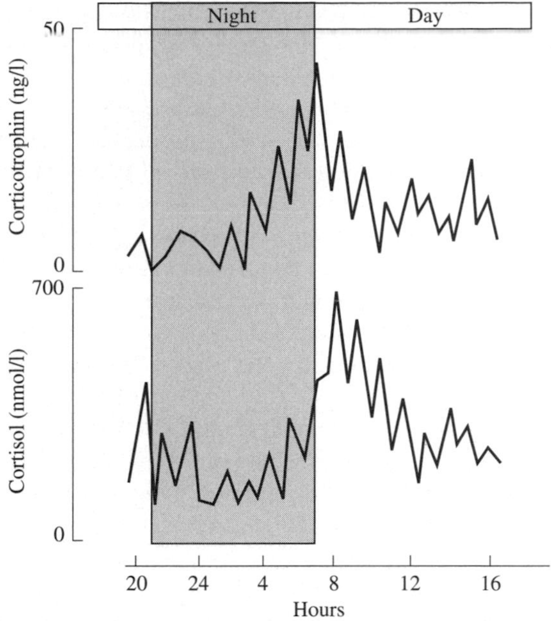

Fig. 5.3. The typical pulsatile pattern of release of the adenohypophysial hormone corticotrophin and the corticosteroid cortisol which it controls. The circadian rhythm, with a peak production of hormone in the morning (around waking) and a minimum production occurring in the middle of the night, is illustrated.

Mineralocorticoids: aldosterone

Actions of aldosterone

The principal effect of aldosterone is to stimulate sodium reabsorption in the kidneys, particularly in the distal convoluted tubule and cortical collecting duct. It also increases sodium reabsorption in the sweat glands, the salivary glands, the gastric glands, and the colon, and may influence the reabsorption of this ion in the renal proximal tubule and the ascending limb of the loop of Henle. Aldosterone-dependent sodium reabsorption along the distal nephron is regulated by a mechanism which involves the active exchange of sodium ions in the tubular lumen for potassium (or hydrogen) ions in the peritubular fluid. The relationship between the ions is not fixed, but is believed to be in a ratio of two sodium ions for one potassium ion. The effects of mineralocorticoids on sodium and potassium transport can be separated from each other, for instance by protein synthesis inhibitors, indicating that the hormone-dependent ion transport mechanisms involve more than one action in the target cell.

Hydrogen ion excretion can also be influenced by mineralocorticoids. In the presence of excess aldosterone, for example, a metabolic alkalosis may develop due to excessive loss of hydrogen ions consequent upon the increased reabsorption of sodium.

The net effect of mineralocorticoid activity in the distal nephron, therefore, is an increased sodium reabsorption and an increased potassium excretion. The plasma sodium ion concentration may then rise and osmoreceptors in the anterior hypothalamus will be stimulated. Consequently, vasopressin, released from nerve terminals in the neurohypophysis, stimulates water reabsorption from the collecting ducts. The plasma solute concentration is then restored to a normal level, and the osmotic stimulus for vasopressin release removed. This chain of events will occur provided that the neurohypophysial system is functioning normally. Thus, the extracellular fluid (ECF) volume is increased as a result of the combined effects of aldosterone on sodium reabsorption and vasopressin on water reabsorption. Furthermore, it is apparent that aldosterone is important in raising the total body sodium level while vasopressin regulates the plasma sodium ion concentration (Fig. 5.4).

The ECF volume rarely increases by more than 15 per cent, however, even when mineralocorticoid activity is increased to abnormal levels such as in primary aldosteronism. Therefore, oedema is not a common symptom in such conditions, because of an 'escape mechanism'. Various factors are probably involved in preventing the excessive expansion of the ECF volume in these situations. These factors include: (1) the glomerular filtration rate (GFR) which may increase as the ECF volume, and hence the arterial blood pressure, rises inordinately; (2) a decreased proximal tubular reabsorption of sodium consequent upon changes in the physical factors which influence this process; and (3) natriuretic hormones which may decrease sodium reabsorption by actions at various renal sites (see below).

Another mineralocorticoid, 11-deoxycorticosterone, has similar effects on sodium reabsorption and potassium excretion but is much less important physiologically. These hormones thus act to conserve sodium and are of importance in maintaining salt homeostasis. It must be remembered that while the primary effect of aldosterone (and other mineralocorticoids) is to increase total body sodium levels, it also has an important function in controlling the potassium level in the plasma.

Mechanism of action of aldosterone

Aldosterone penetrates the cell membrane with relative ease, and once inside the cell it binds to its specific cytoplasmic receptor (known as the type 1 receptor). The hormone-receptor complex enters the cell nucleus where it initiates an increase in mRNA synthesis following its action on the nuclear DNA at the transcription stage (Fig. 5.5). Cytoplasmic proteins are then synthesized on the ribosomes in the cytoplasm. These proteins may then act by increasing the luminal membrane permeability to sodium ions and by stimulating the sodium–potassium exchange pump in the serosal membrane. An increase in permeability of the luminal membrane to potassium ions is also likely. Sodium ions diffuse into the cells from the tubular lumen down their electrochemical gradient, and are then actively transported out of the cells into the peritubular fluid. Potassium ions are actively pumped into the cells at the serosal membrane in exchange for the sodium ions and can then diffuse across the luminal membrane into the tubular fluid, provided that a sufficient concentration gradient is present. Cortisol binds as avidly to the mineralocorticoid receptor as aldosterone itself. Since the amount of cortisol in the blood is vastly

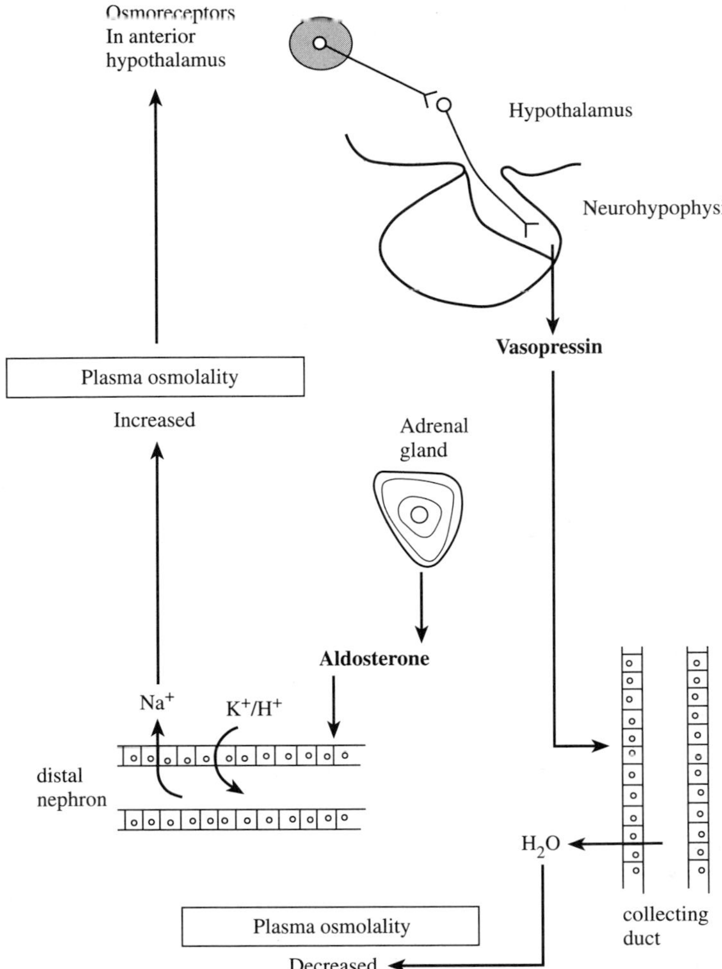

Fig. 5.4. Diagram showing the collaboration between the mineralocorticoid, aldosterone, and the neurohypophysial hormone, vasopressin, in regulating the body's fluid volume.

more than the circulating quantities of aldosterone, it is perhaps surprising that the clinical manifestation of excessive 'mineralocorticoid' activity is not commonplace. The paradox is explained by the presence in the kidneys of an enzyme which converts cortisol to a biologically inactive form (see mineralocorticoid actions of cortisol p. 110).

Recently, evidence for a more rapid action by aldosterone on sodium–hydrogen exchange, which is independent of protein synthesis inhibitors, has been presented for human mononuclear leucocytes and rat vascular smooth muscle cells. This suggests a non-genomic mechanism of action involving different receptors (type 2 receptors) in the cell membranes, and a second messenger system. Indeed, aldosterone appears to stimulate inositol triphosphate generation in human mono-

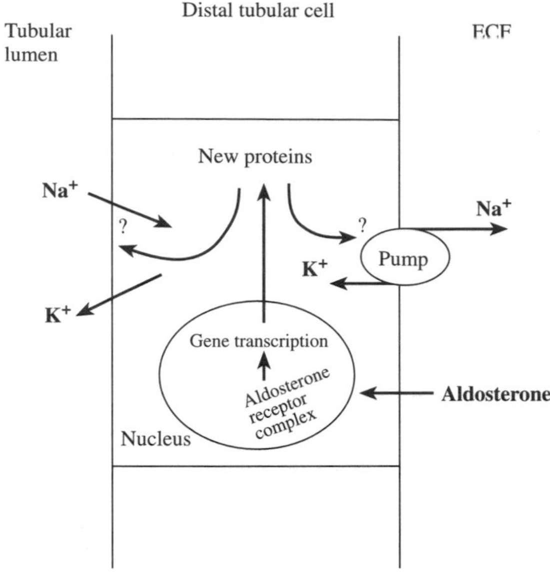

Fig. 5.5. The effect of aldosterone on Na^+ and K^+ transport in the distal nephron by a genomic mechanism involving transcription and protein synthesis.

nuclear leucocytes within one minute, and this may act as part of the second messenger system in these cells.

Control of release of aldosterone

The release of aldosterone is controlled by various factors, including a direct effect of plasma sodium and potassium concentrations. Either a 10 per cent decrease in the plasma sodium or a 10 per cent increase in plasma potassium concentration appears to stimulate the synthesis and release of aldosterone by direct actions on the adrenal cortex. Corticotrophin (ACTH) from the adenohypophysis stimulates the conversion of cholesterol to pregnenolone and therefore has a permissive effect on aldosterone production. However, ACTH is not a major factor in the control of aldosterone production, its primary action being the control of glucocorticoid synthesis and release.

The most important control mechanism for the secretion of aldosterone involves the renin–angiotensin system (RAS). Renin is an enzyme synthesized and stored within secretory granules in cells located along the terminal part of the afferent arterioles entering the renal glomeruli, called juxtaglomerular (JG) cells. Following stimulation of the JG cells, renin is released into the blood where it acts on a plasma protein called angiotensinogen synthesized in the liver, to split off a decapeptide called angiotensin I. This molecule is then rapidly converted to an octapeptide, angiotensin II by converting enzyme found in particularly high concentration in the lungs (Fig. 5.6). Angiotensin II (and its septapeptide metabolite angiotensin III) stimulates the cells of the adrenal zona glomerulosa to produce aldosterone. Angiotensin II is also a potent vasoconstrictor when present in the circulation in large amounts, it acts as a growth factor for arterial smooth muscle, and it stimulates thirst. With regard to this latter action a brain renin–angiotensin system, with all relevant components, has been identified.

One important stimulus for the release of renin from the JG cells is decreased renal perfusion pressure. The decrease in afferent arteriolar blood pressure may be detected directly by the JG cells or by adjacent renal vascular baroreceptors. Haemorrhage, salt and water loss, or abnormally prolonged pooling of blood in the legs when an upright posture is assumed (postural hypotension), all stimulate renin release as a consequence of the generalized fall in arterial blood pressure. Another mechanism for renin release in such situations may be the direct effect of sympathetic stimulation to the kidneys. There is evidence to suggest that the JG cells are directly innervated by adrenergic nerve fibres, and circulating catecholamines can stimulate renin release directly by acting on α-receptors present on these cells.

Another, intrarenal, mechanism for renin release appears to be a change in the concentration of chloride (or sodium) ions in the renal tubular fluid presented to the macula densa. This is an area of modified epithelial cells found at the point where the thick ascending limb of the loop of Henle is adjacent to the afferent arteriolar JG cells (see Fig. 5.6). The macula densa and the arteriolar JG cells together form the juxtaglomerular apparatus (JGA). Under certain circumstances, an increased presentation of chloride (or sodium) ions to the macula densa is associated with a decreased release of renin, while decreased chloride (or sodium) delivery results in an increased release of the enzyme. One consequence of the release of renin by this mechanism may be a decreased GFR brought about by the local contractile action of angiotensin II on the mesangial cells located around the glomerular capillaries.

The neurohypophysial hormone vasopressin suppresses renin secretion (see Chapter 4) and there is also evidence for direct negative feedback effects by angiotensin II and aldosterone on release of the enzyme from the JG cells. Certain prostaglandins have also been shown to stimulate the release of renin.

Atrial natriuretic peptide

Atrial natriuretic peptide (ANP) is another hormone involved in sodium ion regulation which has an inhibitory effect on renin, and thus ultimately on aldosterone, release. This 28-amino acid peptide is synthesized mainly in myocytes located in the atria of the heart, with a minor component coming from ventricular cells. The main stimulus for its release is stretch of the myocytes by an increased atrial volume. Its physiological actions include an increased excretion of salt and water by the kidneys and a decrease in arterial blood pressure. It has an inhibitory influence on the release of various pressor hormone systems including the renin–angiotensin–aldosterone system, catecholamines, and vasopressin.

In addition to ANP other similar molecules have been identified such as brain natriuretic peptide (BNP) and C-type natriuretic peptide (CNP). Other natriuretic

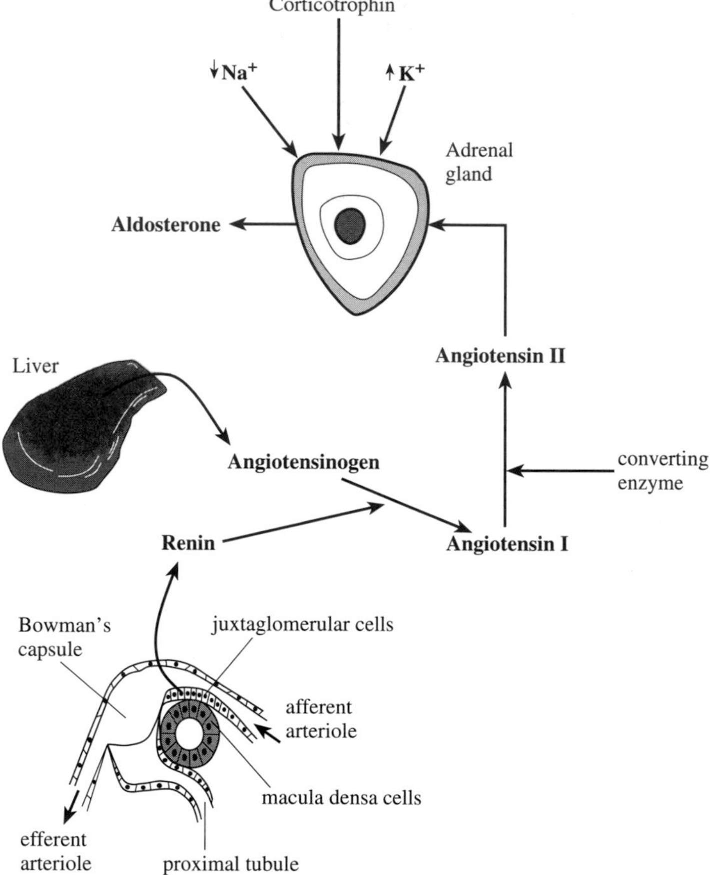

Fig. 5.6. The principal controlling influences on aldosterone production, with particular reference to the renin–angiotensin system.

hormones have been proposed, including a choline-like substance which is present in high concentration in the plasma and hypothalamus of spontaneously hypertensive rats, as well as in the plasma of patients with essential hypertension, and which increases in response to a high sodium intake.

Glucocorticoids

Actions of glucocorticoids

The most important naturally occurring glucocorticoids in humans are cortisol and corticosterone, with the derivative cortisone (itself inactive) being a potentially active steroid since it can be converted to cortisol in the liver and other tissues. The most important physiological effects of glucocorticoids are on carbohydrate,

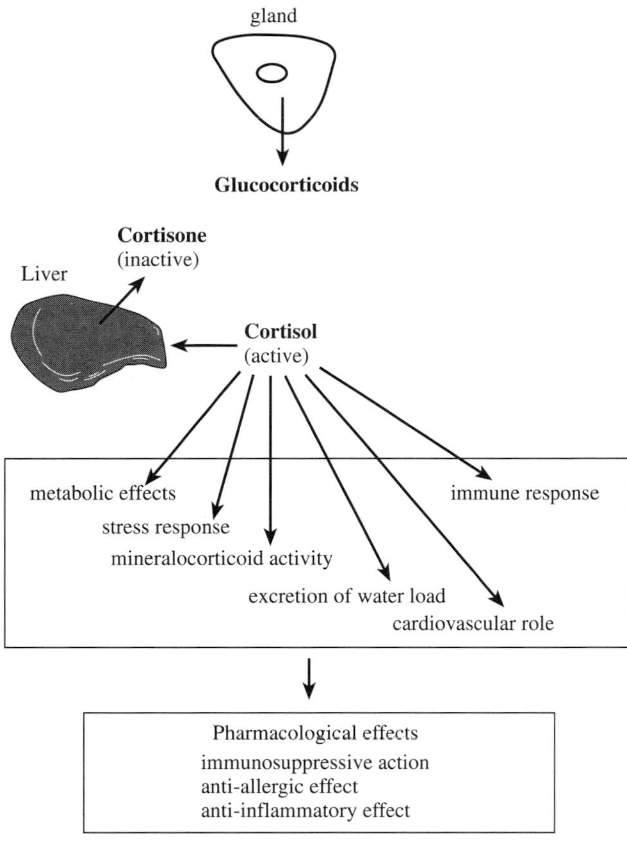

Fig. 5.7. The principal physiological actions of the glucocorticoid cortisol. The pharmacological effects are of clinical importance.

protein, and, to a lesser extent, fat metabolism. They are also essential for resistance to the effects of various noxious stimuli called stressors. When present in the circulation in excessive quantities they exert immunosuppressive, anti-inflammatory, and anti-allergic actions, the effects of which are of great therapeutic value in certain clinical conditions (Fig. 5.7).

Metabolic effects of glucocorticoids

Carbohydrate Cortisol has various effects on carbohydrate metabolism, resulting in the raising of blood glucose concentration. It stimulates hepatic gluconeogenesis (formation of glucose from non-carbohydrate precursors) which initially leads to increased deposition of glycogen in the liver (glycogenesis). Gluconeogenesis is also stimulated indirectly by the increased presentation of glucogenic precursors to the liver, this being another effect induced by glucocorticoids (see following sections). Cortisol also antagonizes the peripheral action of insulin on glucose uptake (see Chapter 11). Any excess glucose produced in the liver cells enters the blood and may produce hyperglycaemia, as seen quite often in the condition of excess glucocorticoid production.

Protein Cortisol inhibits amino acid uptake and protein synthesis in extrahepatic tissues while stimulating these processes in the liver. This hormone is also a potent protein catabolic agent in peripheral tissues such as muscle, skin, and bone. When produced in excess it can cause severe wasting of muscles. The increased quantities of amino acids reaching the liver can serve as gluconeogenic precursors in this organ.

Fat Cortisol influences fat metabolism, particularly when produced in greater than normal quantities. There is an increased mobilization of fatty acids which follows the stimulation of lipolysis in adipose tissue. At least part of this effect may be due to potentiation of the lipolytic actions of other hormones such as somatotrophin and catecholamines. When large amounts of cortisol are secreted by the adrenal cortex, there may be a centripetal distribution of fat (increased deposition in the facial and truncal areas).

The consequences of excess cortisol in the circulation (Cushing's syndrome, see clinical section, p. 120) on the metabolism of carbohydrates, proteins, and fat are responsible for the typical physical features of this condition.

Other effects of glucocorticoids

Mineralocorticoid activity Glucocorticoids have some inherent mineralocorticoid activity, which is normally of minor importance because of the far greater potency of the mineralocorticoids such as aldosterone. However, when cortisol is produced in large quantities, its mineralocorticoid activity assumes greater importance in the regulation of salt metabolism. Interestingly, the type 1 aldosterone receptor appears to bind cortisol as readily as it binds the true mineralocorticoid. Yet, cortisol normally has little mineralocorticoid activity despite it being present in the circulation in much higher concentrations. This apparent paradox is solved by the presence in renal tubular target cells of the enzyme 11α-hydroxysteroid dehydrogenase (11αHSD) which catalyses the conversion of the active cortisol to the inactive cortisone. This mechanism conveniently removes the potentially competing glucocorticoid from the vicinity of the renal mineralocorticoid receptors. The same protective mechanism appears to work in other aldosterone-sensitive target tissues where sodium reabsorption is induced, such as the salivary glands and colon. On the other hand, the same mineralocorticoid receptors are found in the hippocampus in the brain but the 11αHSD enzyme is absent. Here it seems that both cortisol and aldosterone are equally effective in binding to the receptors.

The lack of this renal enzyme results in the clinical condition known as the syndrome of 'apparent mineralocorticoid excess'. One cause of this syndrome is the excess eating of licorice which contains active components glycyrrhizic and glycyrrhetinic acids. These acids inhibit the action of 11αHSD and consequently glucocorticoids remain active in the distal tubular cells and bind to the renal mineralocorticoid receptors inducing hypernatraemia, hypokalaemia, and hypertension.

Water metabolism In the absence of glucocorticoids the ability to excrete a water load is impaired. Part of the action of cortisol on stimulating the excretion of such a water load may be to increase the glomerular filtration rate (GFR). There is evidence to suggest that glucocorticoids increase the glomerular plasma flow rate perhaps as the result of a direct vasodilator effect on the renal vasculature; consequently the GFR increases. Another factor which may be involved in the inability to excrete water loads in glucocorticoid deficiency states is the neurohypophysial hormone, vasopressin, which stimulates water retention. Vasopressin released from nerve terminals in the median eminence acts on corticotrophe cells together with corticoliberin (corticotrophin-releasing hormone, CRH) to stimulate the release of corticotrophin and, consequently, cortisol (see Chapter 4). In the cortisol-deficient state it is possible that any negative feedback effect on vasopressin and CRH is reduced resulting in enhanced release of vasopressin.

Cardiovascular effect Glucocorticoids have been associated with an increased vascular tone, possibly by potentiating the vasoconstrictor effect of other vasoactive molecules such as the catecholamines and even vasopressin.

Growth Glucocorticoids present in excessive quantities in the circulation are associated with an impaired growth rate in children. This effect is partly due to an inhibitory effect of glucocorticoids on somatotrophin release but it also has a direct inhibitory action on insulin-like growth factor I (IGF-I) production (see Chapter 4) and on protein synthesis.

Response to stress Various stressors including severe trauma, haemorrhage, acute hypoglycaemia, febrile and emotional stimuli, are all associated with a dramatic increase in the blood concentrations of corticotrophin and cortisol (see section on control of release of cortisol, p. 115). In hypophysectomized or adrenalectomized animals or humans, even quite mild stress can prove fatal unless adequate replacement doses of glucocorticoids are rapidly administered. The precise nature of the glucocorticoid response to a stress is unknown, but part of the 'tolerance' may be associated with metabolic and cardiovascular effects of these hormones. In addition, there is increasing evidence to suggest that the glucocorticoids regulate the immune system, which can be considered a vital component of the body's response to stressors (see immunosuppressive actions, p. 112).

Pharmacological actions of glucocorticoids

Anti-inflammatory action Cortisol and other glucocorticoids inhibit the normal inflammatory process which occurs when tissue is damaged, but this effect only occurs when the hormones (or synthetic analogues) are present in the circulation in excessive quantities. In the normal process, increased permeability of the capillary walls results in the diffusion of plasma-like fluid into the damaged area together with the migration of leucocytes, by diapedesis, across the capillary membranes. Lysosomal membranes within the leucocytes rupture thus releasing various proteolytic enzymes into the surrounding medium, which then destroy damaged cells and their constituents. Collagen fibres are subsequently formed to repair the original damage. Cortisol blocks all stages of this process thereby preventing the normal repair to damaged tissues. This action by large concentrations of glucocorticoids can be of tremendous therapeutic value in certain inflammatory conditions such as rheumatoid arthritis. It may be the stabilizing action of cortisol on lysosomal membranes which is of particular importance.

Anti-allergic action Large quantities of circulating glucocorticoids have anti-allergic properties, probably due partly to inhibition of the intracellular synthesis of histamine in mast cells and basophils. When an antigen reacts with an antibody on a mast cell, the cell ruptures. The subsequent release of histamine is often associated with the allergic response. For instance, histamine induces capillary dilatation and the membrane permeability is increased, allowing the movement of plasma into the intercellular spaces. The resultant decrease in venous return lowers the blood pressure, this being one feature of anaphylactic shock. In man, the fall in blood pressure is enhanced by the additional arteriolar dilation produced by histamine. Some smooth muscle, in particular bronchiolar muscle, constricts as a result of histamine action, and this effect is probably associated with asthma. It also stimulates salivary pancreatic, gastric, and intestinal secretions. Thus, cortisol, which inhibits the synthesis and release of histamine, alleviates at least some of the allergic responses.

Part of the anti-allergic effect of glucocorticoids may be due to other actions, such as the inhibition of kinin synthesis, the decreased production of antibodies, and the stabilization of lysosomal membranes.

Immunosuppressive actions Another useful therapeutic effect of large quantities of glucocorticoids is the inhibition of the normal immune response. This action results from the gradual destruction of lymphoid tissue which is accompanied by a decrease in antibody production, as well as the decrease in number of circulating lymphocytes, basophils, and eosinophils. This effect is beneficial during transplant and graft operations, although it renders the patient more susceptible to the subversive and uncontrolled spread of an infection throughout the body. Antibiotics are therefore a necessary adjunct to this therapeutic use of large amounts of administered steroids.

It is increasingly clear that the glucocorticoids influence the immune system not only when present in excessively large amounts (i.e. therapeutically, or in the clinical hypersecretory condition of Cushing's syndrome) but also as part of a physiological regulatory influence preventing the immune system from causing damage to the body. For example, when lymphocytes are stimulated to produce toxic substances, such as tumour necrosis factor (TNF), which could cause untold damage to normal, as well as to invading, cells it is vital that the excessive responsiveness of the lymphocytes to the stimulus be kept under rigorous control. An important aspect of this interaction between the hypothalamo–hypophysial–adrenal axis and the immune system is the production of peptide molecules from immune system cells such as macrophages, called interleukins. For example, one of these molecules, interleukin 1 (IL-1), can stimulate the production of CRH and corticotrophin from the hypothalamus and adenohypophysis, respectively. Furthermore, macrophages themselves have been shown to produce corticotrophin when stimulated. This corticotrophin subsequently may act on adrenocortical cells to stimulate the release of cortisol. Therefore, the macrophages can initiate their own 'auto-control' negative feedback system and

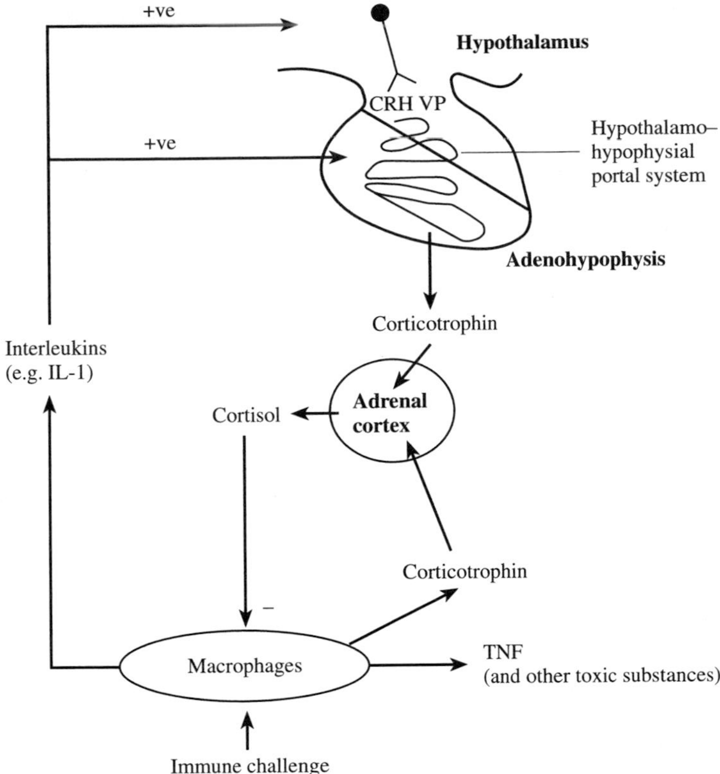

Fig. 5.8. Diagram showing some aspects of the interaction between the hypothalamo–adenohypophysial–adrenal axis and the immune system, represented by the macrophage. The importance of this interaction is now clear. (CRH, corticotrophin-releasing hormone; VP, vasopressin; TNF, tumour necrosis factor.)

at the same time release powerful destructive molecules aimed at invading organisms, for instance. It is likely that this interaction between cortisol and the immune system is an extremely important function of the hypothalamo–hypophysial–adrenal axis (Fig. 5.8).

Effect on blood cells In the presence of maintained, high concentrations of circulating glucocorticoids there is a decrease in the numbers of lymphocytes, basophils, and eosinophils in the blood (see section on immunosuppressive action above). Nevertheless, the total blood cell count actually increases because of increased numbers of neutrophils, erythrocytes, and platelets. It is also worth noting that there is an increase in the plasma protein concentration, due to the stimulating effect of the steroids on hepatic protein synthesis.

Effect on calcium and bone Large quantities of cortisol antagonize the effect of vitamin D metabolites [25(OH)D_3 and 1,25$(OH)_2D_3$; see Chapter 10] on calcium absorption from the gut, but increase the renal excretion of this ion. This latter effect is probably at least partly due to the increase in GFR which the steroids can produce. Since there is some evidence to suggest that somatotrophin release from the adenohypophysis is inhibited by excessive amounts of cortisol this effect, together with those actions influencing calcium metabolism and protein metabolism, probably all combine to cause osteoporesis which is one quite common symptom of excess glucocorticoid production.

Mechanism of action of glucocorticoids

Glucocorticoids, like other steroid hormones, penetrate their target cell membranes and bind to intracellular receptors. The intracellular processes involved in the development of the actions of these hormones are believed to be similar to those described for other steroid hormones in Chapter 2. One intracellular mediator synthesized in response to genomic stimulation by cortisol is the protein lipocortin 1 (LC1). This protein inhibits the activity of membrane-bound phospholipase A_2 thereby decreasing the production of arachidonic acid, the precursor for prostaglandins and leucotrienes. Thus, lipocortin mediates the anti-inflammatory activity of the glucocorticoids. Not only do glucocorticoids influence the intracellular synthesis of LC1 in many target tissues but they can also direct it to the external surface of the cell membrane (e.g. in adenohypophysial and hypothalamic tissue) where it can be exposed to its own receptors (Fig. 5.9). Various lipocortins have now been identified and been shown to belong to a large family of similar proteins.

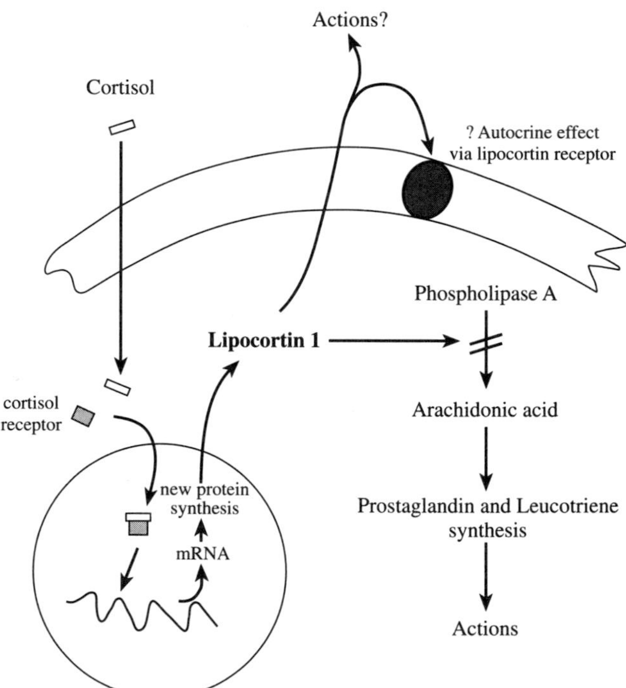

Fig. 5.9. Diagram showing the mechanism of action of cortisol involving the production of the protein, lipocortin 1.

Like aldosterone, it is now appreciated that cortisol can also exert some effects far more rapidly than can be explained on the basis of genome-mediated RNA and subsequent protein synthesis. One example of such a rapid response to cortisol is the acute negative feedback effect on corticotrophin release.

Control of cortisol release

It has been known for some time that hypophysectomy results in a gradual atrophy of the zonae fasciculata and reticularis, and it is now well established that the synthesis and secretion of the glucocorticoids, and to some extent the adrenal sex steroids, are under the control of the adenohypophysial hormone corticotrophin. The diurnal variation in the secretory pattern of cortisol is directly related to the diurnal variation of corticotrophin release, as mentioned earlier in the chapter. The stimulatory effect of corticotrophin is mediated by the activation of adenyl cyclase through a membrane-bound receptor, with a subsequent increase in cAMP concentrations. Cyclic AMP may then stimulate the conversion of cholesterol to pregnenolone, and the various conversions of pregnenolone to progesterone and ultimately to cortisol, by activating the various enzyme systems involved. The release of the adenohypophysial hormone corticotrophin is itself controlled mainly from the hypothalamus through the mediation of the 41-amino acid polypeptide corticortrophin-releasing hormone (CRH), sometimes called corticoliberin. As mentioned in Chapter 4, vasopressin released from nerve terminals in the median eminence into the hypothalamo–hypophysial portal system stimulates corticotrophin release by acting synergistically with CRH. Indeed, CRH and vasopressin have been shown to coexist in parvocellular neurones from the paraventricular nuclei of the hypothalamus, and probably are released together into the primary plexus in the median eminence at least under certain circumstances (see Chapter 4).

Aminergic and cholinergic neurones are involved in the regulation of corticotrophin release, probably by influencing the release of CRH.

Cortisol exerts a negative feedback effect on corticotrophin release by a loop which relates the adrenal cortex to the adenohypophysis. An indirect negative feedback loop relates the adrenal cortex (via cortisol) to the hypothalamus, and/or other parts of the brain (e.g. the hippocampus) to influence the release of the CRH (Fig. 5.10). Three different phases of feedback inhibition have been identified: rapid, early-delayed, and late-delayed phases. Each one probably involves a different mechanism of action. The rapid phase occurs within minutes and is likely to occur through a membrane effect, whereas the early-delayed phase takes place over the following hour and is associated with protein synthesis (likely to be lipocortin 1).

CLINICAL DISORDERS

The introduction of highly sensitive assays has considerably advanced understanding of adrenal cortical disorders and has provided important diagnostic tools. These assays have also allowed a much higher degree of precision in the monitoring of

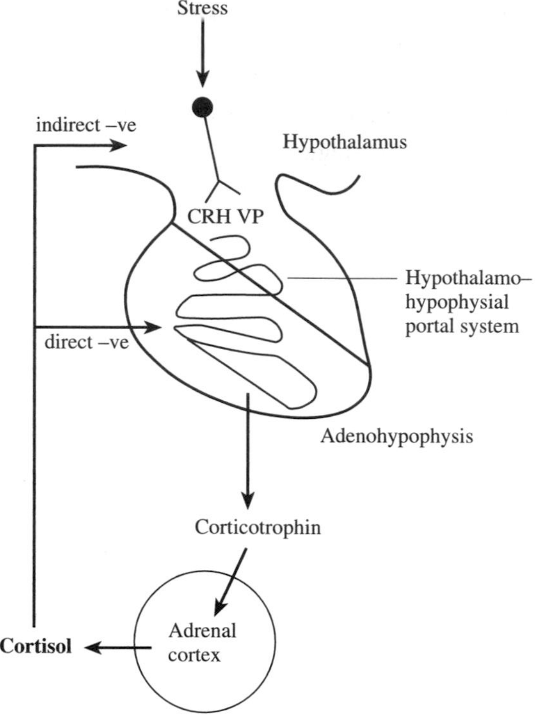

Fig. 5.10. Diagram showing the essential features of the control of cortisol production.

treatment. In aetiology and pathogenesis, however much remains to be clarified and will require substantial advances in molecular biology before genuine understanding replaces conjecture.

Aldosterone

Excess

Hyperaldosteronism refers to a sustained high secretion of aldosterone from one or both adrenal cortices, and can be divided into two categories. In primary hyperaldosteronism, the hyperfunction is due to autonomous adrenal secretion of excessive aldosterone, while in secondary hyperaldosteronism the aldosterone hypersecretion is induced by enhanced levels of angiotensin II, due to a high plasma renin activity (PRA), which in turn may result from a variety of causes. The effects produced in the primary and secondary forms are different.

In the primary situation, the clinical picture is dominated by the pathophysiological actions of aldosterone itself. In the secondary variety, the various causes of raised renin often determine the clinical picture. In both situations the aldosterone level, both in serum and urine, is raised. The important diagnostic biochemical difference is that in primary hyperaldosteronism, angiotensin and renin levels are suppressed, while in secondary hyperaldosteronism they are elevated.

Primary hyperaldosteronism (Conn's syndrome)

This is due in most cases to single or rarely multiple adrenal adenomata arising from the zona glomerulosa. These tumours are almost never malignant and rarely larger than 10 mm. Cases due to bilateral hyperplasia of the zona glomerulosa are being increasingly recognized, and probably outnumber adenoma as a cause of primary hyperaldosteronism: the stimulus either for adenoma or hyperplasia has not been identified, but may be shown to reside in a variety of receptor gene mutations.

Clinical features

Patients usually have hypertension which is based on sodium and water retention, expansion of ECF volume and possibly hyper-reactive arteriolar tone. There are often no secondary effects from the hypertension, and retinopathy and cardiomegaly are usually mild. Peripheral oedema is characteristically rare, due to the 'escape mechanism' referred to in the physiology section earlier in this chapter. Mild hypernatraemia may be present. Hypokalaemia is usually a dominant feature of the clinical presentation, giving rise to symptoms such as muscle weakness and polyuria: this latter symptom is due to partially reversible tubular nephropathy, as a result of which ADH insensitivity occurs, sometimes referred to as nephrogenic diabetes insipidus. There may also be psychiatric changes and cardiac arrhythmias. The frequency of primary hyperaldosteronism probably does not exceed 1 in 500 of the hypertensive population.

Investigations

There is probably no indication for considering the diagnosis unless the serum potassium level is consistently less than 3.4 mmol/l in the absence of diuretic therapy. The entity of normo-kalaemic hyperaldosteronism has been suggested but is extremely rare. Even so, there are many causes of hypokalaemia, including the unrecognized administration of thiazide diuretics and laxatives. Furthermore, hypokalaemia may be a manifestation of the secondary hyperaldosteronism seen in malignant (accelerated-phase) hypertension, other primary renal disorders and in renal artery stenosis.

Following identification of hypokalaemia, ideally with simultaneous evidence of abnormal urinary potassium loss (urine $K^+ > 10$ mmol/l), the diagnosis is established by identifying a high urinary or plasma aldosterone concentration, together with a suppressed plasma renin level. It is important that these samples are taken under standard conditions, both of posture (sitting still for 15 minutes prior to sampling) and adequate dietary sodium, otherwise inconclusive results may be obtained. Hypokalaemia should be corrected before assessing aldosterone secretion, since it has direct inhibitory effects on adrenal aldosterone release, even from adenomas: without correction, a falsely low or normal serum aldosterone may consequently be found.

The diagnosis of zona glomerulosa hyperplasia as a cause of hyperaldosteronism is usually made by exclusion. Negative anatomical localization studies are usual, but a more positive diagnostic phenomenon is the aldosterone response to erect posture, which is usually absent in the presence of single (autonomous) adenoma, but retained or exaggerated in hyperplasia.

The identification of hyper-reninaemic (secondary) hyperaldosteronism is an indication for excluding renal artery stenosis or intrinsic renal disease. Very occasionally, renin-producing renal tumours may be identified by appropriate imaging techniques: a similarly rare disorder named Bartter's syndrome has been described where juxtaglomerular hyperplasia is the pathological hallmark of the hyper-reninaemia which is thought to be responsible for the hypertension.

After establishing the diagnosis biochemically, adrenal vein samples obtained by trans-femoral retrograde catheterization may be used to determine whether the excess aldosterone is unilateral or bilateral in origin. Additional radioisotopic localization using iodo- or seleno-cholesterol may be valuable. Ultrasound is usually unable to localize the small adenoma, but CT scanning of the adrenals as well as MRI may be of value in some tumours associated with primary hyperaldosteronism.

Other causes of apparent mineralocorticoid excess

Liquorice ingestion (containing glycirrizinic acid) and the now infrequently used anti-ulcer drug, carbenoxolone, inhibit 11ß-hydroxysteroid dehydrogenase, inducing endogenous mineralocorticoid excess. Patients consuming large quantities of liquorice may present with weakness due to hypokalaemia.

Glucocorticoid-remediable hyperaldosteronism is a rare cause of mineralocorticoid excess. Instead of being modulated by potassium balance and the renin–angiotensin system, dominant secretory control of aldosterone appears to be transferred to ACTH (which as outlined earlier normally plays only a negligible role in modifying aldosterone release). Accordingly, ACTH-suppressive doses of glucocorticoid (such as dexamethasone 0.5 mg will correct both the hypertension and all abnormal biochemical parameters, including elevated 18-hydroxycortisol and 18-oxocortisol. These latter analytes are the biochemical hallmarks of this rare dominantly inherited disorder.

Similarly rare causes of mineralocorticoid hypertension are the adrenal biosynthetic defects involving 11ß-hydroxylase or 17α-hydroxylase, in both of which hypertension is again responsive to exogenous glucocorticoid administration.

Treatment

The treatment of choice of primary hyperaldosteronism is the surgical removal of the adenoma normally responsible for the clinical syndrome. This usually results in correction of the hypertension: plasma electrolytes revert to normal. In long-standing cases, there may be permanent hypokalaemic tubular and even glomerular damage, with polyuria and uraemia. Management of cases with bilateral disease, either adenoma or hyperplasia, is still controversial. Surgical removal of one and a half adrenal glands has been advocated, but medical treatment with an aldosterone antagonist, spironolactone (50–400 mg daily) provides good long-term control in patients who are unsuitable for surgery either because of diagnostic uncertainty or because of contraindications. Occasional adverse effects, such as gynaecomastia, impotence, and lassitude, may occur with this drug.

Secondary hyperaldosteronism

A rise in circulating angiotensin II levels due to increased renin release, stimulates the adrenal cortex to produce and release increased quantities of aldosterone. This physiological reflex is designed to conserve sodium under conditions such as haemorrhage or salt and water depletion (e.g. diarrhoea and vomiting). In various disease states characterized by hypovolaemia, hypotension and renal underperfusion, this physiological mechanism may become inappropriate, persistent, and exaggerated, simply because sodium and water retention are unable or insufficient to correct the underlying haemodynamic problem. Accordingly, in the nephrotic syndrome, cardiac failure, and in cirrhosis of the liver with ascites, oedema will develop which may be responsive to aldosterone antagonists such as spironolactone. Furthermore, if blood supply to the juxtaglomerular apparatus should be impaired, as in accelerated (malignant) hypertension or in renal artery stenosis, there is enhanced secretion of aldosterone. Nevertheless, the most common cause of secondary hyperaldosteronism is now diuretic therapy. (Table 5.1.)

Deficiency

This is a predictable consequence of adrenalectomy or generalized adrenal cortical destruction, and will be considered later in the chapter. Primary and selective deficiency of aldosterone has been reported as a rare disorder manifest occasionally

Table 5.1. Causes of secondary hyperaldosteronism

Loss of effective blood volume
Dehydration
Haemorrhage
Extravascular loss of sodium and water
Cardiac failure and oedema
Cirrhosis and ascites
Nephrotic syndrome
Salt-losing nephritis
Mechanical obstruction of renal vessels
Accelerated (malignant) hypertension
Fibromuscular hyperplasia
Atheroma
Iatrogenic
Liquorice, glycyrrhizinic acid
Diuretics
Oral contraceptives
Hyperplasia of the juxtaglomeruler apparatus (Bartter's syndrome)
Renin-secreting renal tumour

by hypotension, or more usually asymptomatic hyperkalaemia. Many cases have been associated with diabetes mellitus although the mechanism of this relationship is not known.

Cortisol

Excess (Cushing's syndrome): (see Plate 5.1)

Cushing's syndrome is a rare disease predominantly affecting women in the age group 30 to 50 years. The syndrome is produced by excessive quantities of glucocorticoids secreted by the adrenal cortex. A clinically similar syndrome can be produced by the long-term or high-dose administration of synthetic cortisol analogues, usually employed for immunosuppressive purposes.

Excessive secretion of cortisol may be caused indirectly by increased pituitary corticotrophin (ACTH) production or ectopic ACTH or CRH production by a tumour, which all give rise to adrenal hyperplasia. It may also be caused by independent autonomous hypersecretion of cortisol by the adrenal gland due to adenoma or carcinoma.

The increased frequency of surgical approach to the pituitary fossa in pituitary dependent Cushing's syndrome (usually referred to as Cushing's disease) has revealed micro- and occasionally even macro-adenomata in most cases. Whether these are primary, or secondary to hypothalamic hyperstimulation is still unclear. Some research has supported an activating mutation of the CRH or vasopressin (vlb) receptor genes within the tumour. Adrenal adenomas are the most common cause of ACTH-independent hypersecretion of cortisol; carcinoma of the adrenal is rare in adults, but occurs somewhat more commonly in children. The cause of the rare entity of nodular adrenal hyperplasia in association with Cushing's disease remains obscure. It is possible that fluctuating adrenal stimulation by ACTH in classical Cushing's disease may cause multifocal adrenal nodules to develop, which then become autonomous.

Table 5.2. Causes of Cushing's syndrome (with approximate relative prevalence)

Corticotrophin-dependent Cushing's syndrome	
Cushing's disease	64%
Ectopic ACTH syndrome	13%
Ectopic CRH syndrome	1%
Corticotrophin-independent Cushing's syndrome	
Adrenal adenoma	10%
Adrenal carcinoma	8%
Nodular hyperplasia	2%
Pseudo-Cushing's syndrome	
Depression	1%
Alcoholism	1%

Clinical features

The clinical picture of Cushing's syndrome can range from the florid, easily recognizable patient on the one hand, to individuals with few signs or symptoms on the other (see Plate 5.1). Some of the more common symptoms are proximal muscle weakness (due to steroid myopathy), back pain (due to osteoporosis), gain of weight (due to steroid-induced lipogenesis), acne, and in women, both excessive hair growth (due to associated adrenal androgen release) and amenorrhoea (due to suppression by cortisol of the pituitary–ovarian axis).

The marked wasting of proximal muscles and the associated thin arms and legs give rise to the 'lemon on matchsticks' appearance, while the characteristic red 'moonface' is often a striking feature as are the purple striae found on lower abdomen, upper arms and thighs, and which reflect the catabolic effects on protein structures in the skin. The thinness and easy bruising of the skin are additional manifestations of this process.

Further features which may be present include hypertension (due to sodium retention) and hyperglycaemia (due to steroid-induced gluconeogenesis). On rare occasions when the syndrome does occur in children there is stunting of growth (due to interference by cortisol both with growth hormone release, as well as a direct effect on the bone response to growth factors). In severe forms, hypokalaemia supplements hypernatraemia as direct minerocorticoid effects of cortisol on renal tubular function, and this may contribute to the severe muscle weakness. However, such severe degrees of hypokalaemia are normally associated with ectopic production of ACTH. The anti-inflammatory and immune suppressive effects of steroids together result in increased proneness to bacterial infections. Finally, in ectopic ACTH production, the underlying carcinoma (often bronchial) may give rise to additional signs and symptoms.

Because of their ACTH-dependence, pituitary, ectopic CRH, and ectopic ACTH varieties of Cushing's syndrome may also cause abnormal (Addisonian distribution) pigmentation. This is most striking in ectopic ACTH syndromes (where serum ACTH may be very grossly elevated), and in Nelson's syndrome, where bilateral adrenalectomy for Cushing's disease may be followed by expansion and uncontrolled growth of the causative pituitary adenoma (see below).

Investigations

Precision and cost-saving in diagnosis depends on a two-step approach to the diagnosis.

Confirmation of cortisol excess Stress, depression and obesity may all induce high plasma cortisol levels, so that single random cortisol values are of no diagnostic value. Conversely, patients with Cushing's syndrome may have normal random cortisol levels. Although loss of diurnal cortisol rhythm is frequently found, it is insufficiently discriminating to be used in diagnosis. However, in most states other than Cushing's syndrome, a normal negative-feedback control mechanism between cortisol and ACTH is maintained. Accordingly, as an additional or alternative simple screening test, 2 mg of dexamethasone given at midnight usually suppresses plasma cortisol to less than 200 nmol/l in a sample taken 9–10 hours later (overnight dexamethasone suppression test), but will fail to do so in pathological cortisol excess states. Occasionally, elderly and depressed patients demonstrate a similar abnormality. This test is readily performed on an out-patient basis.

Twenty-four hour urinary excretion of free cortisol is probably the most precise reflection of total cortisol production: providing that urinary collections can be made accurately this is the most effective screening test.

Definitive diagnosis None of the following procedures should be performed unless the screening tests referred to above indicate abnormal values:

1. ACTH concentrations can be accurately determined. This measurement provides the best and most direct way of separating primary adrenal from pituitary lesions. However, although patients with pituitary hypersecretion of ACTH have an inappropriately high plasma level of this hormone, similar or even higher values are found in ectopic secretion: the diagnostic separation of these two identities can be very difficult. Ectopic ACTH cases may have associated high levels of POMC-derived peptides (see Chapter 15) which are useful adjunctive measurements in this difficult differential diagnosis. ACTH levels are low or undetectable in patients with adrenal tumours.

2. Since pituitary-dependent Cushing's disease mostly represents only a partially autonomous abnormality, the administration of dexamethasone 2 mg every 6 hours over a three-day period will usually lower urinary cortisol into the normal range. However, patients with primary adrenal lesions, which are normally totally autonomous, do not exhibit this suppression potential. Nevertheless, both false positive and false negative responses to this test are well documented.

3. Metyrapone (metopirone) interferes with the hydroxylation of 11-desoxycortisol, resulting in a fall in the plasma cortisol level. Administration of this drug to normal patients or those with pituitary-dependent Cushing's disease results in a consequent elevation of ACTH (which can be measured) or an increased secretion of 11-desoxycortisol or its metabolites. Again this reflects comparative non-autonomy. However, if the disorder is a primary autonomous adrenal problem (adenoma or carcinoma) or a source of ectopic corticotrophin, there is usually no such adrenal response.

A similar spectrum of responses is seen with CRH stimulation. As in normal subjects, pituitary-dependant Cushing's disease demonstrates a normal or even exaggerated ACTH response, with no response in patients with autonomous adenomas or ectopic ACTH syndrome.

4. In Cushing's disease, radiography of the skull rarely reveals enlargement of the sella turcica. Either high-resolution CT scanning or MRI usually demonstrates the much more common intrasellar tumour. In addition, the highly specialized technique of selective inferior petrosal venous sinus sampling can be performed to both confirm pituitary aetiology as well as to lateralize the tumour.

5. Radiography of the abdomen may reveal calcification in an adrenal tumour, and CT or MRI scanning may demonstrate the lesion directly. Confirmation may be necessary using transfemoral, transaortic arteriography of the adrenal. Retrograde femoral vein catheterization of the adrenal veins is possible, allowing injection of a contrast medium to delineate the tumour (adrenal venography). This technique also allows sampling of the adrenal vein for cortisol determination in an attempt to demonstrate the high concentration gradient between the adrenal vein and vena cava characteristic of the tumour. Such techniques are usually individualized according to the technical preferences of the department in which the patient is being investigated.

Treatment

Pituitary-dependent Cushing's disease Management of such cases varies greatly between endocrine centres. When a primary pituitary origin of the lesion has been established, a direct surgical approach is increasingly used. A trans-sphenoidal, transnasal surgical approach allows examination of the sella from below, and microadenomas can be selectively removed in early cases without interference with residual pituitary function. More extensive surgery by the trans-frontal route is rarely required.

Other procedures for dealing with the primary pituitary lesion have been evolved, including external irradiation using a cobalt source and delivering approximately 4500 rad (cGy) to the pituitary fossa. Similarly, radioactive implants of yttrium or gold, or external proton bombardment from a cyclotron (which produces a focally increased radiation dose to the tumour) have been used in selected centres. The success rate achieved by these less invasive methods falls short of the direct surgical approach. Furthermore, the risk of irradiation damage to optic nerves and brain may not always be avoidable, and risk of progressive reduction of other pituitary functions is also a long-term consequence. This is probably due to incidental irradiation of the more radiosensitive hypothalamus.

Bilateral adrenalectomy was previously used as standard treatment. However, probably because of consequent pituitary 'release' from the inhibitory feedback of cortisol, there may be enhanced growth of the pituitary adenoma in between 10 and 25 per cent of cases. This results in rapid pituitary fossa expansion by a more infiltrative tumour transformation, as well as increased pigmentation due to escalating ACTH levels (Nelson's syndrome). Although pretreatment with pituitary irradiation may prevent this condition from occurring, adrenalectomy has become progressively less favoured treatment in this type of Cushing's syndrome, except in special circumstances.

On the basis that the primary pituitary ACTH excess may be hypothalamus-dependent, attempts have been made to treat the disorder with a dopamine agonist, somatostatin analogue, or cyproheptadine (a serotonin antagonist), since it has been shown that ACTH release is stimulated by serotonin and inhibited by dopamine. The antifungal drug, ketoconazole, has also been found to have incidental inhibitory effects on adrenal hormone biosynthesis and has been used with some success in pituitary-dependent Cushing's disease.

These approaches are all occasionally used as primary treatment, but more frequently as supplemental management when other approaches have produced incomplete results. Similarly, drugs which more directly inhibit adrenal hormone biosynthesis may be used for temporary control of hypersecretion: these are described in the following section.

Primary adrenal lesions (see Plates 5.2, 5.3) These are normally treated by simple surgical removal using a retroperitoneal (posterior) approach. Although the contralateral adrenal gland may have been temporarily suppressed by negative feedback ACTH inhibition, recovery of function is eventually normal. Carcinoma of the adrenal is normally diagnosed only following removal of the tumour and appropriate histological examination, unless the tumour has already metastasized: the control of the associated Cushing's disease may then be incomplete following surgery, and additional adrenal blocking drugs may be indicated. For this purpose metyrapone (500–750 mg 6-hourly) or an alternative adrenal blocking drug, amino-glutethimide (250 mg 6–8-hourly) may be used separately or together with appropriate monitoring of plasma cortisol levels. Additional responses have been obtained in some cases by the use of a DDT analogue, o'p'-DDD (mitotane). This agent is adrenal-suppressive and cytotoxic and has produced significant but usually temporary remissions in some cases of metastatic adrenal carcinoma, sometimes at the expense of considerable systemic toxicity.

Ectopic corticotrophin production (see Chapter 15)

Pseudo-Cushing's Syndrome

Chronic alcoholism is associated with a number of clinical features suggesting cortisol excess. Central obesity, striae, facial plethora, atrophy of skin, and hypertension are the key elements which may lead to diagnostic confusion. Although the mechanism is not clear, evidence has accumulated that CRH excess is partly responsible, coupled to impaired hepatic clearance of cortisol due to alcohol-induced hepatic dysfunction.

A second form of pseudo-Cushing's syndrome is seen as a consequence of chronic depression, (although this may itself be a feature of patients with Cushing's syndrome). Although other clinical features may be lacking, patients show impaired suppressibility of plasma and urinary cortisol to exogenous steroid, indicative of increased neuroendocrine 'drive' to hypothalamic CRH release. Normal suppressibility returns with successful treatment of the psychiatric state.

Deficiency

Adrenocortical insufficiency may conveniently be divided into two categories: primary deficiency due to disease of the adrenal gland itself (Addison's disease), and secondary insufficiency resulting from absent or low levels of ACTH. The latter cause of adrenal atrophy results from either pituitary disease or from suppression of the hypothalamic–pituitary axis resulting from the previous administration of high doses of exogenous steroids over a long period of time.

An important clinical difference between these two states of adrenocortical deficiency is that in the former there is a decrease in the mineralocorticoid (aldosterone) as well as glucocorticoid (cortisol) hormone concentrations, whereas in the latter, the aldosterone levels are near normal because the zona glomerulosa is not dependant on physiological levels of ACTH.

Adrenal insufficiency may present either as an acute emergency, or as a chronic debilitating disorder which may evade diagnosis for a considerable time: only later may an acute superimposed stress result in the more classical acute and sometimes critical presentation.

Primary adrenal insufficiency (see Plate 5.4)

Clinical features

In the acute state, the usual features of extreme muscular weakness, and dehydration are due to aldosterone deficiency. This leads to hypotension, confusion, and even coma. Such Addisonian 'crises' are fortunately rare due to increased awareness and effective early diagnosis and treatment. In contrast, chronic adrenal insufficiency has an insidious onset, with initial non-specific symptoms consisting of tiredness, weakness, anorexia, vague abdominal pain, and weight loss with occasional dizziness. A more specific sign is increased pigmentation, particularly on the exposed areas of the body, points of friction or in palmar creases. Similar pigmentation may be seen in the buccal mucosa, in scars and in the conjunctiva: such clinical features are a direct result of ACTH-mediated melanocyte stimulation. Some patients may show areas of contrasting depigmentation (vitiligo) reflecting an associated immunological abnormality.

The decreased blood pressure is due to sodium and fluid depletion associated with aldosterone deficiency, while the 'reduced vascular tone' is thought to be the result of low plasma cortisol and aldosterone levels. Postural hypotension results from the volume depletion, and hypoglycaemic episodes are due to the reduced gluconeogenesis which accompanies glucocorticoid deficiency. It is important to stress that an increasing number of cases are being diagnosed in the absence of all the above features: tiredness may be the only clinical symptom.

Although the most common aetiological factor is an autoimmune adrenalitis reflecting part of the thyrogastric autoimmune group of disorders, there are a number of other possibilities set out in Table 5.3. Accordingly, additional clinical features may be present depending on the underlying disease process.

Investigations

Routine investigations may demonstrate the anticipated low plasma sodium and elevated plasma potassium concentration; however, these are not invariably present, particularly in early cases.

The screening criterion for the diagnosis of Addison's disease is the inability of an intramuscular or intravenous injection of the ACTH-analogue, tetracosactrin, to induce a rise in plasma cortisol from a basal level by an increment of at least 250 nmol/l over a 30-minute period to a minimum value of 550 nmol/l. This is a readily performed out-patient procedure. Basal plasma cortisol levels may be

Table 5.3. Causes of primary adrenal insufficiency

Chronic primary adrenal insufficiency (Addison's disease):

- Autoimmune adrenalitis is the most commonest cause, associated in 30% with other autoimmune diseases such as pernicious anaemia and thyroiditis.
- Tuberculosis of the adrenal gland.
- Pneumocystis infection (as a complication of AIDS).
- Rarely, infiltration with metastatic carcinoma, amyloid, fungal infection, haemochromatosis.

Acute primary adrenal insufficiency:

- Any case of chronic primary adrenal insufficiency when stressed by infection or operation.
- Septicaemia with adrenal haemorrhage (Waterhouse–Friderichsen syndrome); often caused by meningococcal septicaemia.
- Following bilateral adrenalectomy without replacement therapy.
- Adrenal haemorrhage either with anticoagulant overdose or with breech delivery.
- Pharmacological steroid therapy, where there is a failure to increase dose in response to stress.

within the normal range, maintained by maximal stimulation of the adrenal cortex by high levels of endogenous ACTH, so that basal, random, diurnal or even 24-hour urinary cortisol levels may lie within the normal range.

Demonstration of an abnormal 'short' tetracosactrin test is normally followed by measurement of plasma ACTH, which provides diagnostically high levels in Addison's disease. Sometimes, attempted prolonged stimulation of the adrenal cortex by tetracosactrin infusion or repeated intramuscular injections is used to confirm the non-responsiveness of the adrenal to maximal stimulation.

In autoimmune adrenalitis a significant titre of adrenal antibodies is demonstrable in 90 per cent of cases, a finding which is rare with other destructive or infiltrative causes.

Finally, other investigations may be necessary to identify the less common aetiologies.

Treatment

The treatment of acute hypotensive Addisonian crisis involves the administration of 2–4 litres of intravenous normal saline over the first 24 hours to correct both the hypovolaemia and sodium deficiency. Hydrocortisone, 200–400 mg daily is given simultaneously by continuous intravenous infusion, gradually reducing as clinical improvement occurs.

Long-term glucorticoid replacement consists of cortisol given in divided dosage between 20 and 30 mg daily, invariably supplemented with the mineralocorticoid fludrocortisone, 0.05–0.2 mg daily. Treatment is often initiated with glucocorticoid doses 2–3 times greater than the basal requirement in order to achieve prompt steroid repletion and more rapid clinical recovery. It is important to avoid excessive long-term replacement dosage in children so as not to impair growth, and in adults to avoid osteoporosis.

The precise choice of replacement doses is difficult, and still depends largely on clinical judgement: essentially the minimum cortisol dose capable of restoring well-being. Attempts have been made to achieve more precise ‘fine-tuning’ using plasma or urinary 24-hour cortisol excretion and/or ACTH day profiles, timing the cortisol doses so as to simulate the normal physiological pattern. However, this often results in net over-replacement with its potential long-term disadvantages. Plasma renin assays can be used to titrate fludrocortisone replacement dosages: again, complete normalization of plasma renin is sometimes associated with hypertension and oedema.

Since patients cannot increase output of adrenal hormones during stress, they are at risk during stressful situations such as infection, operation, or trauma. Accordingly, they are given instructions to increase their steroid replacement dose by a factor of three during such stress periods, and to carry identification cards so that emergency parenteral steroids can be given in the case of an accident. Frequent review and reinforcement of these precautions is necessary. Acute severe illness calls for supplemental intramuscular cortisol in a dose of 100 mg three times daily, or occasionally as a continuous infusion of cortisol.

Secondary adrenal insufficiency: pharmacological steroid effects

Pharmacological steroid therapy represents an important cause of secondary adrenal insufficiency. Since corticosteroid analogues are employed for treatment of a wide range of immunologically based disorders, it is important to be aware both of their endocrine and non-endocrine effects.

The doses of steroids used may be such that partial or complete long-term suppression of the pituitary–adrenal axis is induced, by effects both on the adrenal cortex and pituitary. The use of any dose approximating or exceeding physiological replacement equivalents (5 mg of prednisolone, 0.5 mg of betamethasone or dexamethasone daily) is associated with such suppression, and withdrawal after periods of treatment exceeding 2–3 months can consequently be associated with variable degrees of hypoadrenalism. Although basal steroid requirement on these occasions may be normal, additional stress, such as infection or a surgical procedure, requires short-term supplemental steroid replacement for a considerable period of time. After continuous steroid administration for periods in excess of 18 months to 2 years, pituitary–adrenal recovery is very occasionally incomplete, and lifelong replacement with physiological steroids is then required.

The recovery from the suppressive effects of exogenous steroids appears to be a staged process. Restoration of pituitary ACTH release occurs first, followed after a variable period by recovery of the adrenal cortisol response to ACTH. The pituitary–adrenal axis appears to be unique in its ‘reluctance’ to resume function after such exogenous suppression: both the pituitary–gonadal and the pituitary–thyroid axes recover almost instantly after even 10–15 years of exogenous treatment with the relevant target gland hormone.

Testing of the pituitary–adrenal axis by insulin-induced hypoglycaemia and tetracosactrin provocation has been used to determine the degree of suppression once the decision has been made to discontinue therapeutic corticosteroids: such procedures can provide a guide as to whether steroid replacement is required on a long-term basis. In practice, a more pragmatic approach is used. This involves gradually tailing off any therapeutic steroids to zero dosage, once immunosuppressive treatment is no longer required. If subsequently symptomatic (tiredness, anorexia, and hypotension), patients are recommenced on physiological steroid replacement (ideally hydrocortisone 10 mg 12-hourly) for a further 4–6 months, and then discontinued. On the other hand, once asymptomatic, patients are not maintained on continuous basal replacement, but advised to use physiological stress-level dosage (e.g. prednisolone 5 mg 8-hourly) only during any intercurrent medical, surgical, or emotional stress episode over a subsequent period of 6–12 months. After this period of time it is generally considered that normal pituitary–adrenal function will have been restored.

Adverse effects of therapeutic-dose corticosteroids

Apart from pituitary-adrenal suppression, a number of significant adverse effects are regularly encountered with corticosteroid therapy. These simulate the clinical profile of Cushing's syndrome, with the more significant features listed below: the majority are both dose- and duration-dependent.

1. Peptic ulceration, with proneness to haemorrhage and silent perforation: use of H_2 or proton pump inhibitors prevent this complication.
2. Osteoporosis may be precipitated, occasionally within a 12 month interval (See Chapter10).
3. Diabetes and hypertension may be triggered or aggravated: there are no specific preventive manoeuvres.
4. Growth may be impaired in children (See Chapter13).
5. Wound healing and infection responses are inhibited.
6. Avascular necrosis (usually of the femoral head) may be triggered.
7. Psychiatric problems (especially depression and psychosis) may be precipitated.
8. Myopathies may occur, usually affecting proximal lower limb girdle muscles.

Attempts have been made to minimize the risks of the above complications in situations where long-term treatment is unavoidable. The type of steroid appears not to influence the risk, although longer-acting analogues are more likely to cause problems and deflazacort may have preferential benefits. Alternate day therapy has also been shown to benefit some patients. Individual complications can be minimized by simultaneous use of other drugs: for example editronate to reduce osteoporosis risk and H_2 receptor blocking drugs to reduce peptic ulcer risk.

Disorders of adrenal steroid synthesis

Clinical disorders may arise due to congenital enzyme defects which impair the synthesis of cortisol and aldosterone. These syndromes are rare, although minor degrees of abnormality may evade clinical recognition.

There are two consequences of such defects. First, deficiency of hormones distal to the biosynthetic block (usually involving the cortisol pathway), results in triggering negative feedback of ACTH release. Secondly, consequent on the increased plasma ACTH concentration, there is a stimulation of other ACTH-dependent pathways unaffected by the block, leading (usually) to excess androgen and mineralocorticoid production and release (see Fig. 5.2). In addition, there is an associated hyperplasia of the gland resulting from prolonged ACTH hyperstimulation, giving rise to the diagnostic term 'congenital adrenal hyperplasia (CAH)'. The clinical features are dependent on the severity of the particular defect, which may be so mild that in order to establish biochemical diagnosis, stimulation with exogenous corticotrophin may be necessary.

The abnormalities are almost exclusively due to single gene defects transmitted as an autosomal recessive trait. In the case of the common 21-hydroxylase defect, the causative mutant genes occur with a frequency of 1 in 50. The chance of two heterozygotes intermarrying is therefore 1 in 2500. With a 1 in 4 probability of producing a homozygous offspring, the prevalence of this type of congenital adrenal hyperplasia will be approximately 1 in 10 000 births. Modification of activity of crucial P-450 microsomal and mitochondrial enzymes (each responsible for one step in cortisol biosynthesis) by relevant gene deletions creates the biochemical block. Once an affected offspring has been genetically 'finger-printed' the gene carrier status can be verified by chorionic villus sampling in subsequent pregnancies. This allows diagnosis (and institution of therapy) at the earliest possible time: indeed, it has been shown that corticosteroid therapy during pregnancy can prevent the *in utero* development of ambiguous genitalia.

21-Hydroxylase deficiency (see Plate 5.5)

This defect is responsible for 95 per cent of all cases of congenital adrenal hyperplasia and for a similar proportion of all cases of females with ambiguous genitalia. The gene which encodes the 21-hydroxylase enzyme (CYP21B) is located on the short arm of chromosome 6, closely linked to the genes encoding HLA-B and HLA-DR. The homozygous state results in a severity of enzyme deficiency causing a failure of 17α-hydroxyprogesterone and progesterone conversion to 11-desoxycortisol and 11-desoxycorticosterone, respectively, with consequent glucocorticoid and a variable degree of mineralocorticoid deficiency. The excess of substrate is thus channelled into enhanced synthesis and secretion of androgens in direct response to the increased ACTH drive.

Clinical features

In severe cases, a female infant is born with apparently male external genitalia resulting in incorrect gender assignment. Within a few days, vomiting and dehydration occur due to cortisol deficiency, and unless rapidly diagnosed and treated with steroid replacement, the condition may be fatal. A similar course of events but without significant genital changes occurs in affected male infants.

In less severe cases the lack of metabolic disturbance may result in considerable delay in recognition. In the female, androgen-induced clitoral hypertrophy and labial fusion simulate normal male external genitalia: the more proximal external urethral opening (hypospadias) may be easily missed. Such cases may only be diagnosed later when muscular hypertrophy, voice deepening and excessive hair growth develop in a female (pseudo-hermaphroditism). In fact, some cases are so completely androgenized that they are reared as males: the diagnosis is only made when they present with infertility! In the male, precocious puberty may be the only manifestation.

The most subtle clinical presentation in females consists of hirsutism alone with minimal or no clitoral enlargement, and presenting with amenorrhoea in the late-teens or early-twenties. In the male, infertility may be the only manifestation of this minimal biosynthetic defect. Both these minor presentations probably represent the heterozygous form of the disorder.

Investigations

1. Severe, salt-losing cases are hyponatraemic and sometimes hyperkalaemic. Cases with less severe mineralocorticoid deficiency may be evaluated using plasma renin activity.

2. A stained buccal smear to identify the nuclear Barr bodies found in the female (XX) genotype and peripheral leucocyte cell culture with karyotype determination is carried out on any infant in whom there is doubt about gender.

3. The plasma 17α-hydroxyprogesterone concentration, and excretion of its urinary metabolite, pregnanetriol are elevated, and both demonstrate complete suppressibility into the normal range following physiological doses of exogenous corticosteroid.

In less florid cases, usually in older girls presenting with hirsutism, the heterozygous state is reflected by normal or minimally elevated 17α-hydroxyprogesterone levels which demonstrate hyper-responsiveness to ACTH stimulation as the only definable abnormality.

4. Less specific investigations, such as bone age, will demonstrate skeletal age advancement in keeping with abnormally increased androgen production.

Treatment

In emergency cases, rehydration with intravenous saline and corticosteroid administration are life-saving. This treatment is later replaced by orally administered glucocorticoids and sometimes mineralocorticoids (fludrocortisone 0.05–0.1 mg daily).

In milder cases presenting later in life, cortisol is used in doses of 10–50 mg daily, with a slightly higher proportion given in the evening to suppress the dominant overnight physiological release of ACTH.

In post-pubertal cases, the longer acting dexamethasone (0.25–0.75 mg daily) provides more effective corticotrophin suppression. In younger children, the drug is contraindicated since pituitary-suppressive doses may also be associated with suppression of growth.

Replacement doses are monitored by measurement of serum 17α-hydroxyprogesterone or urinary pregnanetriol levels, which are reduced into the normal range by appropriate doses of glucocorticoid. Cases presenting with salt loss at birth will later in life sometimes require ongoing treatment with fludrocortisone in the doses mentioned above. However, in a proportion of children the enzyme defect 'matures', so that mineralocorticoid replacement is no longer necessary.

All patients are advised to triple their glucocorticoid dose during intercurrent stress, since the potential hazards are the same as those of the adrenocortical deficiency found in Addison's disease. Normal lifespan and fertility are usually achieved, although plastic surgery to the genitalia is sometimes necessary in late-diagnosed cases. Later presenting 'compensated' cases, with already established gender identity, usually do not justify therapy of any type, and are capable of enhancing adrenal function normally in response to stress states.

11β-Hydroxylase deficiency

In this disorder, cortisol and aldosterone synthesis are both decreased. The resulting higher level of ACTH stimulates the available metabolic pathways resulting in excess androgen production. Mineralocorticoid excess results from the enhanced secretion of 11-desoxycorticosterone.

Clinical features

The clinical picture is again one of virilism, presenting in childhood or early adult life. Salt loss is not a feature but hypertension is almost invariable.

Investigations

There is usually a lesser elevation of 17α-hydroxyprogesterone than seen in the 21-hydroxylase deficient patients. Plasma 11-desoxycortisol is increased together with increased urinary excretion of its tetrahydro derivative.

Treatment

Glucocorticoid is given as for the 21-hydroxylase defect. Both virilism and hypertension are reversed with optimal replacement doses.

Other rare enzymatic defects

17-Hydroxylase deficiency results in reduced levels of cortisol, androgens, and oestrogens, but with ACTH-promoted excessive synthesis of mineralocorticoids. This results in clinical hypogonadism in either sex, coupled to hypertension and occasionally hypokalaemia. Corticosteroid administration results in correction of the hypocortisolism and normalization of the blood pressure. However, the defect in sex hormone production in the male usually requires adphyiditional androgen replacement.

3β-Dehydrogenase deficiency results in reduced synthesis of all major corticosteroids: cortisol, aldosterone, testosterone, and oestrogens. There is hypotension, volume depletion, and hyponatraemia. Survival is uncommon.

Apparently non-functioning adrenal adenomas

With the increased use of CT and MRI scanning, so-called 'incidentalomas' of the adrenal are sometimes identified in the course of abdominal imaging for an unrelated condition. The diagnostic and therapeutic approach to these findings is difficult. Almost invariably, there is neither clinical nor biochemical evidence of adrenal dysfunction (although systematic screening for aldosterone, cortisol and catecholamine excess is usually performed). Repeat imaging in 6–12 months is normally recommended: approximately 25 per cent of cases eventually come to surgery, either because of enlargement of the lesion, or the patient's (or physician's) concern. The findings are usually those of a non-functioning benign adrenocortical adenoma.

Systematic autopsy assessments have historically provided evidence of an approximate 10 per cent prevalence of such benign tumours not only in the adrenal, but also in the pituitary gland.

FURTHER READING

PHYSIOLOGY

Gutkowska, J. and Nemer, M. (1989). Structure, expression and function of atrial natriuretic factor and extraatrial tissues. *Endocrine Reviews*, **10**, 519–536.

Jacobson, L. and Sapolsky, R. (1991). The role of the hippocampus in feedback regulation of the hypothalamic-pituitary-adrenocortical axis. *Endocrine Reviews*, **12**, 118–34.

Skott, O. and Jensen, B.L. (1993). Cellular and intrarenal control of renin secretion. *Clinical Science*, **84**, 1–10.

Walker, B.R. and Williams, B.C. (1992). Corticosteroids and vascular tone; mapping the messenger maze. *Clinical Science*, **82**, 597–605.

CLINICAL

Bockman, R.S. and Weinerman, S.A. (1990). Steroid-induced osteoporosis. *Orthop. Clinics North America*, **21**, 97–107.

Derksen, J., Nagesser, S.K., Meinders, A.A., *et al.* (1994). Identification of virilizing adrenal tumours in hirsute women. *New England Journal of Medicine*, **331**, 968–73.

Edwards, C.R.W. (1991). Lessons from liquorice. *New England Journal of Medicine*, **325**, 1242–3.

Gordon, R.D. (1994). Mineralocorticoid hypertension. *Lancet*, **344**, 240–3.

Migeon, C.J. and Donohue, P.A. (1991). Congenital adrenal hyperplasia caused by 21-hydroxylase deficiency: its molecular basis and remaining therapeutic problems. *Endocrinology Metabolism Clinics North America*, **20**, 277–96.

Miller, W.L. (1994). Genetics, diagnosis and management of 21-hydroxylase deficiency. *Journal of Clinical Endocrinology and Metabolism*, **78**, 241–6.

Oelkers, W, Diederich, S., and Bahr, V. (1992). Diagnosis and therapy surveillance in Addison's disease: ACTH test and measurement of plasma ACTH, renin and aldosterone. *Journal of Clinical Endocrinology and Metabolism,* **75**, 259–64.

Orth, D.N. (1995). Medical progress: Cushing's syndrome. *New England Journal of Medicine*, **332**, 791–803.

Osella, G., Terzolo, M., Borretto, G., *et al.* (1994). Endocrine evaluation of the incidentally discovered adrenal mass (incidentalomas). *Journal of Clinical Endocrinology and Metabolism*, **79**, 1532–9.

Reznek, R.H. and Armstrong, P. (1994). The adrenal gland: imaging procedures. *Clinical Endocrinology*, **40**, 561–76.

White, P.C. (1994). Disorders of aldosterone biosynthesis and action. *New England Journal of Medicine*, **331**, 250–8.

Yanovski, J.A. (1994). Glucocorticoid action and the clinical features of Cushing's syndrome. *Endocrinology Metabolism Clinics North America*, **23**, 487–509.

6

The adrenal medulla

PHYSIOLOGY

The adrenal medulla is the central part of the adrenal (suprarenal) gland, one of which lies on the superior pole of each kidney. It secretes catecholamines of which, in man, 80 per cent consists of adrenaline (epinephrine) the remainder being noradrenaline (norepinephrine) and small amounts of dopamine. The adrenal medullae are not essential for life since their function can be compensated for by increased sympathetic activity.

Anatomy, histology, and development

The adrenal medulla is embryologically derived from the neural crest, and consists of granule-containing cells which are called chromaffin cells. There is histological evidence to suggest that there are two types of cells, each synthesizing its specific hormone, adrenaline or noradrenaline. Approximately 80 per cent of the chromaffin cells in human adrenomedullary tissue appears to be of the type which synthesizes adrenaline.

The arterial blood supply to the adrenal gland reaches the outer capsule of the gland from branches of the renal and phrenic arteries, although there is a less important arterial supply from the aorta. From the capillary plexus on the outer adrenal capsule most of the blood enters sinusoids which descend through the adrenal cortical tissue, perfusing the cells on the way. Thus, most blood reaching the adrenal medulla is partly deoxygenated, but contains relatively high concentrations of hormones secreted by the adrenocortical cells. There are also small medullary arteries which descend directly to the adrenal medulla from the outer capsule, and which provide a supply of true arterial blood. Venous blood enters a central adrenal vein, which passes along the axis of the gland. The adrenal medulla is innervated by preganglionic sympathetic fibres which terminate directly on the chromaffin cells. Thus, the main stimulus for release of the adrenomedullary hormones is the preganglionic sympathetic neurotransmitter acetylcholine.

Functional significance of the adrenal medulla

The physiological importance of the adrenal medullae remains uncertain since they can be extirpated without any apparent deterioration in the general maintenance of homeostasis. Indeed, sensitivity of tissues to sympathetic nervous activity appears to increase in this situation. Nevertheless the ability of the adrenal medullae to release catecholamines into the general circulation suggests an important reinforcing mechanism which would not only prolong the direct effects of general sympathetic activity, but would also increase the blood concentration of energy substrates through the metabolic effects of circulating adrenaline. These metabolic effects are of particular relevance to the catecholamines since they emphasize the difference between a hormone, such as adrenaline, which can reach all cells of the body through the circulation, and noradrenaline which is mainly released at nerve endings and which acts on those cells with sympathetic innervations.

The release of catecholamines from the adrenal medulla as part of general sympathetic stimulation is probably of particular importance in conditions of emergency and stress (the 'fear–fight–flight' situation first described by Cannon in 1920).

The catecholamines

Synthesis, storage, and release

The catecholamines (dopamine, noradrenaline, and adrenaline) are synthesized in the brain, at sympathetic postganglionic nerve endings, and at the sites of chromaffin tissue such as the adrenal medullae. The synthesis pathway originates with the amino acid tyrosine (derived mainly from the diet, although hydroxylation of phenylalanine in the liver is also important). Tyrosine is hydroxylated to L-dopa and this is then decarboxylated to dopamine, which is further hydroxylated to form noradrenaline. Noradrenaline can be converted to adrenaline by methylation, brought about by the enzyme phenylethanolamine-*N*-methyl transferase which is found only in adrenomedullary tissue, the organ of Zuckerkandl, and, in minute amounts, in the brain (Fig. 6.1). Extremely high local concentrations of glucocorticoids from the adrenal cortex via the sinusoidal system stimulate the methylation reaction in the adrenal medulla.

The catecholamines are stored in granules within the chromaffin cells of the adrenal medullae and their release by exocytosis is stimulated by acetylcholine from the preganglionic sympathetic nerve endings. The chromaffin cells may therefore be considered as specialized postganglionic sympathetic nerve fibres which can release their catecholamines directly into the bloodstream.

Direct electrical stimulation of certain areas in the hypothalamus which elicit general sympathetic discharge (with the release of noradrenaline at the postganglionic sympathetic nerve endings for a local effect) also induces the release of catecholamines into the general circulation through stimulation of the adrenal medulla. In humans, the principal catecholamine released from this gland is adrenaline whereas at the postganglionic sympathetic nerve endings noradrenaline is released. It is interesting to note that direct electrical stimulation of selected parts of the hypothalamus associated with the release of catecholamines has been claimed to be selective with respect to the actual catecholamine released from the adrenal medulla; certain areas when stimulated appear to be associated with

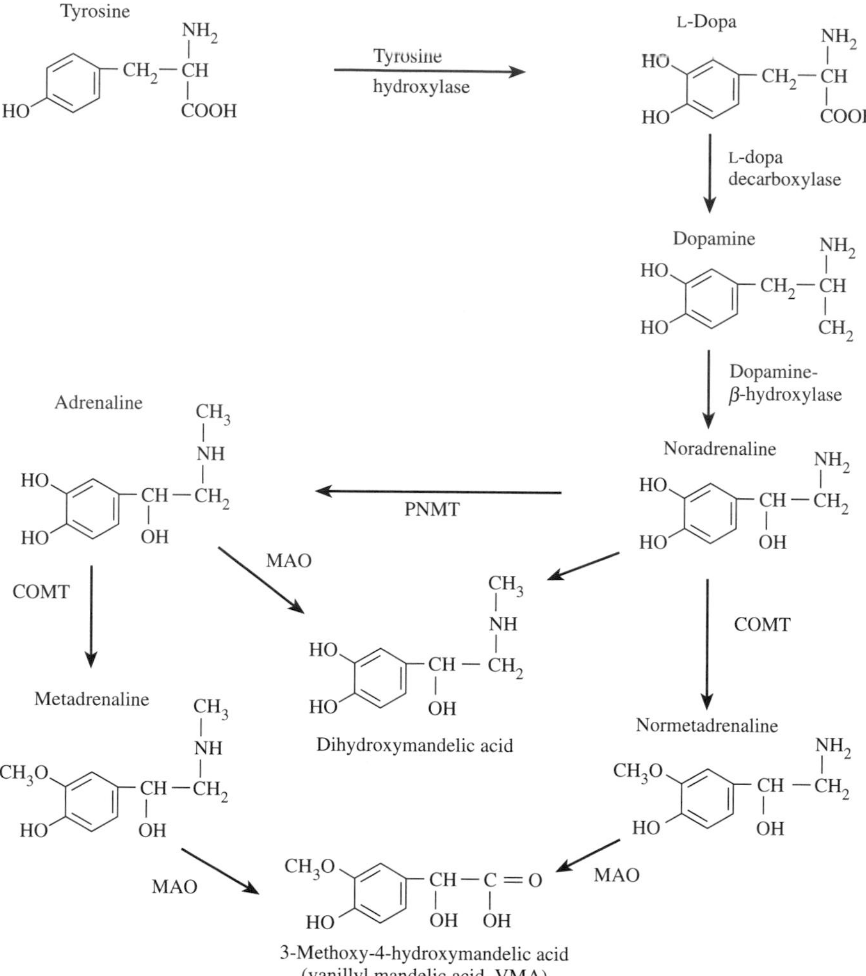

Fig. 6.1. Diagram showing the synthesis of the adrenomedullary catecholamines adrenaline and noradrenaline, and their degradation products (COMT, catechol-*O*-methyl transferase; MAO, monamine oxidase; PNMT; phenyl ethanolamine-N-methyl transferase.)

the release of noradrenaline alone, whereas other areas appear to be related to the selective release of adrenaline. These observations indicate separate neuronal pathways relating the hypothalamus to the different cells in the adrenal medulla associated with the release of either one of the catecholamines from this endocrine gland.

Other biologically active peptides have been identified in chromaffin cells, including the enkephalins, neuropeptide Y, galanin, and vasopressin. These substances appear to coexist with the catecholamines, and presumably are released from the same granules following the action of acetylcholine on the chromaffin cell membranes.

Actions

The effects of adrenomedullary stimulation and sympathetic nerve stimulation are generally similar. There are, however, certain tissues in which adrenaline and noradrenaline produce different effects. The existence of at least two different types of receptor, α and β, with different sensitivities for the various catecholamines accounts for the different responses. According to this classification system the α-receptors are equally sensitive to both adrenaline and noradrenaline; the β-receptors respond more to adrenaline, and are in general relatively less sensitive to noradrenaline. However, this is an over-simplification. A more recent classification identifies different α and β subtypes, so that there are α_1 and α_2 subtypes and β_1, β_2, and β_3 subtypes of catecholamine receptor. The principal body systems which respond to adrenaline and/or noradrenaline are considered individually.

Cardiovascular system

(1) *heart rate*: increased by both adrenaline and noradrenaline (positive chronotropic action involving β_1-receptors which bind both catecholamines);

(2) *force of contraction of heart muscle*: increased by both adrenaline and noradrenaline (positive inotropic action also involving β1-receptors);

(3) *coronary blood flow*: in man it is uncertain whether adrenaline or noradrenaline increase coronary blood flow.

(4) *blood vessels of skin*, *mucous membranes*, and *splanchnic bed*: vasoconstriction, by adrenaline and noradrenaline; and

(5) *blood vessels of skeletal muscle*: vasoconstriction by noradrenaline (via α_1-receptors), but chiefly vasodilation by adrenaline (via β_2-receptors).

As a result of the general vasocontriction of blood vessels by noadrenaline, peripheral resistance to blood flow is increased. This increase in peripheral resistance together with the increased stroke volume results in increased systolic and diastolic pressures such that the mean arterial blood pressure rises. An increased mean arterial blood pressure following the administration of noradrenaline stimulates the baroreceptors in the carotid sinus and aortic arch. The receptors in turn stimulate the medullary cardio-inhibitory centre which then reflexly inhibits the heart rate through the vagus, overcoming the initial tachycardia. The actions of adrenaline on the heart are such that the systolic pressure increases but the diastolic pressure may decrease; the mean arterial blood pressure following the administration of adrenaline therefore may not change, or if it does then only by increasing slightly. Since this catecholamine induces a vasodilatation in skeletal muscle, its vasoconstictor effect on the blood vessels of the skin and splanchnic bed is counteracted; the peripheral resistance therefore may actually decrease. However the diastolic pressure may not fall because the stroke volume is increased. Although the baroreceptors normally respond to a raised pulse pressure by increasing their phasic frequency, the tachycardia induced by the direct effect of adrenaline on cardiac muscle is still observed as the stimulus is insufficient to cause a reflex decrease in the heart rate.

Respiratory system
Both sympathetic stimulation (or the administration of noradrenaline) and adrenaline induce dilatation of the bronchi and bronchioles by relaxing the bronchial and bronchiolar muscles. However, adrenaline is a more potent bronchodilator than noradrenaline, and this is because of its relatively greater effect on β_2-receptors.

Gastrointestinal tract
Adrenaline and noradrenaline relax the smooth muscle of the gastrointestinal tract (decreased tone) and inhibit peristalsis: the pyloric and ileocolic sphincters contract.

Central nervous system
Adrenaline activates the ascending reticular system (induces arousal). In man it also appears to initiate anxiety, stimulation of breathing, and coarse tremors of the fingers. Noradrenaline appears to be much less potent in producing these effects.

Blood
Adrenaline increases coagulation time (perhaps by increasing the activity of factor V). It also increases the red blood cell count, the haemoglobin concentration, and the plasma protein concentration. It is believed that these increases are due to simple haemoconcentration because of movement of fluid out of blood into the intercellular spaces. Adrenaline also reduces the eosinophil count, although this effect may be mediated by cortisol from the adrenal certex (see Chapter 5). Noradrenaline does not appear to produce these various effects on the blood system.

Metabolism
Carbohydrate Adrenaline is a potent hyperglycaemic agent, due mainly to its actions on the liver and also on the pancreas (see Chapter 11). In the liver it promotes glycogenolysis and gluconeogenesis. Because of the presence in hepatic tissue of a phosphatase which can hydrolyse the glucose-6-phosphate (formed by glycogenolysis) to glucose, the glucose can then diffuse into the bloodstream. Adrenaline also stimulates glycogenolysis in skeletal muscle, but because this tissue does not have the phosphatase, lactic acid is formed from the metabolism of glucose-6-phosphate. The lactic acid reaches the liver where it becomes converted to glucose.

While noradrenaline has little direct effect on carbohydrate metabolism, both the catecholamines can inhibit the glucose-induced secretion of insulin from the β-cells of the islets of Langerhans in the pancreas (see Chapter 11), and this effect is believed to be mediated by catecholamine α-receptors. Indeed it appears that β-receptor stimulation on the islet cells results in a subsequent enhanced release of insulin by other stimuli.
Fats Adrenaline and, to a lesser extent, noradrenaline stimulate lipolytic activity in adipose tissue (and muscle), with a resultant increase in the plasma free fatty acid concentration. This is via β2-receptor stimulation. Adrenaline increases the total oxygen consumption (calorigenic action) and increases the basal metabolic rate.

The eye

Adrenaline (and to a lesser extent noradrenaline) dilates the pupil of the eye by stimulating the contraction of the radial smooth muscle.

Metabolism and excretion

Circulating catecholamines are mainly taken up by postsynaptic nerve endings (where they may either be stored in granules or inactivated) and by the liver and kidneys (where they are inactivated). The two principal enzymes involved in the inactivation of the catecholamines are monoamine oxidase (MAO) and catechol-*O*-methyl transferase (COMT). The first of the enzymes (MAO) is located in the mitochondria of the nerve axons, while COMT is present on the postsynaptic cell membranes and in the liver and kidneys. The catecholamines are converted to metadrenaline and normetadrenaline by COMT. Both of these metabolites may be excreted directly in the urine or following conjugation, as glucuronides and sulphates, or following oxidation, via an intermediate aldehyde, as 3-methoxy-4-hydroxy mandelic acid (vanillyl mandelic acid, VMA). A somewhat smaller proportion of the intermediate aldehyde is reduced to 4-hydroxy-3-methoxyphenylglycol (HMPG). MAO is responsible for formation of the aldehyde and it may also act directly on the catecholamines, with COMT acting secondarily on the degration products. 2–13 per cent of the catecholamines are directly excreted in the urine, mostly as conjugates. When large quantities of adrenaline are secreted from chromoffin cells, for example when a phaeochromocytoma is present, the COMT inactivation mechanism is the more important. This results in a disproportionately high urinary concentration of metadrenaline, although other degradation products, particularly VMA, which is widely used as a diagnostic aid, are present (see Fig. 6.1).

Interaction with other hormones

Various hormones appear to interact with the catecholamines. The thyroid iodothyronines, for example, when present in excess are associated with various clinical manifestations of excessive catecholamine production; and the hyperactivity effects, such as tachycardia, can be blocked partially by β-receptor blockers such as propranolol. There is some evidence to suggest that the iodothyronines may stimulate the synthesis of certain catecholamine receptors in the tissues. Another example of an interaction between catecholamines and other hormones is indicated by the effects of adrenaline and noradrenaline on insulin production by the islet β-cells.

CLINICAL DISORDERS

Hyposecretion of catecholamines due to adrenal medullary damage is rarely encountered in clinical practice: however, defective catecholamine release from nerve endings is the basis of the rather more common clinical picture of autonomic neuropathy. This entity is not dealt with in this book, except in the context of diabetic neuropathy (Chapter 11). A variety of other causes, including the Shy–Drager and Guillain–Barré syndrome are associated with dysautonomia. A rare congenital syndrome of dopamine-ß-hydroxylase deficiency has been described, in which low adrenaline and noradrenaline levels are coupled to correspondingly raised levels of dopamine.

Where bilateral adrenal medullary damage does occur, for example with tuberculous or malignant destruction of the adrenal glands, or following adrenalectomy, no symptoms or other clinical features occur, since catecholamine production from sympathetic nerve endings satisfies all normal biological requirements.

Drugs that induce intracellular glucopenia, such as 2-deoxyglucose or insulin, can induce an acute release of adrenal medullary adrenaline and noradrenaline, and can thereby be used to identify adrenal medullary destruction or dysfunction. This test is occasionally of value in determining the primary cause of adrenocortical insufficiency: in infective and infiltrative lesions, the medulla is involved as well, while in the immunologically based disorder of primary adrenocortical insufficiency (see Chapter 5) the adrenal medulla is spared.

Hypersecretory states are confined to two types of tumour: phaeochromocytoma and neuroblastoma.

Phaeochromocytoma

This tumour occurs predominantly in the 25–55 age group, and is a rare cause of hypertension and other catecholamine-related symptoms. In about 30 per cent of cases it is familial, and is associated with one or more abnormalities found in a condition known as multiple endocrine neoplasia (MEN) type II: this is considered in detail in Chapter 16. Approximately 5 per cent of phaeochromocytoma are associated with neuroectodermal lesions such as neurofibromatosis.

The vast majority (about 85 per cent) occur within the adrenal medulla, are sometimes multiple (10 per cent) and malignant (5 per cent). The tumour may also occur in other locations, such as the sympathetic ganglia of the truncal region; a common site is the organ of Zuckerkandl. Although phaeochromocytoma accounts for less than 1:1000 cases of hypertension, it is of clinical importance, since removal of the tumour results in a restoration of normal blood pressure in the majority of instances: untreated, the prognosis for life is poor. Although it commonly produces large amounts of catecholamines, clinical features stemming from this over-production are often disproportionately small: accordingly, phaeochromocytoma is often diagnosed for the first time at autopsy in patients previously and erroneously considered to have had essential (primary) hypertension. It has also been identified for the first time following peri-operative collapse (and often death): a high index of suspicion at the time of diagnosis of hypertension might have been life-saving.

Clinical features

Hypertension, which is the cardinal sign, may be intermittent or persistent, depending on the secretory pattern of the tumour. As indicated above, it is also now appreciated from autopsy data on hypertensive patients that asymptomatic cases exceed those with symptoms. If no other suggestive symptoms are present, the true diagnosis may remain unsuspected and undiagnosed. Typically, in intermittent catecholamine secretors, the patient complains of attacks which may be precipitated by emotion, physical exercise, or even meals, and which consist of pounding headaches, sweating, pallor, pain in the chest or abdomen, and apprehension to the point of fear of imminent death. Paraesthesiae, nausea, and vomiting may also occur.

If observed during an attack, there is sweating and the skin is pale from cutaneous vasoconstriction. Pupils are dilated, limbs feel cold, and there is hypertension and occasionally pyrexia. After an attack there is often marked weakness. Hypertensive 'crises', which can be fatal may be induced by anaesthesia and operation in patients with previously unrecognized tumours. Postural hypotension is a common clinical finding, with or without symptoms. It is more frequent in cases with persistent hypertension and is due to catecholamine-induced hypovolaemia.

One of the major differential diagnoses is simple anxiety. Understandably, the clinical features are similar, including the paroxysmal hypertension. A careful history is an essential element but psychosocial factors may be very similar in the two conditions. Most laboratories report only one positive phaeochrmocytoma case identified for every 400–500 patients who are biochemically screened. (Table 6.1.)

Children with phaeochromocytoma sometimes have distinctive clinical features: nausea, vomiting, polyphagia, polyuria, and polydipsia are comparatively rare in adults but occur in up to 20 per cent of children.

Investigations

The most commonly employed screening test is a 24-hour urine assay for catecholamine metabolites (VMA). Although frequently used because it is comparatively inexpensive, this screening assay fails to diagnose about 30 per cent of phaeochromocytomas. Metadrenaline assay provides a lower incidence of false negative diagnoses. Many centres consider that measurement of urinary or plasma adrenaline and noradrenaline is the only approriate screening investigation, and is ideally performed on three consecutive days. The justification for performing such tests in otherwise asymptomatic hypertensive patients is difficult to establish. In paroxysmal hypertension the indications are clear. In persistent hypertension, the

Table 6.1. Differential diagnosis of phaeochromocytoma

Hyperventilation
Anxiety episodes
Menopausal flushing
Hypoglycaemia
Hyperthyroidism
Alcohol or other drug withdrawal
Acute porphyria
Caffeine excess
Temporal lobe epilepsy or diencephalic seizures

low yield of positive results suggests that screening tests should only be performed in young patients, particularly in the absence of a family history of hypertension. It also needs to be excluded where hypertension is severe, associated with one or more of the characteristic symptoms mentioned above or refractory to conventional treatment.

Localizing the biochemically confirmed tumour is an important pre-operative exercise. Imaging of the adrenal has become simplified with the advent of high resolution ultrasound (US), CT, and MRI scanning. More than 90 per cent of tumours can be localized by one of these methods. Failing this, scanning using the adrenal medullary cell-seeking isotope MIBG-131 is often helpful (see Fig. 6.2). False negativity is as low as 10 per cent and approaches zero for malignant tumours: false positive results are extremely rare. Previously, retrograde trans-femoral venous catheterization of the adrenals with multiple sampling for plasma catecholamines was used, but this has been largely superseded by the less invasive imaging methods mentioned above.

Pharmacological tests aimed at stimulating catecholamine release (and a blood pressure rise) are now probably only of historic interest: histamine and tyramine have been shown to produce relatively large rises in blood pressure in phaeochromocytoma. These diagnostic approaches are at best unreliable, and at worst dangerous. However, pharmacological suppression tests in patients with borderline catecholamine elevation are sometimes useful. Clonidine, an α_2-agonist, fails to reduce the catecholamine levels of genuine phaeochromocytoma into the normal range. Similarly pentolinium, a short-acting ganglion blocker suppresses non-tumour catecholamine levels, but not those of phaeochromocytoma cases.

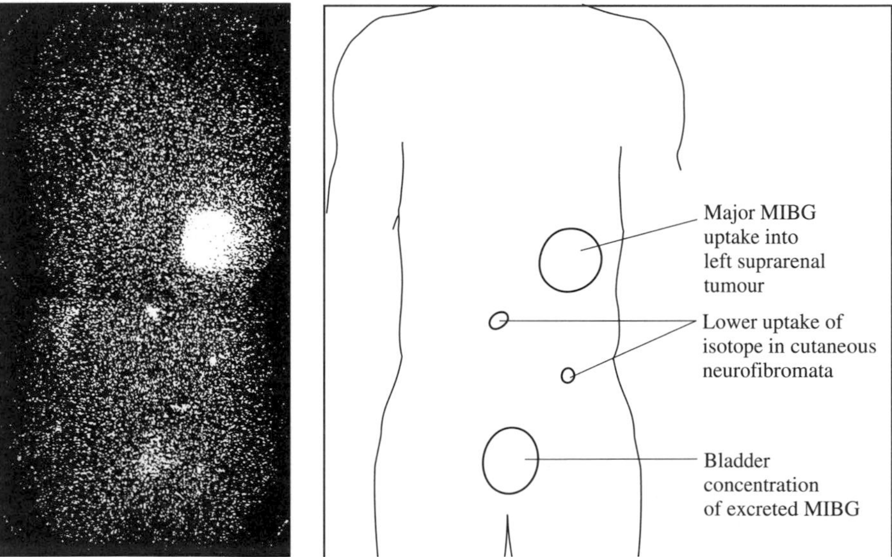

Fig. 6.2. Isotope scan using MIBG-131 in a patient with phaeochromocytoma (arrow). The patient also had neurofibromatosis, the larger lesions of which also concentrate isotope.

Treatment

This is normally achieved by surgery following localization of the tumour. Catecholamines may be released due to surgical manipulation of the gland, and it is therefore essential that the patient be adequately prepared prior to surgery. Such preparation involves the use of phenoxybenzamine (20–60 mg per day for several days) as an alpha blocker, and in some patients the addition of beta blockers (e.g. propranolol 40–160 mg per day). It is generally considered desirable to ensure that hypovolaemia has been reversed either using the above drugs (which may take up to two weeks), or with pre- or intra-operative volume repletion. These procedures significantly reduce the likelihood of hypotension after removal of the tumour.

Occasionally, phaeochromocytoma is malignant and even multiple. In these instances, surgery, radiotherapy, and chemotherapy have all been used with variable success. High-dose tumour-seeking isotope (MIBG-131) is sometimes effective in achieving isotopic ablation of tumour masses. Although theoretically sound, this approach is at best only palliative. In inoperable tumour cases or where surgery is contraindicated, long term control of hypertension and other symptoms can be achieved with combined alpha- and beta-adrenergic blockade.

Neuroblastoma (sympathoblastoma) — ganglioneuroma group

This tumour spectrum ranges from the highly malignant neuroblastoma to the relatively benign ganglioneuroma, with its significantly higher incidence in childhood. Symptoms may include episodic hypertension, sweating attacks, pallor, and occasionally diarrhoea, which is probably due to the associated over-production of vasoactive intestinal peptide (VIP). Extreme peripheral catecholamine effects are probably negated by the extensive amine degradation which occurs within the tumour.

FURTHER READING

PHYSIOLOGY

Fedida, D., Braun, A.P., and Giles, W.R. (1993). 1α adrenoceptors in myocardium: functional aspects and transmembrane signaling mechanisms. *Physiological Review*, **73**, 469–87.

CLINICAL

Bouloux, P.M.G., Perrett, D., and Besser, G.M. (1985). Methodological considerations in the determination of plasma catecholamines by high performance liquid chromatography coupled to electrochemical detection. *Annals of Clinical Biochemistry*, **22**, 194–203.

Elliott, W.J. and Murphy, M.B. (1988). Reduced specificity of the clonidine suppression test in patients with normal plasma catecholamines. *American Journal of Medicine*, **84**, 419–24.

Kuchel, O. (1985). Phaeochromocytoma. *Hypertension*, **7**, 151–8.

Lehnert, H., Weber, P., Nagele-Wohrle, B., *et al.* (1988). Intra-operative localization of phaeochromocytoma by I-123 MIBG single probe measurement. *Klinische Wochenschrift*, **66,** 61–4.

Medeiros, L.J., Wolf, B.C. Balogh, K., and Federman, M. (1985). Adrenal phaeochromocytoma: a clinico-pathological review of 60 cases. *Human Pathology*, **16**, 580–9.

Modlin, I.M., Farndon, J.R., Shepherd, A., *et al.* (1979). Phaeochromocytoma in 72 patients: clinical and diagnostic features, treatment and long-term results. *British Journal of Surgery*, **66,** 456–65.

Ross, E.J. and Griffith, D.N.W. (1989). The clinical presentation of phaeochromocytoma. *Quarterly Journal of Medicine*, **266,** 485–96.

Sheps, S.G., Jiang N.S., Klee, G.G., and Van Heerden, J.A. (1990). Recent developments in the diagnosis and treatment of phaeochromocytoma. *Mayo Clinic Proceedings*, **65**, 85–95.

7

Male reproductive endocrinology

PHYSIOLOGY

The endocrinology of the gonads is considered in two chapters. This chapter discusses the male gonads (the testes), and the following (Chapter 8), the female gonads (the ovaries), including such relevant topics as pregnancy, the fetoplacental unit, parturition, lactation, and the menopause. Since genetic sex differentiation and early embryonic gonadal development are two topics which are fundamental and closely related to the testes and the ovaries, these are considered first.

Genetic sex differentiation

Every human cell contain 46 chromosomes in pairs, 22 pairs being somatic (autosomal), the twenty-third being the sex determinant chromosomes. The female sex is genetically determined by a pair of X chromosomes, while the male has one X chromosome and one Y chromosome. Cell division of a parent germ cell by meiosis (first and second meiotic divisions) results ultimately in the separation of the chromosomes in each pair. Thus, the daughter cells formed each have half the total number of chromosomes (i.e. 23 chromosomes). Propagation of the species therefore depends on the fusion of two daughter cells each with half the number of chromosomes (haploid) to form a new cell with the full complement of 46 chromosomes (diploid). One daughter cell comes from the mother and the other from the father. The formation of daughter cells (gametes) by meiosis is called gametogenesis. The new cell with the XX sex chromosomes develops into a genetic female, while the cell with the XY chromosomes develops into the genetic male, the Y chromosome being ultimately the genetic sex determinant (see Fig. 7.1).

Early embryonic development of the gonads

In the embryo, primordial germ cells migrate from the yolk sac to the genital ridge of mesoderm on the dorsal wall of the developing abdominal cavity. Proliferation of the cell of the genital ridge, incorporating the primordial germ cells, results in the development of the primitive gonads beside the mesonephros. These primitive gonads are initially identical in both sexes. Up to the sixth week of intrauterine life both Müllerian (female) and Wolffian (male) primitive genital tract systems develop and it is only after the sixth week that the gonads begin to differentiate into either testes or ovaries. Testicular formation is consequent upon the existence, and influence, of the Y chromosome. On this chromosome an RNA transcription factor, known as 'sex-determining region of the Y chromosome' protein (sry

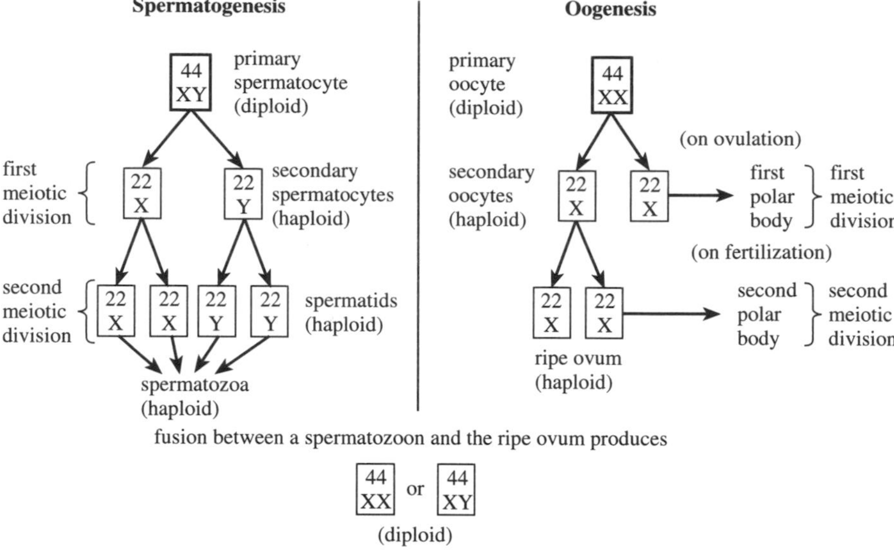

Fig. 7.1. The production of spermatozoa (spermatogenesis) and a ripe ovum (oogenesis).

protein), stimulates the expression of the Müllerian inhibiting factor (MIF) in the fetal Sertoli cells. MIF inhibits the further development of the female (Müllerian) genital tract and causes its regression. Furthermore, the sry protein simultaneously represses expression of the cytochrome P-450 aromatase gene, and consequently testosterone is not aromatized to oestradiol. Instead, testosterone induces the development of the Wolffian tract into the epididymis, vas deferens, and seminal vesicles. Thus, development of the testes and male genital tract requires the positive influence of the Y chromosome; in its absence, by default, the primitive gonads become ovaries and the female genitalia develop as the Wolffian ducts regress.

The testes

Anatomy, histology, and development

From the sixth week of intrauterine life the Sertoli cells of primitive testes suppress the further development of the female Müllerian system by secreting the peptide Müllerian regression (or inhibiting) factor. Sex cords which contain the germ cells develop from the coelomic epithelium covering the genital ridge to become the seminiferous tubules. The development of interstitial cells from the surrounding mesoderm results in the production of androgens, primarily testosterone, which then stimulate the formation of the epididymis, vas deferens, and seminal vesicles from the Wolffian duct, and also probably influence the development of the brain. Should failure of primitive testicular function occur and the Müllerian duct system remain, an outwardly normal but incomplete female genital tract system develops in a male genotype.

From the seventh to eight months of intrauterine life the testes normally begin to descend into a sac outside the body called the scrotum, an effect which is controlled by various factors including Müllerian inhibiting factor and the androgens produced by the fetal gonads. The adult testes are therefore maintained at a temperature which is about 2° C lower than normal body temperature; this process is necessary, some maintain, for normal spermatogenesis.

The two adult testes are ovoid glands approximately 4 cm long and 2 cm wide each with a volume of approximately 15–20 ml. The framework of each gland is provided by the fibrous tunica albuginea, the whole being surrounded by the serous tunica vaginalis. The walls of the coiled seminiferous tubules consist of Sertoli cells outside which lie several layers of spermatogenic cells, some of which become closely associated with them. The interstitial cells of Leydig form clumps between the tubules. The seminiferous tubules open into the rete testis from which the vasa efferentia ducts drain seminiferous fluid into the coiled epididymis. This becomes the vas deferens which, unlike the previous ductile components, contains no smooth muscle (Fig. 7.2). Ultimately, the vasa deferentia from the testes open into the urethra in the penis. Arterial blood is supplied by the testicular artery; venous blood collects in a plexus which drains into the testicular vein. The right testicular vein drains into the inferior vena cava and the left drains into the left renal vein. Each testis is supplied with lymphatics which drain the para-aortic nodes, and is innervated by sympathetic nerve fibres. The nervous and vascular

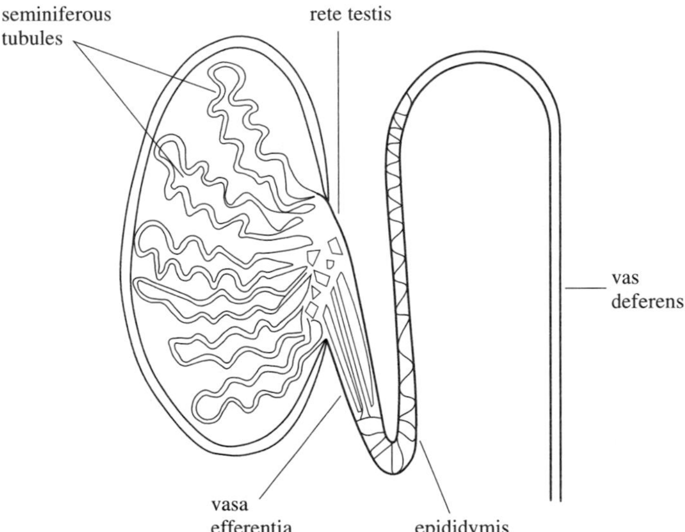

Fig. 7.2. Diagram showing the principal structures of the adult testis and reproductive tract.

supplies enter and leave the testis via the spermatic cord. The capillaries in the testes have membranes which are not fenestrated.

Testicular functions

In the adult male, the testes have two important, closely related functions: the production of mature male gametes (spermatogenesis); and the production of steroid hormones (steroidogenesis). The testes have usually developed sufficiently to perform both the functions by puberty which usually begins between the ages of 12 and 14.

Spermatogenesis

The process of spermatogenesis takes place in association with coiled seminiferous tubules, and is continuous from puberty to old age. It begins with the formation of spermatogonia by mitotic division from activated germ cells, in the germinal epithelium which lies outside the Sertoli cell 'barrier' lining of the seminiferous tubule (see Fig. 7.3). From each clone of spermatogonia formed, most become activated to progressively develop into primary and subsequently (by first meiotic division) secondary spermatocytes. However, a few return to the quiescent phase to be activated later on, thus providing the means by which males can produce large numbers of mature cells continually throughout life. The developing primary spermatocytes push between adjacent Sertoli cells by disrupting the tight junctions which link them to each other, and enter the adluminal compartment. Each short-lived secondary spermatocyte then undergoes a second meiotic division to produce two haploid spermatids.

The Sertoli cells are intimately involved in the later stages of development since secondary spermatocytes and spermatids both become enveloped by these structural cells and form specialized junctions with them. The Sertoli cells contain high concentrations of glycogen and one of their functions is probably to provide an energy source for the developing spermatids. The spermatids are released into the seminiferous tubules where they finally mature into spermatozoa.

The whole spermatogenic process takes approximately 60 days, and at any instant all stages of development are present within the seminiferous tubules. Indeed, a longitudinal cross-section through a seminiferous tubule would reveal the various stages of cell development repeated in a regular pattern all along the length of the tubule (the spermatogenic 'wave'). Furthermore, examination of a cross-section through a seminiferous tubule on a time lapse would illustrate the synchronized development of clones through the different cell types which is called the spermatogenic 'cycle'. The continuous production of gametes in the male is different from the corresponding process in the female in whom the number of oocytes is predetermined before birth (see Chapter 8). Spermatogenesis is under endocrine control, involving the hypothalamus and the anterior pituitary (adenohypophysis), and this will be described in a later section.

As mentioned above, the Sertoli cells appear to be intimately involved in the maturation process. Ultrastructural studies have demonstrated that the Sertoli cells envelop the developing spermatocytes and spermatids, and provide nutritional,

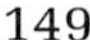

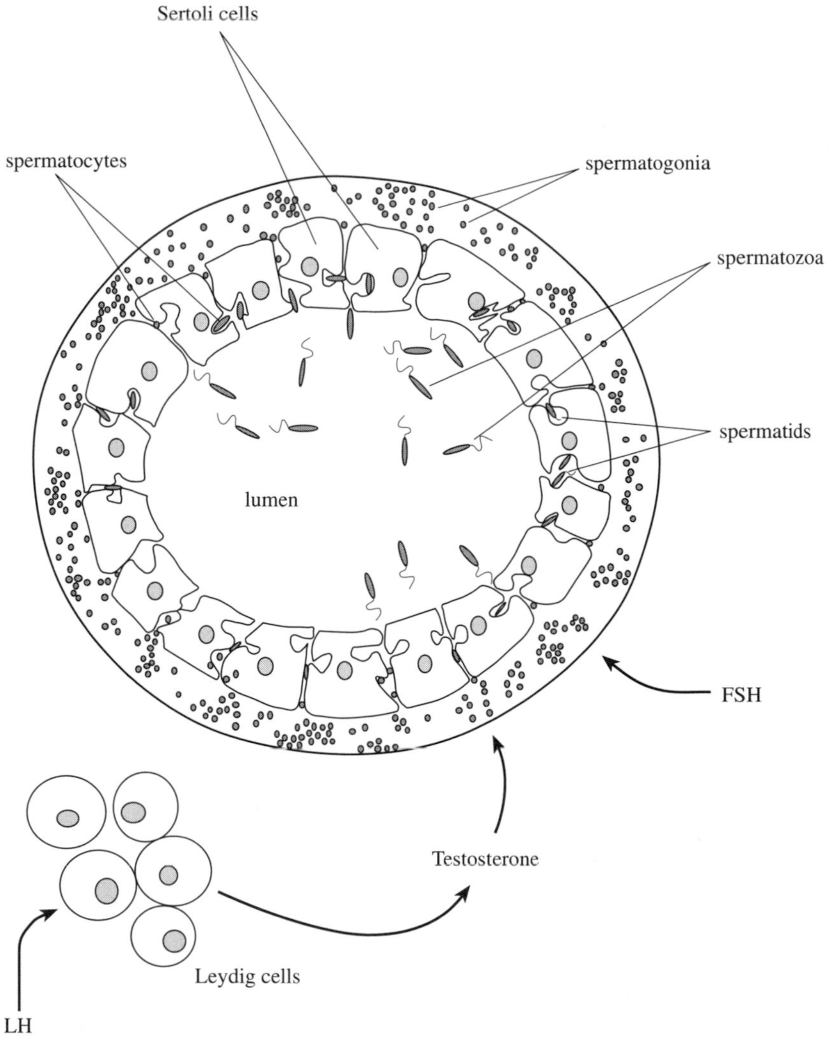

Fig. 7.3. Diagram of a cross-section through a seminiferous tubule with the various stages of spermatogenesis indicated. (FSH, follicle-stimulating hormone; LH, luteinizing hormone.)

mechanical, and other forms (as yet undefined) of support for the maturing gametes. The Sertoli cells also appear to be linked to each other by tight and gap junctions, the latter possibly allowing intercellular communication. The Sertoli cells secrete various substances into the luminal compartment of the seminiferous tubules. Another function of the Sertoli cells is endocrine, and this is discussed in a following section.

Steroidogenesis

The second function of the testes is the synthesis of steroid hormones which are vital to the development and maintenance of male reproductive capability. The hormones which induce growth and maintain the development of the male genital tract are called androgens. The principal sources of androgens in the male are the interstitial cells of Leydig situated between the seminiferous tubules. The testicular androgen produced in the greatest quantities is testosterone of which 95 per cent is synthesized in the Leydig cells, the remainder being of adrenocortical origin (see Chapter 5).

In both testis and adrenal cortex the biosynthetic pathway is similar, the initial precursor being cholesterol which can be either derived from the plasma low-density lipoprotein component or be synthesized in the glands from acetate. The rate-limiting step in testosterone synthesis is the conversion of cholesterol to pregnenolone, and this is under hormonal control by luteinizing hormone (LH) (see later). The Leydig cells, unlike the adrenals, only have the 17α-hydroxylase enzyme so that the key intermediate molecule, pregnenolone, formed from cholesterol is only hydroxylated at position 17 before side-chain cleavage to form dehydroepiandrosterone (DHEA) in the presence of 17,20-desmolase. These enzyme activities are now believed to exist in a single cytochrome P-450 enzyme. Some pregnenolone may alternatively be converted to progesterone which can also be hydroxylated before being converted to a ketosteroid although this pathway is not commonly followed in humans. Androstenedione is the common final precursor in the series of reactions resulting in testosterone synthesis (see Fig. 5.2).

Testosterone not only has androgenic effects of its own but can be converted to a much more potent androgen called dihydrotestosterone (DHT) in many target cells. This peripheral conversion of one hormone to a more potent one is of tremendous importance, and is due to the activity of the cytoplasmic enzyme 5α-reductase which is found in the target cells. Tissues in which this conversion takes place include the seminiferous tubules, the prostate gland and the skin. The brains of some mammals (e.g. rats) are also capable of converting testosterone to DHT. Some DHT is also produced by the Leydig cell directly.

Another conversion which testosterone undergoes in some peripheral tissues as well as in the testicular Leydig cells is aromatization to 17β-oestradiol. Small quantities of this hormone, and indeed the progesterone also secreted in small amounts by the Leydig cells, are continually produced as by-products, but their role in the development and maintenance of male reproductive function is at present obscure.

The normal daily secretion of testosterone in adult males is between 4 and 9 mg. Once secreted, approximately 98 per cent of the testosterone is plasma protein-bound, either to albumin (40 per cent) or to a β-globulin which is specific for gonadal hormones (i.e. it also binds oestrogens) and is called sex-hormone-binding globulin (SHBG). Total plasma levels of testosterone are approximately 13–30 nmol/l in adult males and 0.5–2.5 nmol/l in adult females. There is little change in the plasma concentration of testosterone with increasing age in healthy men, the values usually lying within the normal range for young adults. However, there may be a smaller testosterone response to LH stimulation which may be associated with a decrease in the number of Leydig cells with age.

Actions of androgens

Androgens are defined as hormones which stimulate the growth and development of the male genital tract. This includes the testes, the entire male duct system, and the accessory organs. The latter include the various secretory glands (such as the prostate, the seminal vesicles and the bulbourethral glands) and the penis, all of which are involved in the conveyance of spermatozoa or in the production of certain constituents which are required in the seminal fluid. During the growth phase at puberty androgens also stimulate the increase in scrotal capacity to accommodate the growing testes. The scrotum becomes wrinkled and pigmented as a result of pubertal androgenic activity.

Testosterone is also vital for normal spermatogenesis. This androgen is believed to enter the seminiferous tubules by facilitated diffusion after it has been produced in the interstitial Leydig cells. Within the seminiferous tubules it is bound to an androgen-binding protein produced by the Sertoli cells as well as being bound to intracellular receptors within these cells. The testosterone can then be converted to oestrogens or dihydrotestosterone (DHT) within the cell. While the function of the testicular oestrogen is unknown, the testosterone, and particularly the DHT, are necessary for the maintenance of spermatogenesis and in the absence of these androgens, the process is arrested at the primary spermatocyte stage.

The spermatozoa produced in the seminiferous tubules have very little cytoplasm of their own and therefore depend on the secretions of the accessory sex glands for nourishment and for the medium which provides their optimal environment. The seminal fluid is rich in fructose, which is the principal source of metabolic energy for the spermatozoa, and is secreted by the seminal vesicles. The prostate gland secretes a dilute fluid which is rich in calcium citrate, fibrinolysin, acid phosphatase, and prostaglandins. The bulbo-urethral glands secrete mucus. The thick, slightly yellow seminal fluid which is therefore produced from the secretions of these various glands provides most of the seminal volume, and is necessary for the maintenance of viable and motile spermatozoa.

Androgens are also necessary for the appearance and development of the secondary sex characteristics of the male. These include the male physique which results from the muscular development and linear growth which are induced mainly by stimulation of protein synthesis. Androgens are important anabolic agents which also stimulate cellular division. They therefore stimulate linear growth at puberty, acting in conjunction with somatotrophin (growth hormone) from the pituitary, but also bring about its cessation due to the fusion of the epiphyses to the shafts of the long bones. Androgens stimulate the growth of facial and body hair, recession of the scalp line, and the lowering of the voice pitch due to the thickening of the vocal cords and enlargement of the larynx. The androgens probably develop and maintain libido and influence behavioural development, but the relative importance of a hormonal effect compared with possible environmental stimuli (social conditioning, role assignment, etc.) is a subject of controversy at present. It would seem that behavioural attitudes often associated with the male, such as aggression, are due to a combination of hormonal and environmental influences.

A possible behavioural role for androgens in the fetus has been suggested by experiments on species such as the rat. What is interesting in these animals is that the 'masculinizing' effect of androgens will only result if the androgens are first converted to oestrogen by aromatization in the brain soon after birth. There is no conclusive evidence for a conversion of testosterone to oestrogen in human brain at present.

Other actions of androgens include the stimulation of sebum secretion by the sebaceous glands (often producing acne in pubertal males) and the mild retention of various ions (including sodium, potassium, and calcium) and water by the kidneys.

Control of androgen production

The production of testosterone by the Leydig cells of the testes is controlled indirectly by the hypothalamus, an influence which is mediated from the adeno-

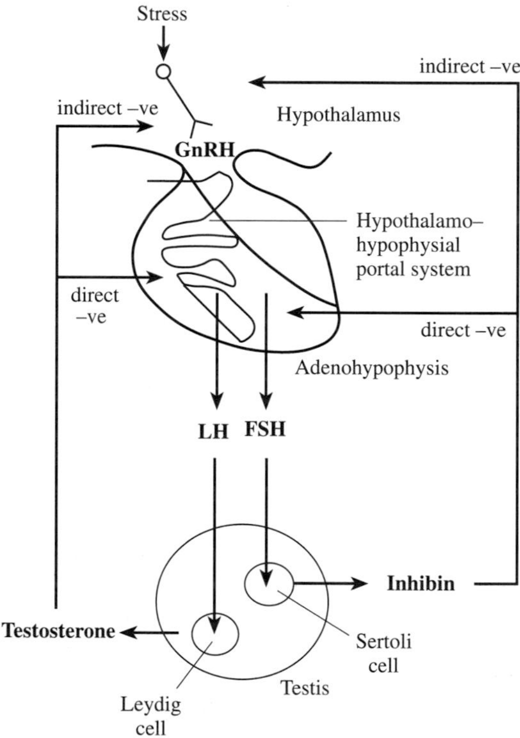

Fig. 7.4. Control of testicular function by the hypothalamo–adenohypophysial axis. (FSH, follicle-stimulating hormone; GnRH, gonadotrophin-releasing hormone, LH, luteinizing hormone.)

hypophysis. This control system therefore functions in two stages, the first relating the central nervous system (the hypothalamus) to the adenohypophysis and the second relating the adenohypophysis to the testes (Fig. 7.4).

Certain hypothalamic neurones in the arcuate and ventromedial areas, when stimulated, release a neurosecretion into the hypothalamo–hypophysial portal system which then conveys it to the adenohypophysis. This neurosecretion is a decapeptide called gonadotrophin-releasing hormone (GnRH) which, as its name implies, stimulates the gonadotrophe cells of the anterior pituitary. The GnRH is secreted in pulses which, in turn, drive the pulsatile release of luteinizing hormone (LH) and follicle-stimulating hormone (FSH) from the adenohypophysis. It is the gonadotrophin LH which stimulates steroidogenesis in the interstitial Leydig cells of the testes.

Evidence for negative feedback by androgens on LH release includes the observation that the plasma LH concentration increases markedly after castration. This negative feedback involves a direct loop to the adenohypophysis, and part of the feedback response may involve the conversion of testosterone to DHT within the adenohypophysial tissue. There is also evidence for an indirect negative loop relating the plasma androgen concentration to the production of GnRH. Testosterone decreases the frequency of LH pulses, and this is generally believed to indicate a negative feedback at the hypothalamic level.

Physiological concentrations of plasma androgens appear to exert their principal negative feedback effects on LH release, but not FSH release. Since the hypothalamic GnRH influences the release of both of the gonadotrophins (see Chapter 4), differential secretion is probably controlled mainly at the adenohypophysial level. However, the hypothalamus might also secrete a specific FSH-releasing factor, although no evidence for such a substance has yet been obtained.

Control of spermatogenesis

Spermatogenesis requires the presence of testosterone for normal function. It is therefore influenced by the hypothalamo–adenohypophysial–Leydig cell system relating GnRH, LH, and androgens. In addition, it is dependent on the other adenohypophysial gonadotrophin, FSH, which is believed to act on the Sertoli cells in the seminiferous tubules. The importance of the Sertoli cells in relation to spermatogenesis has been mentioned earlier, and is probably due to the close intercellular association between them and the developing spermatocytes and spermatids.

Since the plasma FSH concentration increases with LH levels after castration, and yet physiological levels of plasma androgens have little effect in inhibiting FSH release, it would appear that some other testicular substance is involved in the negative feedback regulation of FSH. Indeed, a protein synthesized by the Sertoli cells exerts a negative influence on FSH production and has been named 'inhibin'. The synthesis of inhibin is stimulated by FSH itself, so that as it is produced it then inhibits by direct negative feedback the further release of FSH. Inhibin may have an additional indirect negative feedback on the hypothalamus. The potential use of this protein or an agonist derivative as a male contraceptive remains to be developed.

Thus, the release of the adenohypophysial gonadotrophin FSH in the male is controlled by its target hormone (inhibin) in the same way that LH is controlled by androgens.

CLINICAL DISORDERS

Excess

Androgen excess states in the adult male are uncommon, and when they occur remain unrecognized in most instances, since normal androgenization of the male covers such a wide spectrum. Primary tumours of either adrenals or the testes may give rise to excessive androgen production in childhood, then resulting in precocious puberty, which is considered in Chapter 13. Primary germ cell tumours (seminoma or teratoma) or non-germinal (interstitial or Sertoli cell) tumours may also cause androgen excess and often present as a testicular swelling. This can be further investigated by testicular ultrasound, coupled to the measurement of a variety of tumour markers. Such tumours are frequently metastatic by the time diagnosis is reached.

Congenital adrenal hyperplasia has been dealt with previously: in male children, the common 21-hydroxylase variant (see Chapter 5) will result in precocious puberty. Less severe heterozygous enzyme defects (corresponding to the late-onset form manifest in women by hirsutism and oligomenorrhoea) are likely to go unnoticed in men for reasons mentioned above. There is, however, a higher risk of infertility in affected males, which is potentially reversible by corticosteroid therapy.

Most hyperandrogenism currently encountered is iatrogenic. The syndrome is produced by the administration of conventional or substituted androgens (anabolic steroids) for body building purposes. There is no doubt that they are effective as anabolic agents, but carry with them the significant side-effect of infertility consequent on gonadotrophin suppression: depending on duration and doses used, this is not always fully reversible. Hyperlipidaemia, prostatic hypertrophy, and a rebound loss of libido may also occur, as well as the other side-effects of androgen therapy mentioned later in this chapter.

Deficiency

Deficiency syndromes result logically either from primary testicular defect or damage, or occur secondary to hypothalamo–adenohypophysial dysfunction. Whatever its aetiology, the major clinical manifestations of androgen deficiency depend upon the age of onset.

The prepubertal male displays a delay in the development of secondary sex characteristics. Longitudinal growth is subsequently not punctuated by the pubertal growth spurt (which is both somatotrophin- and androgen-dependent). Furthermore, growth will continue beyond the usual 16–18 years, because of the delay in epiphyseal fusion which is androgen- (and oestrogen-) dependent. Body habitus is then described as 'eunuchoid', implying a disproportionate length of limbs compared to the trunk. This is manifest by an arm span exceeding the height by more than 5 cm, and a sole–pubis measurement which is often more than 5 cm in excess of pubis–vertex.

Hypogonadism after puberty results in muscular atrophy and the disappearance of body hair, sexual libido, and often potency, but little or no change in voice. The skin often develops a wrinkled parchment-like texture which in severe forms is quite characteristic: as in the case of reduced bone density which develops long term, this is based on the lack of anabolic androgen action. There is often a loss of the androgen-dependent assertiveness and a more subtle loss of well-being. On the positive side, there is evidence of relative protection from atherosclerosis, and both benign prostatic hypertrophy as well as prostatic malignancy occur less commonly.

Primary testicular disorders

Klinefelter's syndrome

This is an example of primary testicular failure associated with a chromosomal abnormality. Forty-seven chromosomes are present due to an additional X chromosome (XXY karyotype), most commonly arising by non-dysjunction during meiosis. The clinical features are variable. The diagnosis is usually made in late pubertal or early adult life because of a lack of sexual development and small and characteristically firm testes which histologically show Leydig cell hyperplasia and hyalinization of seminiferous tubules. The frequently associated gynaecomastia, which is far less common in other forms of hypogonadism is not adequately explained, although in part it is probably gonadotrophin-dependent (and yet unresponsive to androgen replacement therapy): there is also an increased oestrogen: androgen ratio which may be relevant. Infertility is almost invariable. The disorder is common, affecting 0.2 per cent of all males, and is found in a rather higher proportion of individuals who are educationally subnormal or suffering from chronic psychiatric disorder. Clinical subtypes less frequently associated with gynaecomastia are due to mosaicism (XXY/XY, XXY/XYY and other variations), and these cases are very occasionally fertile. Conversely, in some patients with Klinefelter's syndrome, infertility is the only feature, and accordingly the diagnosis may be entirely missed during life.

Typically, as in all cases of primary testicular disorder, serum testosterone levels are reduced and gonadotrophin levels markedly elevated, although these findings are less striking in mosaic forms. The diagnosis is confirmed by a suitably stained buccal smear of squamous cells which reveal Barr bodies (nuclear membrane inclusions found normally in female XX cells) and which confirm the supernumerary X chromosome. A karyotype following leucocyte culture, which displays all the component chromosomes, may demonstrate 47-XXY complement, or indeed multiple cell lines in mosaic variants. Skin fibroblast culture, to determine other tissue karyotypes, may be necessary to clearly define the more obscure mosaics.

Treatment involves correction of the hypogonadism by hormonal replacement as outlined later in this chapter, and surgical correction of the gynaecomastia (which does not respond to androgen replacement). The abnormal testes do not represent an abnormal malignancy risk. However, cosmetically and aesthetically, it is sometimes desirable to insert testicular prostheses into the scrotum, a comparatively minor procedure.

Reifenstein's syndrome

This condition has some homology with Klinefelter's syndrome in terms of the features mentioned above. However, there is hypospadias, a chromatin-negative buccal smear, and karyotype reveals a normal XY pattern. This rare condition is a variant of testicular feminization, reflecting a partial end-organ resistance to the effects of testosterone and dihydrotestosterone.

Testicular agenesis

This rare condition of complete failure of testicular development represents prenatal failure. As anticipated, laboratory findings of severe hypogonadism are present. The principal differential diagnosis is cryptorchidism (undescended testes). In contrast to agenesis, however, this condition is characterized by a positive response of plasma testosterone to chorionic gonadotrophin given in a dose of 1500 units a day for five consecutive days.

Myotonic dystrophy

In this condition, in addition to classical features of frontal balding, lens opacities, skeletal muscle weakness, cardiomyopathy, and myotonia, multiple organ abnormalities often include testicular atrophy. Normally, only seminiferous tubules are affected. If assayed, serum inhibin levels are low, and FSH correspondingly raised: plasma testosterone and LH are usually normal. The disorder is inherited as an autosomal-dominant.

Cryptorchidism

The testes normally enter the scrotum by the seventh month of intrauterine life, although approximately 10 per cent of males have an empty scrotum at birth. Nevertheless, in this latter group only approximately 1 per cent are still undescended by the fifth year of life. Failure of testicular descent may be apparent rather than real, due to abnormal retractility stimulated by environmental cold or anxiety (placing the patient in a warm bath will almost always reverse this retractility).

True failure of testicular descent may be due either to anatomical abnormalities in or superior to the inguinal canal (which will not be dealt with in detail in this chapter), or occasionally due to LH/FSH deficiency. In a number of cases where non-descent has occurred, fertility is impaired due to the warmer environment of testicular development in the undescended and particularly abdominal position. Accordingly, it is generally advised that therapeutic action be taken before the age of 9 years, and sometimes earlier, to ensure optimal seminiferous development and to avoid the slightly greater risk of testicular tumours which result from the untreated cryptorchid state.

When doubt exists about bilateral non-descent, human chorionic gonadotrophin can be given in a dose of 1500–2000 units twice weekly for six weeks, followed by exploratory and corrective surgery (orchidopexy) if no response is obtained. The balance of evidence suggests that cryptorchid testes may have some impairment of endocrine as well as seminiferous function, and supplemental androgens may be required in later life to ensure full and normal pubertal development and maintenance of a normally androgenized state in adulthood.

Bilateral mumps orchitis

When mumps occurs in the postpubertal period, testicular involvement is present in approximately 20 per cent of cases usually with considerable pain and swelling. In a small percentage of cases, infertility results from seminiferous damage due to direct viral damage: there is some evidence that hypogonadism due to Leydig cell involvement may also occur. Corticosteroid therapy during the acute phase may be of benefit, but no clear evidence exists that this reduces the risk of ultimate seminiferous failure.

Primary hypogonadism occurs as a minor feature in a variety of other rare conditions and syndromes, including haemochromatosis and amyloidosis.

Secondary testicular disorders

Whereas in primary testicular disorders serum testosterone and inhibin are reduced but gonadotrophin levels elevated, in this secondary group both serum gonadotrophins and target gland hormones are reduced.

The cause may be part of a generalized reduction in adenohypophysical hormones (panhypopituitarism) often due to a space-occupying pituitary adenoma, craniopharyngioma, or other invasive lesion. Alternatively, isolated deficiencies of FSH or LH have been described with the appropriate clinical manifestations, either due to tumour or without any apparent anatomical abnormality. The site of lesion in this latter group is not clear. However, administration of repeated daily doses of synthetic GnRH results in a measurable increase in LH and/or FSH in many cases, suggesting that the primary defect is at the hypothalamic level (see Chapter 17).

One of the most important causes of hypogonadism in males is prolactinoma. Because of the short-loop negative feedback, hyperprolactinaemia suppresses both LH and FSH (see Chapter 4), resulting in hypogonadism and infertility, together with reduced libido which is probably a direct cerebral effect of prolactin excess.

Kallman's syndrome is an uncommon disorder based on FSH and LH deficiency, usually associated with reduced sensation of smell: hyposmia or anosmia (see also Chapter 4).

A variety of other disorders can affect the pituitary–adrenal axis, resulting in either hypogonadism or infertility: chronic illness of any type, especially hepatic or renal disease, chronic alcohol excess, and opiates.

Management of hypogonadism

The approach to treatment depends on the age of the patient at diagnosis and the primary or secondary nature of the gonadal disorder. When diagnosed at puberty, primary hypogonadism is carefully treated with testosterone esters or the long-acting oenanthate in a dose of 100 mg monthly, monitoring growth velocity and bone age (see Chapter 13). Once longitudinal growth has been completed and the risk of accelerated and premature epiphyseal fusion is no longer present, testosterone oenanthate 250 mg every 3–4 weeks (or alternative androgens in equivalent doses) may be used. Testosterone implants may also be used, with effectiveness lasting between 3 and 6 months. Compliance with oral preparations tends to be less satisfactory, and these formulations also appear to be less effective clinically. Testosterone-impregnated skin patches have recently been introduced into clinical practice. Compliance and effectiveness appear to be satisfactory.

The age until which androgen replacement should be continued is debatable, but the failure to replace androgens over the normal reproductive lifespan of the male usually results in waning libido and potency, and the patient will usually request continuation. Bone density and muscle strength also suffer in adult androgen deficiency. The controversial evidence to suggest that development of atherosclerosis is retarded in hypogonadal males may also effect the decision to treat. Introduction of androgens to males with late-diagnosed hypogonadism may be unwise: stimulation of libido after prolonged sexual abstinence can result in emotional conflict and marital disharmony. It is important to stress that in primary gonadal failure, no form of therapy will restore fertility.

Side-effects of androgen therapy include polycythaemia and occasional gynaecomastia, due to aromatization of androgen to oestrogen. The methyl-testosterone derivative sometimes used for oral replacement may be associated with hepatic cholestasis and benign tumour formation, and some physicians recommend regular hepatic screening by ultrasound. In secondary hypogonadism, it may appear logical to use gonadotrophin or GnRH therapy rather than treatment with androgens. However, such an approach is more expensive and less convenient and is normally only employed for the management of the associated infertility (see below).

Infertility

Approximately 10 per cent of couples are infertile, and in approximately one-third of such cases the male is the responsible partner. The common causes of infertility are shown in Table 7.1.

Investigation involves endocrine profiling for circulating gonadal hormones, gonadotrophins and prolactin. Seminal analysis of three ejaculates is required in a totally fresh state. Motility, abnormal forms and absolute sperm count as well as fructose and other biochemical constituents are evaluated. Occasionally, testicular biopsy is required to confirm the extent of involvement of the seminiferous tubules. Complete hyalinization precludes any successful therapy, while certain forms of maturation arrest or a more normal appearance indicate at least some potential for medical or surgical treatment respectively.

Management of male infertility is usually unrewarding. In a patient with oligo- or azoospermia, together with a raised serum FSH level, correctable infertility can be confidently excluded: a reduced inhibin level consequent on disabled seminiferous function is the basis of the raised FSH, activated by negative feedback. Approximately 10 per cent of all cases appear to ‘recover’ spontaneously, without reversal of any identifiable disorder, and sometimes even in the course of inves-

Table 7.1. Major causes of infertility

Endocrine
Chromosome disorders: Klinefelter's syndrome
Hypopituitarism: selective FSH/LH deficiency
Primary testicular failure (auto-immune endocrinopathy)
Hyperprolactinaemia
Hypothyroidism
Non-endocrine
Maturation arrest of spermatogenesis: no obvious cause
Retrograde or absent ejaculation
Specific antisperm antibodies
Previous testicular irradiation or cancer chemotherapy
Previous tuberculous, gonorrhoea, mumps, prostatitis
Varicocoele or spermatic duct obstruction
General ill-health due to systemic disorders
Previous cryptorchidism, trauma, or torsion

tigation! In the remainder, the identification of a pituitary problem provides the best prognosis: either GnRH or gonadotrophins can be used, depending on the site of the underlying defect: fertility can be restored in around 30 per cent. Such treatment may need to be continued for many months: from initiation of therapy and the subsequent re-induction of spermatogenesis to the appearance of the first sperm in the ejaculate alone takes three months.

In the remaining cases, appropriate surgery where an anatomical abnormality exists (varicocoele or spermatic cord obstruction) may be successful. In the presence of maturation arrest a number of other drugs, including gonadotrophin, corticosteroids, or high-dose androgen administration, have been used: however, the response in these cases is well below 10 per cent. Eventually, one may need to resort to some form of artificial insemination. Aspiration cytology of the testis has been recently introduced as a helpful diagnostic aid. Certain cytological characteristics predict those cases in whom it is worth considering attempted harvesting of sperm by epidydimal aspiration. Such sperm can then be used for artificial insemination or in vitro fertilization (IVF).

Disorders of libido and potency

Lack of sexual libido is only occasionally due to hypogonadism. Hyperprolactinaemia may cause a direct inhibitory effect on libido, as well as acting via its short-loop gonadotrophin suppressive action. However, in the majority of cases, anxiety, depression, or other functional or psychiatric disorder is the fundamental cause and a solution is not to be found in endocrine therapy.

Impotence is again frequently due to psychogenic disorders involving stress and anxiety. However, in some instances androgen deficiency may be present, and in others autonomic neuropathy due to a variety of causes, including diabetic autonomic neuropathy and spinal disease. Venous valve incompetence in the draining veins of the penis is an uncommon but surgically correctable abnormality.

Typically, functional/psychological impotence is abrupt in onset, quite variable in severity, and sometimes temporally related to stress situations (conversely improved during holiday periods, etc.): nocturnal erections are also often maintained. Organic causes have a more gradual onset and unremitting course.

A full discussion of the treatment of disorders of libido and potency is complex and outside the scope of this text. Apart from identifying any of the uncommon endocrinopathies and correcting them, sexual counselling and various forms of psychological intervention have much to contribute: careful discussion and identification of social amd personal pressures and tensions is all-important.

Various vacuum systems have been developed for inducing and maintaining erections. These somewhat cumbersome techniques are not always very acceptable to patients. The intracavernosal injection of papaverine prostaglandins or phentolamine often induces very satisfactory (but occasionally protracted) erections. Initially performed by a urologist, even a single injection in patients with psychogenic impotence may restore confidence, and subsequent spontaneous erections can be restored. In the usually more persistent case, whether functional or organic, the technique is comparatively easily mastered by the patient himself.

'Blind' administration of androgens, in the absence of demonstrable endocrinopathy has often been tried. Except for transient improvement, which is more likely to be due to placebo effect, there is no evidence of sustained benefit.

Gynaecomastia (see Plate 7.1)

This term is applied to hypertrophy of the breast in males. The endocrine development of the breast is complex, under the effect of gonadotrophins, growth hormone, and oestrogens. Additionally, progesterone and prolactin probably play a part. Gynaecomastia is a common but self-limiting phenomenon at birth, occurring as a result of transplacental transfer of oestrogens. It is less often found during puberty, due to selectively enhanced oestrogen pathways in the maturing testis. In old age, gynaecomastia also occur 'physiologically', possibly due to waning androgen and maintenance of previous oestrogen levels. The most common cause is a late pubertal form, which sometimes persists for 5 to 10 years before slowly resolving: the cause of this type of gynaecomastia remains unknown at present, and is rarely clarified even by extensive endocrine profiling. Table 7.2 includes the more common conditions responsible for gynaecomastia.

Management involves removal of the underlying factor, if possible. Either prolactin inhibition using dopamine agonists (such as bromocryptine) or anti-oestrogens (such as clomiphene or tamoxifen) have been tried in some cases, on the basis of removing factors permissive to breast tissue hypertrophy: benefits have been neither striking nor lasting. If embarrassment and self-consciousness dictate, surgical correction can be obtained by means of a minimal operation involving an ultimately inconspicuous subareolar incision, a procedure normally performed by a plastic surgeon.

Table 7.2. Principal causes of gynaecomastia

'Physiological' (neonatal, pubertal, ageing)
Primary and secondary hypogonadism (all causes)
Testicular tumours (HCG and steroid producing)
Ectopic (non-endocrine) HCG production
Klinefelter's and Reifenstein's syndromes
Partial peripheral androgen resistance syndromes
Systemic illness
Hyperthyroidism
Renal failure
Cirrhosis
HIV infection
Spinal cord injury
Re-feeding
Drugs
Oestrogens
Spironolactone
Cimetidine
Ketoconazole
Digoxin
Phenytoin
Phenothiazines
Idiopathic

Delayed puberty (see Chapter 13)

Male menopause

Although serum androgen levels reduce with age, such changes are more gradual than in women. Although there is a wide range of organ system functions which decline with age, there is still little evidence to show that such decline is necessarily related to circulating androgen levels. Bone density is as relevant to fracture proneness in males as in females, but there is as yet no information to show that androgen supplementation will reduce fracture rate (as it does in women). Nevertheless, hypogonadal males have been shown to have reduced bone density. Although beneficial effects of androgen supplementation on a variety of mood and cognitive functions has been demonstrated, it is not known whether the benefits accrue from physiological replacement or pharmacological surfeit.

There are potential adverse effects of androgen 'replacement' in the male, which are not seen in a parallel situation in the female. The prostate is exceedingly androgen-sensitive, and the occurrence of accelerated benign prostatic hyperplasia as well as carcinoma is likely: since up to 10 per cent of 'normal' ageing prostates contain microscopic cancer foci, such potential adverse effects must be fully

Oogenesis and the menstrual cycle

The first menstrual cycle (menarche) usually begins in girls aged between 9 and 12 years of age, and it indicates the beginning of female reproductive capability. Each menstrual cycle usually lasts for approximately 28 days, although there is tremendous individual variation in its actual duration. In some women it can be as short as 20 days while in others it can be as long as 40 days. Usually, between the ages of 45 and 55 years the cycles become increasingly infrequent and finally cease completely. The period of increasing ovarian failure, known as the climacteric, culminates in the complete cessation of menstruation (the menopause).

By convention, each menstrual cycle begins with the first day of menstruation (day 1) when the endometrial lining of the uterus from the previous cycle is shed with the loss of blood (up to 400 ml over the menstrual period). Menstruation usually lasts for approximately 5 days, and this is followed by a phase of growth and development during which ovarian follicles mature and the cells of the endometrium proliferate. This phase generally lasts for 8–9 days in an average 28-day cycle. By the end of this phase of the cycle, one follicle (rarely more) has reached the final stage of growth, and the ovum is released by a process called ovulation. This is a mid-cycle event which usually takes place during days 14–15 of the average cycle. During the subsequent 10 days the endometrium is maintained in a state of readiness for possible implantation by a fertilized ovum. If the ovum is not fertilized, implantation will not occur and hormonal support for the maintenance of endometrial activity is withdrawn. Necrosis of uterine tissue at the end of the cycle leads to the subsequent loss of the endometrial lining (menstruation) which marks the beginning of another menstrual cycle.

Each menstrual cycle therefore involves regular changes in the ovaries and in other parts of the body, particularly the uterus. The cyclic changes in the ovaries (the ovarian cycle) are under hypothalamo–adenohypophysial hormone control, and include the ripening of the follicles, the process of ovulation, the formation of the corpus luteum, and the production of ovarian hormones. The uterine changes are related to the ovarian cycle by the ovarian hormones and these cyclic changes involve the preparation of the endometrium for possible implantation by a fertilized ovum (the endometrial cycle) (Fig. 8.1).

The ovarian cycle

Each ovarian cycle comprises two component phases, the follicular and luteal phases, separated by the process of ovulation.

Follicular phase

At the beginning of each menstrual cycle, some ovarian follicles begin to grow and develop. Initially, each follicle consists of an outer layer of thecal cells and an inner layer of granulosa cells which surround the ovum. In the maturation process the ovum increases in size and both groups of cells proliferate under hormonal influence. The thecal cells form two distinct layers: an outer fibrous capsule (the theca externa) and an inner glandular, and vascular, layer (the theca interna). The granulosa cells secrete a fluid (follicular fluid) which gradually fills and enlarges

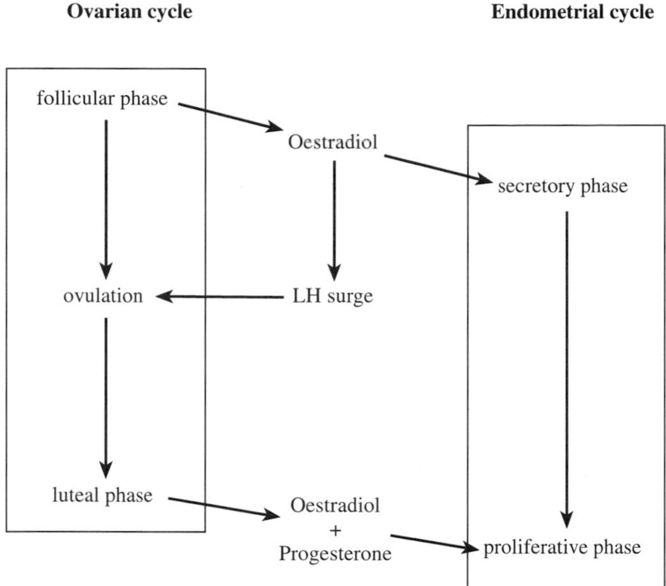

Fig. 8.1. Diagram showing the phases of the ovarian and endometrial cycles and the endocrine links between them. (LH, luteinizing hormone.)

the intrafollicular space (the antrum) so that those cells surrounding the ovum become separated from the outer layer of granulosa cells with connection between them only being maintained by a narrow stalk. The development and growth of the pre-antral follicles which may, or may not, become antral follicles depends on the synthesis of specific hormone receptors coinciding with the presence of adequate levels of the relevant hormones, the adenohypophysial gonadotrophins luteinizing hormone (LH) and follicle-stimulating hormone (FSH). Thecal cells synthesize LH receptors while granulosa cells initially synthesize receptors for FSH and oestrogen. Only those follicles which have reached this stage of development and have the necessary receptors at the precise time when the adenohypophysial gonadotrophins are present in the requisite quantities now continue to ripen. All other potential follicles will regress at this stage and be absorbed into the stroma, the degenerative process being called atresia (Fig. 8.2).

The binding of LH to its thecal cell receptors stimulates these cells to synthesize androgens, primarily androstenedione, partly by regulating the rate-limiting conversion of cholesterol to pregnenolone. As in the Leydig cells in the testis, this is achieved by activating the specific cytochrome P-450 cholesterol side-chain cleavage enzyme. Meanwhile, FSH binds to the granulosa cells which, while being incapable of synthesizing androgens themselves, do have a powerful aromatizing enzyme capable of converting thecal cell androgens to oestrogens. This aromatizing enzyme, the cytochrome P-450 aromatase, is stimulated by FSH. Only limited oestrogen synthesis occurs within the thecal cells. Thus, LH stimulates the thecal

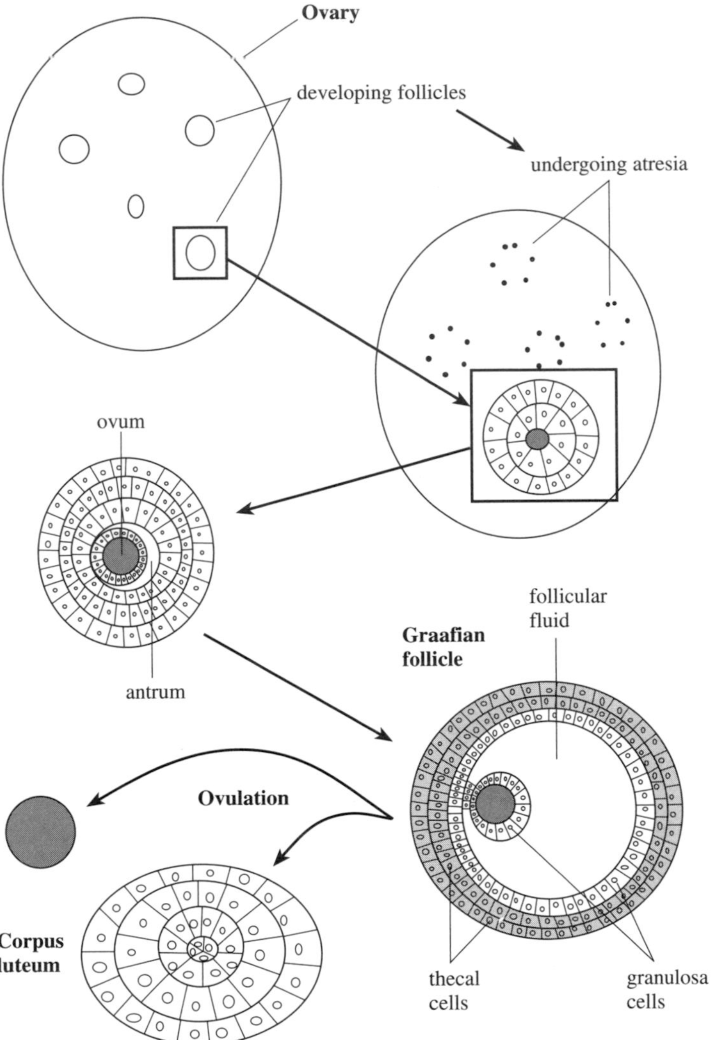

Fig. 8.2. The stages of growth and development of the ovarian Graafian follicle culminating in the process of ovulation and the formation of the corpus luteum.

cells to synthesize androgens while FSH stimulates the aromatization of androgen to oestrogen (principally 17β-oestradiol) in the granulosa cells — a perfect example of collaboration between adjacent cells (Fig. 8.3).

The presence of oestrogen receptors in the granulosa cells results in the follicular oestradiol now also acting directly on these cells, leading to further proliferation and growth. This is an example of an autocrine action by a hormone. Consequently, more oestradiol is produced, and this intraovarian stimulation results in a local positive feedback loop at the cellular level. Insulin-like growth

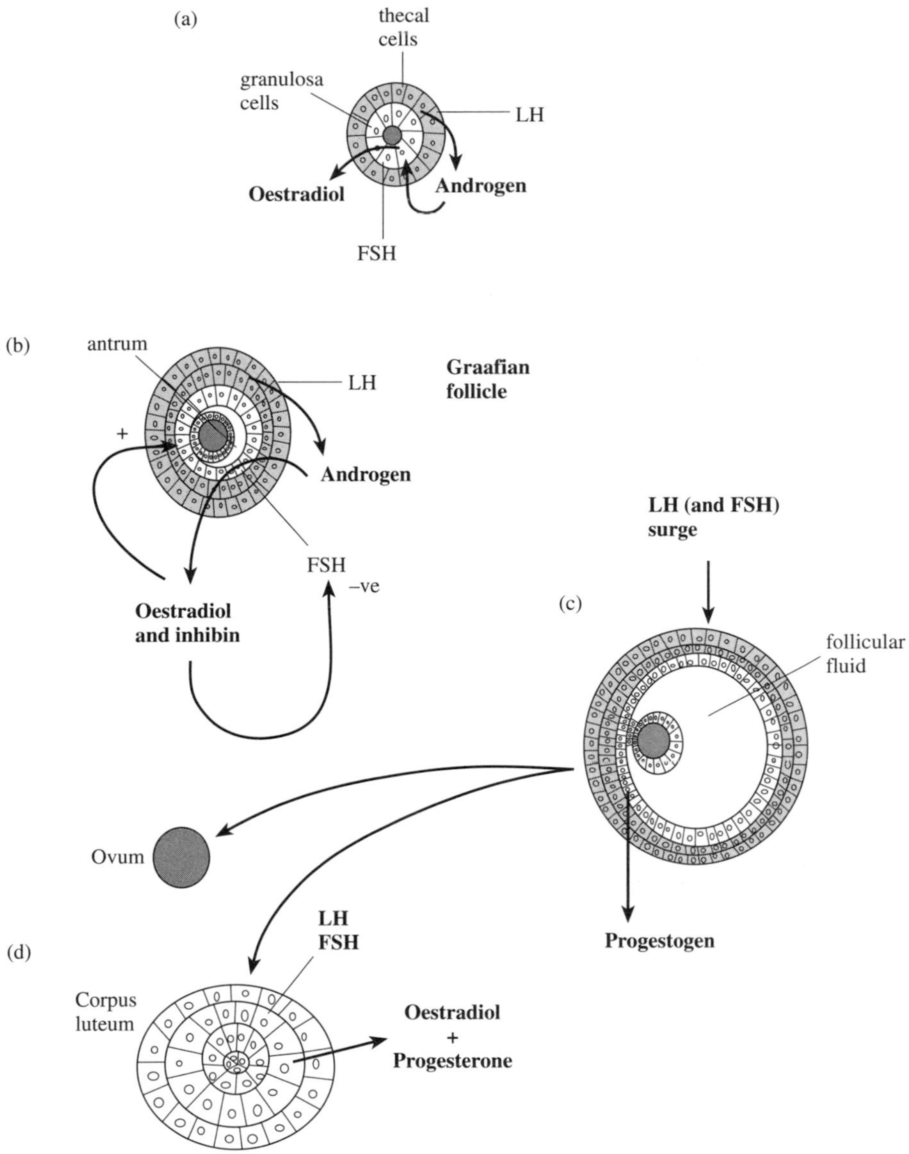

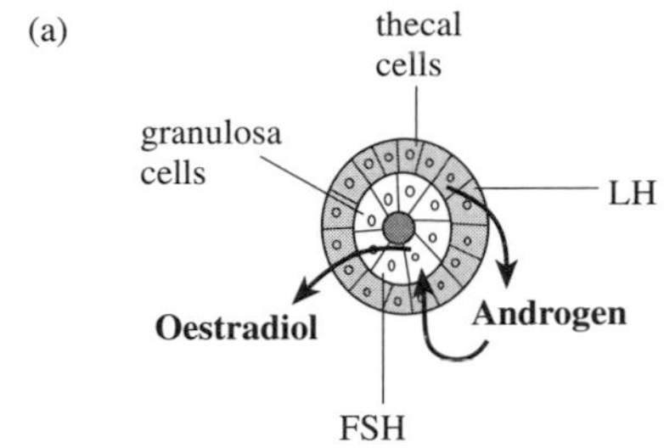

Fig. 8.3. The relationship between ovarian hormones and the stages of the ovarian cycle. (a) preantral phase, (b) early antral phase, (c) late antral phase (graafian follicle), (d) formation of corpus luteum after ovulation. (FSH, follicle-stimulating hormone; LH, luteinizing hormone.)

factor IGF-I is another hormone which is produced by the growing follicles and it probably plays an important role in the growth and development process.

As the plasma oestradiol level rises during the mid-follicular phase, a selective negative feedback by the oestradiol on FSH production occurs. This effect, together with the inhibitory action of the protein heterodimer hormone, inhibin, produced by the FSH-stimulated granulosa cells, results in a decrease in the plasma concentration of this adenohypophysial hormone. Any antral follicles still FSH-dependent at this stage now fail to develop any further and regress by atresia. In the maintained basal presence of FSH, together with the increasing quantities of oestrogen, the outer layers of granulosa cells of the remaining (Graafian) follicle now synthesize receptors specific for LH. This Graafian follicle is now capable of further maturation under the influence of its own oestrogens alone, and has no further need for FSH. It enters the final maturation process which consists of the terminal growth of the follicle and the release of its ovum into the peritoneum by a process called ovulation. The stimulus for this event is a sudden surge in LH which is accompanied by a smaller surge in FSH.

The above description of events related to FSH and LH is almost certainly far too simplistic since numerous other molecules are present in follicular fluid which may influence mitosis, atresia, and other crucial components of the ovarian cycle. Many of these molecules are non-steroidal factors better known for other endocrine effects in the body and include oxytocin, vasopressin, catecholamines, prostaglandins, as well as the insulin-like growth factors (IGFs) mentioned above. Gonadal steroid concentrations are generally far higher in the follicular fluid than in the blood; oestrogen and progesterone levels are particularly high in the larger follicles while the androgen concentration in the smaller follicles is generally higher than in the larger follicles. Thus, actual control of the various stages of follicular development probably involves many factors, steroidal and non-steroidal, present in the microenvironment of the follicular fluid.

Just prior to ovulation, as a consequence of the LH peak and the synthesis of LH receptors on the outer granulosa cells, these cells begin to synthesize progestogens (mainly 17α-hydroxyprogesterone at this stage) instead of converting androgens to oestrogens. These cells also have reduced capacity to respond to oestrogens and FSH during this short, pre-ovulatory phase.

Luteal phase

Following ovulation there is now a significant rise in progesterone production by the outer granulosa cells which is sufficient to cause a small increase in the basal body temperature (of the order of 0.3–0.6° C). This is a useful clinical indicator that ovulation has actually taken place.

Conversion of the follicular remnants to a corpus luteum is brought about by the LH surge. Some thecal cells become incorporated within the corpus luteum which is composed principally of hypertrophied granulosa cells. These cells contain high concentrations of lipids and are rich in mitochondria, and their transformation to luteal cells is associated with an increasing production of progesterone as well as oestradiol. If pregnancy occurs, the corpus luteum persists and continues to secrete steroids until the fetoplacental unit can assume this function usually by the twelfth week. The corpus luteum also produces various non-steroidal factors such as oxytocin, relaxin, inhibin, and prostaglandins. If pregnancy does not occur the high plasma concentration of progesterone exerts a powerful negative feedback on the hypothalamo–hypophysial axis, in addition to any negative feedback by oestradiol and other luteal factors such as inhibin. Consequently LH (and FSH) support is withdrawn, the corpus luteum degenerates (luteolysis), and ovarian steroid production decreases.

The luteolytic process in humans may also be influenced by the oestrogens produced by the luteal cells themselves. The possibility that these oestrogens act by stimulating the luteal synthesis of prostaglandin $F_{2\alpha}$ in very high concentrations locally, and that this prostaglandin then stimulates luteolysis, requires further investigation. Other luteolytic factors produced by the corpus luteum itself, such as oxytocin, may well be involved also.

A maintenance role for prolactin on the corpus luteum, while shown to be important in some species, has not been identified in humans.

The endometrial cycle

Proliferative phase

Once the endometrial lining from the previous cycle has been shed (by day 5), the underlying endometrial cells undergo proliferation and growth. This phase coincides with the increasing production of oestrogens from the developing ovarian follicle. The oestrogens stimulate the growth of secretory glands and blood vessels which penetrate the thickening endometrium. The glands enlarge and become tortuous while the blood vessels become coiled (Fig. 8.4).

At the same time as the endometrium is growing, the cervical epithelium begins to secrete a mucus which becomes progressively more watery as the circulating

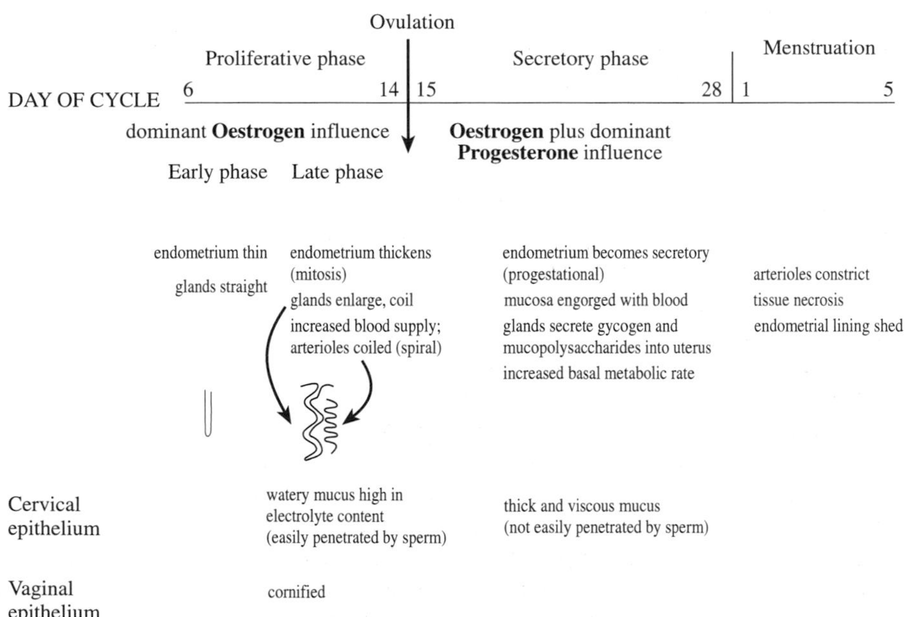

Fig. 8.4. The endometrial changes during the menstrual cycle.

oestrogen level reaches its preovulatory peak. This watery mucus is easily penetrated by spermatozoa introduced into the cervix so that the increased likelihood of a spermatozoon reaching the uterus and the Fallopian tubes coincides with the timing of ovulation.

Oestrogens induce the synthesis of intracellular progesterone receptors in the uterus so that by the beginning of the secretory phase the uterus is also responsive to this hormone.

Secretory phase

Following ovulation and the establishment of the corpus luteum, progesterone is secreted in increasing quantities in addition to oestradiol. In the presence of progesterone the endometrium undergoes progestational changes which are preparatory for possible implantation by a developing blastocyst should fertilization of the ovum have occurred. The mucosa becomes engorged with blood and the glands now secrete a thick viscous fluid which is not readily penetrated by spermatozoa. The secretion contains large supplies of nutrients such as glycogen to the uterus which would then be available for the developing blastocyst. Progesterone induces the further coiling and folding of the various secretory glands and blood vessels as well as stimulating gland secretory activity.

This phase is maintained until around day 25 when hormonal maintenance begins to be withdrawn, unless fertilization has occurred. Menstruation, beginning on day 1 of the following cycle, starts with the constriction of spiral arteries in the endometrium. Ischaemia in the tissues is followed by the dilatation of the arteries probably due to the accumulation of vasodilator substances from the necrotic tissue. The necrotic walls of the vessels rupture producing haemorrhage and sloughing of the cells. Blood shed into the uterus clots and is subsequently liquefied by enzymes. The bleeding ends when the spiral arteries again constrict after approximately five days, and this is followed by the generation of a new endometrial lining at the beginning of the next proliferative phase.

The ovarian hormones

Oestrogens

Synthesis, storage, and release

While the developing ovaries of a female fetus may not produce hormones, the granulosa cells (and to a lesser extent thecal cells) of the follicles in the adult ovaries synthesize oestrogens which are 18-carbon steroids. Other sites of oestrogen production are the corpus luteum, the fetoplacental unit during pregnancy, and to a minor extent the adrenal glands.

The biosynthesis of ovarian oestrogens involves the formation of androgens (androstenedione, which can be converted to testosterone) from the precursor progesterone. This latter steroid is synthesized from pregnenolone which is derived from cholesterol. As described above, the androgens formed by the thecal cells of the follicle are aromatized to oestrogens in the granulosa cells which are thus the principal source of these hormones during the follicular phase. The main oestrogen

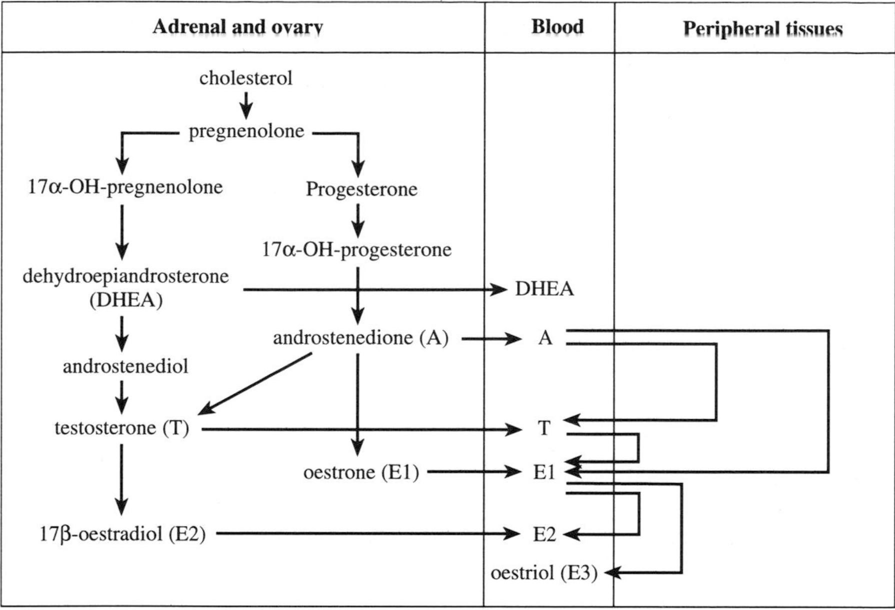

Fig. 8.5. Diagram showing the principal synthesis and conversion pathways for the androgens and oestrogens.

synthesized by the granulosa cells is 17β-oestradiol, with small quantities of another less potent oestrogen called oestrone also being produced. Oestrone can itself be converted to 17β-oestradiol. In the general circulation another even less potent oestrogen can be derived from oestrone, and this is called oestriol (Fig. 8.5). During the luteal phase, oestrogens are synthesized by cells of the corpus luteum.

It is important to appreciate the role played by adipose tissue as a site for steroid conversion, principally in the direction of androgen (chiefly androstenedione) to oestrogen (oestrone). Thus, adipose tissue in menopausal women, when the ovaries cease to produce oestrogens, provides much of the circulating oestrogen. Indeed, obese menopausal women can have normal or even raised circulating oestrogen levels compared with normal weight premenopausal women, because of the tremendous capacity of the fatty tissues to convert androstenedione to oestrone, compensating for the loss of ovarian oestradiol.

The degradation of 17β-oestradiol to its less potent derivatives and excretory products occurs chiefly in the liver. The principal excretory products are the more water-soluble conjugates with sulphuric or glucuronic acids. The sulphates and glucuronides are then excreted into the bile or the urine.

Over 70 per cent of circulating oestrogens are bound to a plasma protein called sex-hormone-binding globulin (SHBG) which also binds testosterone. Another 25 per cent is bound to the plasma albumin. Plasma oestrogen concentrations vary throughout the menstrual cycle. During the follicular phase the 17β-oestradiol level is initially of the order of 75–300 pmol/l (20–80 pg/ml) rising to a pre-ovulatory peak of 750–1800 pmol/l (120–480 pg/ml). The level then falls before rising to a second, usually lower peak of 350–1100 pmol/l (95–300 pg/ml) in the middle of the luteal phase.

Actions

Oestrogens are necessary for the development and maintenance of the uterus, the Fallopian tubes, the cervix, the vagina, the labiae minora and majora, and the breasts. The role of oestrogens in the growth of the endometrium during the proliferative phase and their important effect in stimulating the synthesis of progesterone receptors in uterine tissue has been discussed previously (see endometrial cycle).

These ovarian hormones increase the motility of the Fallopian tubes and raise the threshold of excitability of uterine muscle, the latter effect being associated with spontaneous pacemaker potentials. They act on the cervical mucosa to stimulate the secretion of a watery, more alkaline, mucus which is favourable to the survival and transport of spermatozoa. At ovulation, the mucus is at its thinnest and a cervical smear made at this stage will show a fern-like pattern (ferning). Oestrogens also cause changes in vaginal cytology, including a tendency for the epithelium to cornify due to increased keratin formation.

Oestrogens may induce mild salt and water retention, at least partly by stimulating angiotensinogen production in the liver. Also, movement of electrolytes and water from blood vessels into the extravascular space may be stimulated by oestrogens. These effects may be associated with the increase in body weight and the specific changes, such as increased breast tenderness, before menstruation which could contribute to the irritability and tension associated with this premenstrual phase (premenstrual tension).

The oestrogens are mild anabolic agents, but they induce a decrease in circulating cholesterol levels by a mechanism which has not been completely elucidated but which may involve an increase in high-density lipoprotein (HDL) synthesis and a decrease in low-density lipoprotein (LDL) synthesis. HDL and LDL are linked to a protective and a contributory effect on heart disease, respectively. This could be one of the factors responsible for the lower incidence of atherosclerosis and heart disease recorded for menstruating women. This protective effect of oestrogens is lost to some extent in postmenopausal women. Another protective effect of oestrogens, which is lost at menopause, is the maintenance of bone mass through an action which is unclear but may involve other factors.

The relationship between oestrogens and androgens is indicated by the development of the female secondary sex characteristics such as broad hips, the accumulation of fat in the breasts and buttocks, and the high ratio of scalp to body hair, all of which depend at least partly on oestrogens acting in the absence of large amounts of circulating androgen. It is quite possible that androgens as well as oestrogens act on the central nervous system, and that both groups of steroids contribute to the maintenance of sexual libido and various other aspects of behaviour in women. Certainly, oestrogen, androgen, and progestogen receptors have been localized to various parts of the brain. The involvement of these hormones on the development of the brain and behavioural effects is the subject of much research at present.

Oestrogens stimulate the growth and development of the ductile system in the breasts, an effect which is of particular relevance to pregnancy and lactation. Also during pregnancy, oestrogens are important stimulators of myometrial growth (increased glycogen and actinomysosin content) and they sensitize the myometrium to the action of oxytocin (see section on parturition, p. 186).

Finally, oestrogens play a crucial role in regulating the events of the menstrual cycle by their negative and positive feedback effects on the adenohypophysis and, probably, the hypothalamus.

Mechanism of action

The oestrogens are lipophilic and cross their target cell membranes readily. Their identified receptors are intracellular phosphoproteins, with phosphorylation possibly involved in the subsequent activation process. Hormone-binding to the receptor thus produces an active configuration which binds to the hormone-responsive element on the nuclear DNA. Consequent interaction with the transcriptional apparatus results in activation of target gene expression.

Progestogens

Synthesis, storage, and release

The most potent naturally occurring progestogen in women is progesterone. It is a 21-carbon steroid which is not only important for its own endocrine effects but also because it is a precursor molecule in the synthesis of steroids in all tissues which produce them. Progesterone is secreted primarily by the corpus luteum during the luteal phase of the menstrual cycle, and by the fetoplacental unit during pregnancy. However, it is also produced in small quantities by the adrenal cortices in both sexes. The principal progestogen secreted by the outer granulosa cells of the ripening follicle during the late follicular phase is 17α-hydroxyprogesterone.

Progestogens are transported in the blood bound to transcortin (the plasma globulin that also binds corticosteroids, see Chapter 5) and albumin, with approximately 2 per cent present in the free, unbound, state. Progesterone has a half-life of approximately 5 minutes in the blood, and its principal degradation product, pregnanediol, is formed mainly in the liver. This product is conjugated in hepatic tissue, and the glucuronide is the principal urinary excretory product.

During the follicular phase of the menstrual cycle, the plasma progesterone concentration is normally less than 5 nmol/l (1.5 ng/ml). During the luteal phase, the plasma level rises to a peak value of approximately 40–50 nmol/l (12–16 ng/ml). In men, the plasma concentration is approximately 1 nmol/l (0.3 ng/ml).

Actions

Progesterone is primarily responsible for the secretory (progestational) changes in the endometrium, which have been briefly mentioned in the section on the endometrial cycle. The secretions from the cervical and vaginal epithelia also change, with the mucus becoming thicker and less easily penetrable by spermatozoa. The effect of progesterone on the myometrium, particularly during pregnancy, is antagonistic to that of oestrogens, so that the excitability of cells decreases as does their sensitivity to oxytocin. It may act by hyperpolarizing the cell membranes, and decreasing spontaneous pacemaker activity. Progesterone stimulates the growth and development of the alveolar system in the breasts, an effect which is of particular relevance to the lactation process.

Progesterone has a natriuretic effect when present in high concentrations, and it is believed that this effect occurs because the hormone can bind firmly to renal aldosterone receptors, so that aldosterone can no longer stimulate sodium reabsorption. As a consequence of the natriuresis aldosterone release is stimulated so that sodium balance can be restored to normal levels. It has been suggested that this compensatory effect, together with the salt-retaining properties of oestrogens, may contribute to the characteristic symptoms of the premenstrual period in some women.

Progesterone is associated with the rise in basal body temperature (0.2–0.5° C) that occurs immediately after ovulation and which persists during most of the luteal phase, until the plasma progesterone level begins to fall. This effect is often ascribed to a direct action by the steroid on the hypothalamic temperature regulatory centre, but this is now disputed. The increase in basal body temperature is nonetheless a useful indication that ovulation has taken place.

Other effects of progesterone on the central nervous system, such as involvement in development and behaviour, are likely although they remain ill-defined. Certainly, progesterone receptors have been localized to specific areas of the brain. Also, behavioural and other mental changes associated with the premenstrual syndrome have been liked to alterations in progesterone production.

Finally, progesterone has a negative feedback effect on the adenohypophysis, and possibly on the hypothalamus, and this contributes to the hormonal regulation of the menstrual cycle. The possibility that it has a positive feedback effect, or that it facilitates the oestrogen-induced LH-surge just before ovulation, is considered in a later section (see control of the menstrual cycle, p. 175).

Mechanism of action of progesterone

Progesterone diffuses into its target cell and binds to specific phosphorylated protein receptors probably located within the cell nucleus. Here, the hormone-receptor complex binds to a specific identifiable target gene following which protein transcription occurs. The subsequent synthesis of intracellular proteins, which can mediate the specific effects of the hormones (by acting as enzymes, for example), is the ultimate step in the mechanism of action. A more detailed consideration of the mechanisms of action of hormones at the chromosomal level is given in Chapter 2.

Androgens

The production of androgens in the female is normally low compared to males, the principal source being the adrenal glands. Nevertheless, it appears that the plasma androgen level rises during the menstrual cycle (it is synthesized by the thecal cells of the follicle during the follicular phase at least), although effects due to the androgens during the cycle are unknown. The essential role of the ovarian androgens, notable androstenedione, as precursors for oestrogen synthesis is shown in Fig. 8.5. If the androgen to oestrogen ratio rises to an abnormally high value in females, certain masculinizing changes can develop. For instance, virilization and hirsutism can occur, and the menstrual cycle will be disrupted. A possible causal role for excessive androgenic effects in the condition of polycystic ovaries (PCO) and its associated syndrome has been indicated.

The plasma testosterone concentration in women is normally in the region of 0.5–2.5 nmol/l (0.15–0.7 ng/ml), rising to values of 3–6 nmol/l (0.9–1.7 ng/ml) during pregnancy.

Control of the menstrual cycle

It is now apparent that numerous steroidal and non-steroidal factors are almost certainly involved in the fine control of the events of the menstrual cycle. Nevertheless, the key elements are undoubtedly the hormones of the hypothalamo–hypophysial–gonadal axis. Thus, the menstrual cycle is associated with the secretion of the ovarian hormones (the oestrogens and progestogens) which in turn is associated with the release of gonadotrophins (FSH and LH) from the adenohypophysis, and gonadotrophin–releasing hormone (GnRH) from the hypothalamus. Not only is control of the menstrual cycle related to the feedback effects of hormones but also to central nervous influence via the hypothalamus.

Control of ovarian hormone secretion

Follicular phase

At the beginning of each menstrual cycle the concentrations of ovarian steroids in the general circulation are basal and hence any negative feedback effect on adenohypophysial gonadotrophin release is minimal. Under the influence of the rising levels of FSH and LH, the primary follicles begin to develop. The combined effects of LH on the thecal cells to produce androgens, and of FSH on the granulosa cells to aromatize the thecal androgens to oestrogens, result in slowly rising oestrogen levels in the blood. As the plasma oestrogen concentration increases it begins to exert a negative feedback on FSH production which falls around day 9 of the follicular phase. The ovarian production of the polypeptide inhibin is probably also related to the inhibition of FSH production. The other gonadotrophin LH does not show any marked fall in production at this stage presumably because it is less sensitive to the negative feedback influence of oestrogens at these concentrations and mainly because inhibin has no effect on LH production. The removal of the FSH stimulus on follicular growth results in the regression of those antral follicles which are still FSH-dependent (Fig. 8.6).

The plasma oestrogen concentration now increases sharply over the following four to five days as the remaining Graafian follicle continues to ripen. The follicular androgen production also increases during this late follicular phase. The raised oestrogen level, if maintained at a sufficiently high concentration for a minimum period of 36 hours, now has a positive feedback effect on the hypothalamo–adenohypophysial system. Consequently, there is a sudden rapid surge in

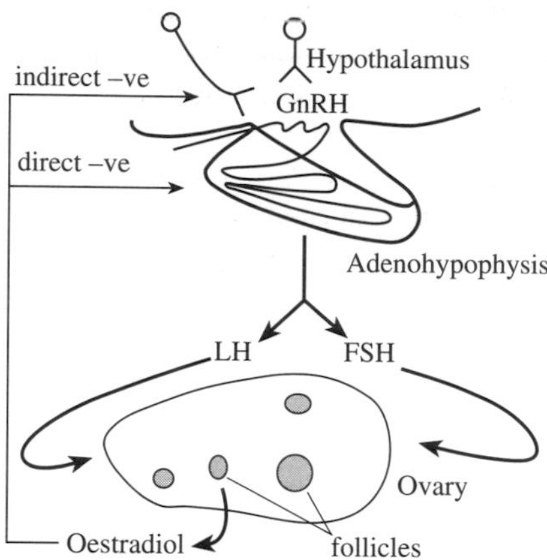

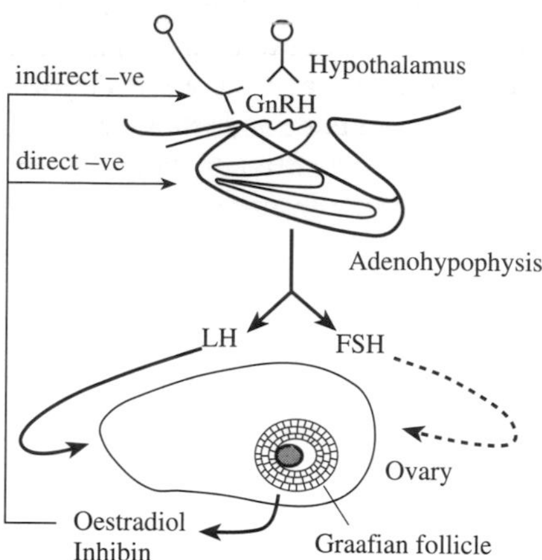

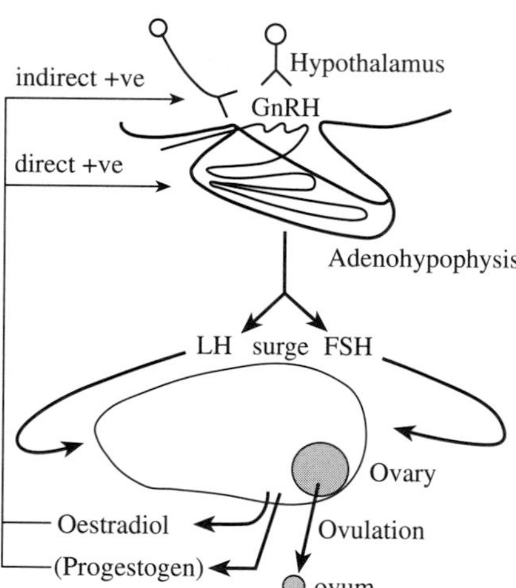

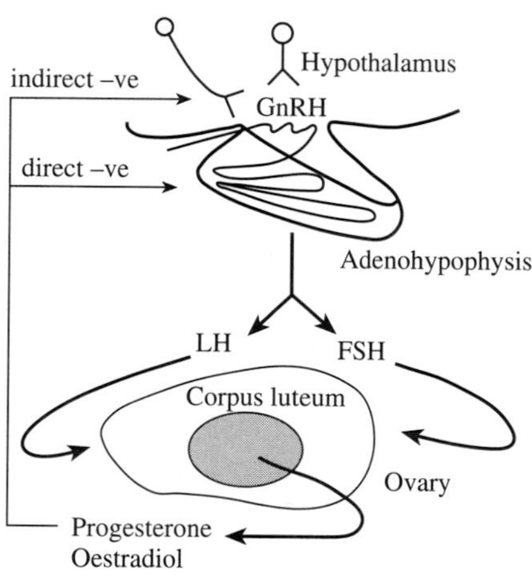

Fig. 8.6. The endocrine control of the menstrual cycle. (FSH, follicle-stimulating hormone; GnRH, gonadotrophin-releasing hormone; LH, luteinizing hormone.)

LH, and to a lesser extent FSH, production. These surges of gonadotrophin, particularly of LH, induce the final stage of maturation of the Graafian follicle. This final ripening stage includes a decreased stimulation of the thecal cells to produce androgens and oestrogens but an increased stimulation of the granulosa cells which now synthesize progestogens. The small but increasing quantities of follicular progestogen released prior to ovulation may enhance the positive feedback by oestrogens on gonadotrophin production and/or may exert a direct positive feedback effect of their own. In addition, it has been suggested that another component which contributes to ovulation is the inhibition of a non-steroidal surge-attenuating factor which may be present during the earlier part of the follicular phase. This factor would normally inhibit the LH surge.

The ultimate effect of the gonadotrophin surge is to cause the follicle to rupture (probably due to activation of enzymes, such as collagenase, which digest the follicular wall) and the process of ovulation culminates in the release of the ovum into the peritoneal cavity.

Luteal phase

The decrease in oestrogen production at ovulation removes the positive feedback influence of these steroid hormones on gonadotrophin release. The LH and FSH levels now fall, quite sharply at first, but remain sufficiently high to stimulate the newly formed luteal cells to secrete progesterone and oestrogens. Approximately eight days after ovulation, the plasma progesterone concentration reaches a peak and this coincides with a second, usually lower peak of oestrogens. The effect of these raised steroid levels is a profound negative feedback on the production of gonadotrophins which then fall to basal levels. The dominant negative feedback influence at this stage is probably the raised progesterone level which not only exerts a direct effect of its own but is capable of inhibiting any possible positive feedback influence by oestrogens should these latter hormones reach sufficiently high plasma levels for at least 36 hours.

Unless pregnancy is initiated by the implantation into the prepared uterus of a blastocyst, the corpus luteum now degenerates following the withdrawal of gonadotrophin support. Oestrogen and progesterone levels decrease in consequence, and the negative feedback effect on the hypothalamo–adenohypophysial system is removed. Following the loss of the old endometrial lining during menstruation because of the diminished steroid hormone support, the rising levels of LH and FSH initiate the follicular events of the following cycle.

The plasma concentrations of ovarian and adenohypophysial hormones throughout the menstrual cycle are shown in Fig. 8.7.

The influence of prolactin on ovarian function

The adenohypophysial hormone, prolactin, also influences ovarian function. Pathological hyperprolactinaemia can have a profound inhibitory effect on the menstrual cycle and is now believed to account for up to 20 per cent of all infertility cases in women. Physiological hyperprolactinaemia occurs during pregnancy and during the first months of intense lactation, and this is probably the reason why menstrual cycles are not immediately re-established after parturition. It is important to note that prolactin release is pulsatile in form, and this may account for the occasional pregnancy which can arise during lactation due to an escape from the natural contraceptive effect of this hormone.

High plasma prolactin concentrations may act by inhibiting the effect of gonadotrophins on the ovaries, and/or may inhibit the release of the gonado-

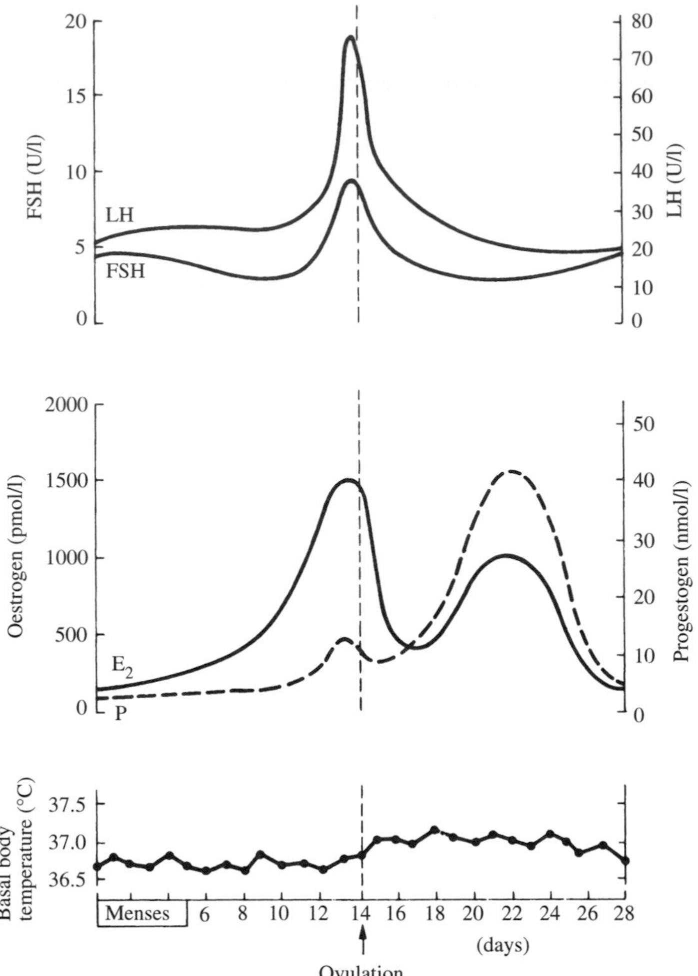

Fig. 8.7. Graphs showing the typical pattern of changes in plasma concentrations of follicle-stimulating hormone (FSH), luteinizing hormone (LH), 17β-oestradiol (E_2) and progestogen (P), and in the basal body temperature of a women with normal ovulatory cycles. Note that the small pre-ovulatory increase in progesterone is in fact due to 17α-hydroxyprogesterone.

trophins from the adenohypophysis by a central action, possibly via the hypothalamus. Another proposed mechanism of action is that prolactin might stimulate a corticotrophin-induced production of adrenal androgens.

There is also some evidence for a facilitating effect by low concentrations of prolactin on the LH-stimulated production of progesterone from the proliferating granulosa cells during the late follicular phase, at least in some species.

Control of gonadotrophin secretion

The control of LH and FSH release from the adenohypophysis is primarily directed from the hypothalamus, and modulated by feedback loops involving the ovarian steroids (see Chapter 4).

Hypothalamic control

An essential element in the control of release of the adenohypophysial gonadotrophins is the pulsatile secretion of the hypothalamic gonadotrophin-releasing hormone (GnRH) into the local portal blood system. The production of this decapeptide in neurones of the arcuate nucleus is itself controlled, at least partly, by neurotransmitters released from nerve terminals synapsing with the GnRH–producing fibres, and arising from other parts of the brain. Some of these neurones appear to be adrenergic, dopaminergic, cholinergic, or serotoninergic on the basis of their neurotransmitters. Noradrenaline and acetycholine can stimulate the pulsatile secretion of GnRH by either increasing frequency or amplitude of release, whereas dopamine appears to suppress GnRH secretion.

In addition to the nervous control of GnRH by neurones from other areas of the brain, the ovarian steroids can influence its release by effects in the hypothalamus. The oestrogens exert their positive feedback effect partly by increasing GnRH release, while their negative feedback influence is also probably mediated partly by a hypothalamic action. The mechanisms by which these effects are produced are uncertain, but may involve the mediation of the adrenergic and other neurones which influence GnRH release and are probably directed at changing the frequency or amplitude of the GnRH pulses. The pulsatile nature of GnRH release is an essential component in the control of normal menstrual cycles. Continuous infusions of GnRH or one of its long-acting agonists is associated initially with increased gonadotrophin secretion but after a few days production is decreased and gonadal function is reduced. Furthermore, the frequency of the GnRH pulses may at least partly determine the ratio of LH to FSH released by the gonadotrophes of the adenohypophysis.

Direct hormonal feedback control

Postmenopausal women have basal levels of plasma oestrogens and raised concentrations of plasma LH and FSH. This observation together with the finding that an injection of oestrogen will reduce the LH and FSH levels, suggests that oestrogen exerts a negative feedback effect on gonadotrophin release. In fact, the principal influence of oestrogens on LH (and FSH) release is a negative one. The exception is when plasma oestrogen levels rise sharply by more than 40 pmol/l (10 pg/ml), are maintained at very high levels (e.g. above 800 pmol/l) for at least 36 hours, and in the absence of a raised plasma progesterone concentration. Such a situation occurs during the late follicular phase, and under these conditions, the oestrogens exert a powerful positive feedback effect on LH (and to a smaller extent FSH) release. The induced LH surge then elicits the final stage of maturation of the Graafian follicle and initiates the process of ovulation.

In a sense, progesterone has the reverse effect, with peak concentrations exerting a negative feedback on gonadotrophin release, part of this response probably being due to an enhancement of the normal negative feedback effect of oestrogens when present in high (but not above 800 pmol/l) concentrations. This enhancing effect by progesterone of the oestrogen-induced negative feedback is seen during the luteal phase. On the other hand, low progestogen levels can exert a positive feedback effect on LH and FSH release, either by a direct action of their own or by potentiating the positive-feedback influence of oestradiol. Thus 17α-hydroxyprogesterone participates in the preovulatory LH and FSH surges.

At least part of the effect of ovarian hormones on gonadotrophin release appears to be by a direct action on the gonadotrophe cells of the adenohypophysis. For example, oestrogens can alter the sensitivity of the gonadotrophes to GnRH in certain situations.

The role of inhibin on the hypothalamo–adenohypophysial axis has been indicated in an earlier section (p. 167).

Control of prolactin secretion

Prolactin is believed to influence its own release from the adenohypophysis by a short negative feedback loop on the hypothalamus. It is believed to stimulate the release of the prolactin inhibitory hormone, dopamine, which then reaches the adenohypophysis by the local portal blood system. Dopamine may not only inhibit the release of prolactin but may also inhibit gonadotrophin secretion by a direct action on the gonadotrophes. One prolactin-releasing factor from the hypothalamus is the tripeptide TRH (thyrotrophin-releasing hormone).

PREGNANCY

Fertilization

The process of reproduction is essentially concerned with the preservation of genes from the male and female alike. The first step in this process is, therefore, the merger of the male haploid cell (the spermatozoon) and the female haploid cell (the released ovum). Regarding the various extremely interesting aspects of human sexual behaviour and the mating process itself, the reader is directed to a specialized text on reproductive physiology. Here, let it suffice that we identify the important processes of arousal in both sexes, and the erection of the reproductive organs again in both sexes although erection of the male penis is of far greater significance with regard to the actual deposition of spermatozoa within the female vagina. Of the many millions of spermatozoa deposited (normal concentration approximately 50×10^8/ml), very few spermatozoa normally reach the ovum in the Fallopian tube and of these only one succeeds in fertilizing it.

Implantation

Once the ovum has been fertilized it undergoes cell division as it passes down the Fallopian tube to the uterus. It reaches the uterus three to four days after ovulation

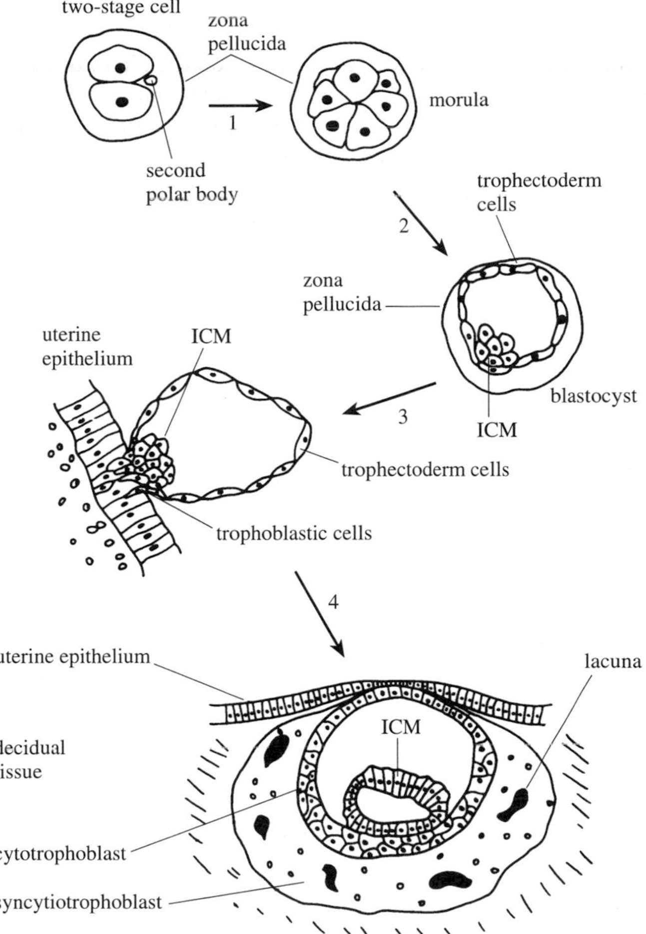

Fig. 8.8. Diagram showing the development of the fertilized egg from the two-cell stage to the morula (1), to the developing blastocyst (2), which implants (3) and finally to the growing embryo (4). (ICM, inner cell mass.)

by which time it has reached the 32–64 cell stage and become a blastocyst. The blastocyst consists of two types of cell, an outer rim of trophectoderm cells, and a cluster of cells called the 'inner cell mass' (ICM). Most of the ICM is surrounded by a fluid-filled cavity (Fig. 8.8). Once within the uterus the blastocyst continues to grow and develop for approximately six days before 'fusing' with a section of the endometrium (implantation). During the unattached phase, the blastocyst receives its nutrients and oxygen from the surrounding intrauterine environment. The initiation of implantation is believed to be the stimulation of adjacent uterine tissue by the trophectoderm cells, although the nature of the stimulus is unknown. It is believed that the stimulus is non-specific but it may cause the release of chemicals within the uterine epithelium which then spread to the underlying stromal tissue. Histamine and prostaglandins have been implicated in this process, and they may induce the profound changes in the endometrium initiated by the implanting blastocyst. These changes include an increased vascular permeability in the stroma which leads to a local oedema, changes in the composition of the intercellular matrix, and a growth of capillaries towards the implanting blastocyst, all of which are part of a process called 'decidualization'.

In order that the endometrium responds to the stimulus for decidualization, it is necessary that oestrogens are superimposed on the progesterone background of the luteal phase. A progesterone-dominated uterus in the absence of oestrogen remains hostile to implantation. Oestrogens appear to be necessary for inducing endometrial responsiveness to the initial blastocyst stimulus.

The first stage of the implantation process therefore involves intimate contact between the trophectoderm cells of the blastocyst and the adjacent uterine epithelium. The trophectoderm cells become trophoblastic and invade the decidual tissue. The outer layer of trophoblast cells loose their cell membranes and form a syncytium (the syncytiotrophoblast), while the inner trophoblast cells form the cytotrophoblast. As the trophoblast destroys the decidual tissue, the phagocytic cells release nutrients which can then pass to the inner cell mass by a developing vascular system. As the blastocyst implants deeply into the endometrium, the uterine epithelium fuses over it.

The trophoblast gradually develops a vascular system, which lies in close proximity to the developing maternal vascular system, and the two together form the placenta. The inner cell mass has meanwhile also been growing and develops into the fetus. In many ways the developing fetus and placenta function together as a fetoplacental unit.

The fetoplacental unit

The placenta is the site where fetal and maternal blood circulations are closely associated with each other although the two systems are physically separate. Most of the gaseous and metabolic exchanges between fetus and mother takes place in this region of close proximity, although the placenta also functions as a barrier to the transfer of large molecules (e.g. proteins) and cells. The placenta is therefore a site of selective exchange in both directions.

However, the fetus and placenta function together with respect to their endocrine function in maintaining the pregnancy and in preparing the mother for the processes of parturition and lactation.

Human chorionic gonadotrophin (HCG)

One of the earliest functions of the implanting trophoblast is the synthesis of human chorionic gonadotrophin. This two-chain glycoprotein is synthesized in the syncytiotrophoblast and is released into the material circulation. It stimulates the corpus luteum in the ovary which then continues to produce the oestrogens and progesterone which are necessary for the maintenance of pregnancy. The HCG therefore replaces the adenohypophysial LH which by day 24 of the menstrual cycle is only being secreted in small, basal quantities because of the steroid feed-

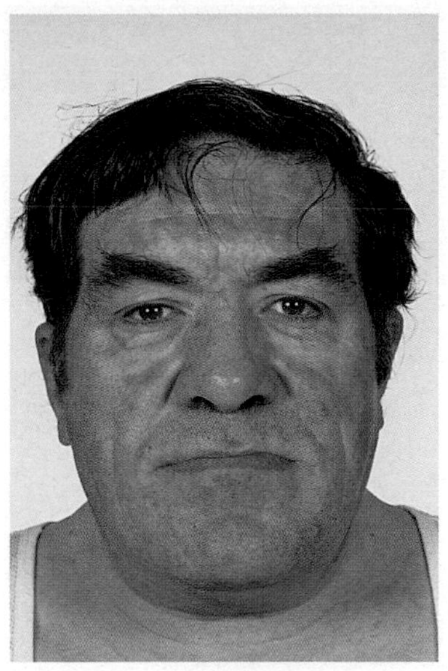

Plate 4.1 Male age 40 with acromegaly: coarse features with mild prognathism. Presented with polyarthropathy and carpal tunnel syndrome and treated by trans-sphenoidal adenomectomy and post-operative radiotherapy.

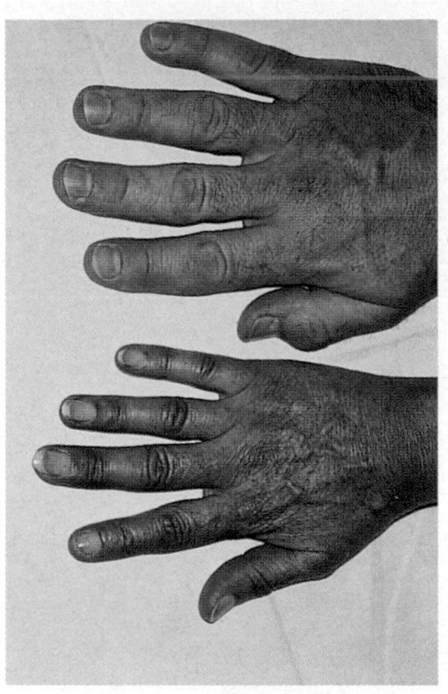

Plate 4.2 Same acromegalic male as plate 4.1: patient's hand with comparison hand of unaffected male of same age. Patient was unaware of any change in hand size.

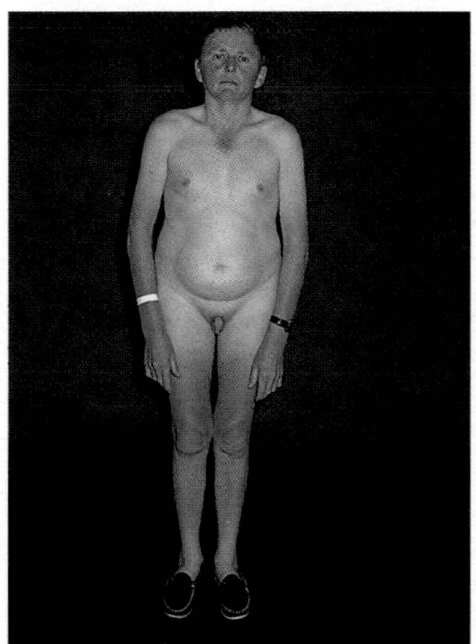

Plate 4.3 Idiopathic (presumed auto-immune) pan-hypopituitarism: loss of body hair, muscle wasting and regression of secondary sex characteristics. Patient presented with progressive fatigue. MRI pituitary scan normal.

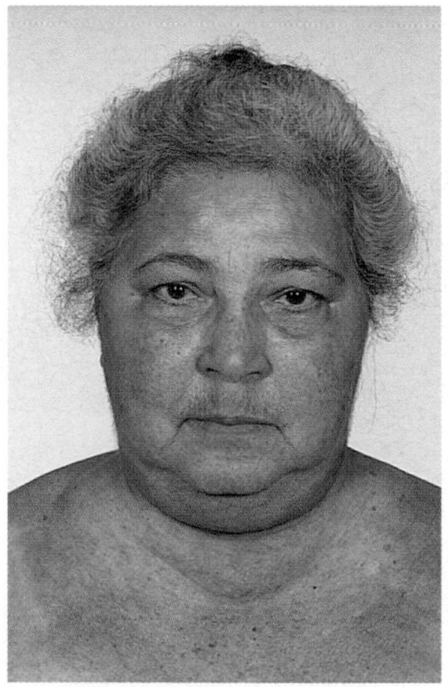

Plate 5.1 Pituitary-dependent Cushing's disease: facial plethora and striking upper truncal obesity. Patient presented with back pain (osteoporosis) and hypertension: ultimately treated by trans-sphenoidal removal of 4 mm pituitary adenoma.

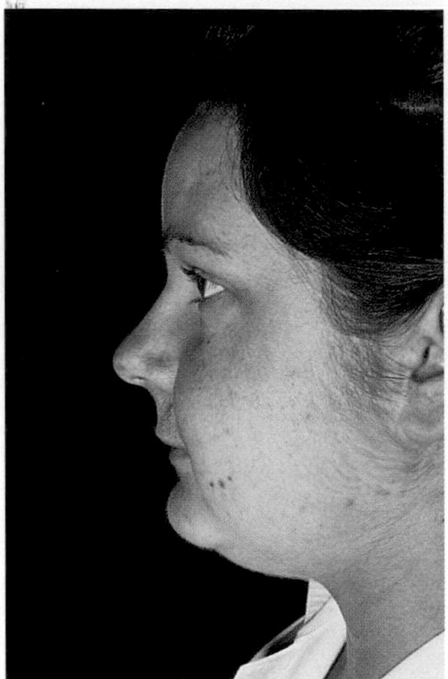

Plate 5.2 Cushing's syndrome due to unilateral adrenal adenoma: hirsutism, acne and facial obesity. Presented with fatigue and progressive weight gain. Treated with unilateral adrenalectomy, following biochemical confirmation and CT localization.

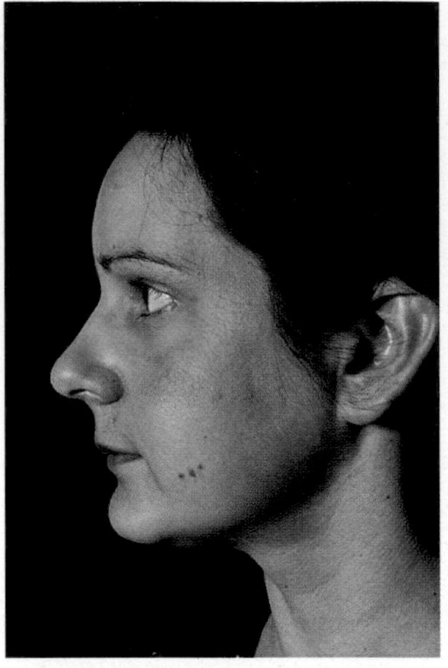

Plate 5.3 Same patient six months postoperatively: rapid regression of all abnormal clinical features and independent of steroid replacement (temporarily steroid dependent for two months due to feedback suppression of contralateral adrenal).

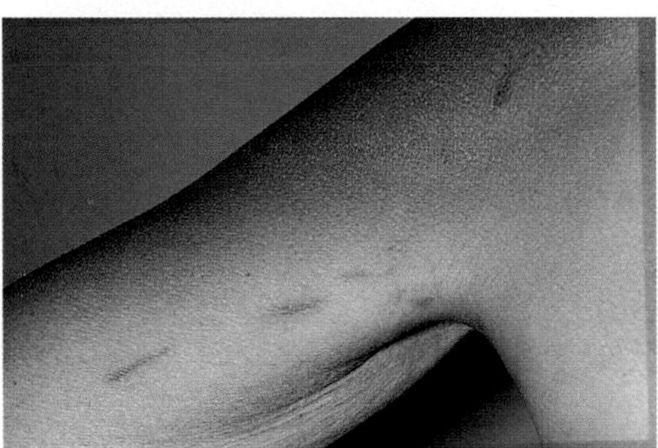

Plate 5.4 Addison's disease (adrenocortical failure): pigmentation in scars. Abnormal pigmentation was also present on buccal mucosa and appendectomy scar. Patient presented with fatigue, weight loss and postural hypotension.

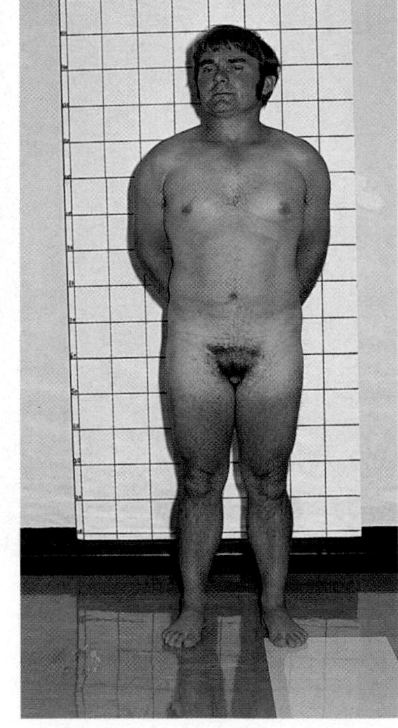

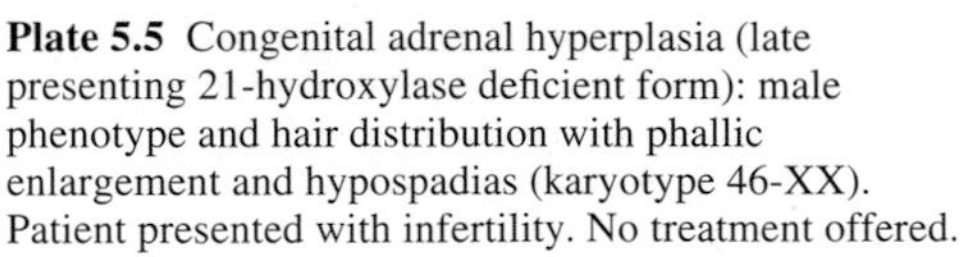

Plate 5.5 Congenital adrenal hyperplasia (late presenting 21-hydroxylase deficient form): male phenotype and hair distribution with phallic enlargement and hypospadias (karyotype 46-XX). Patient presented with infertility. No treatment offered.

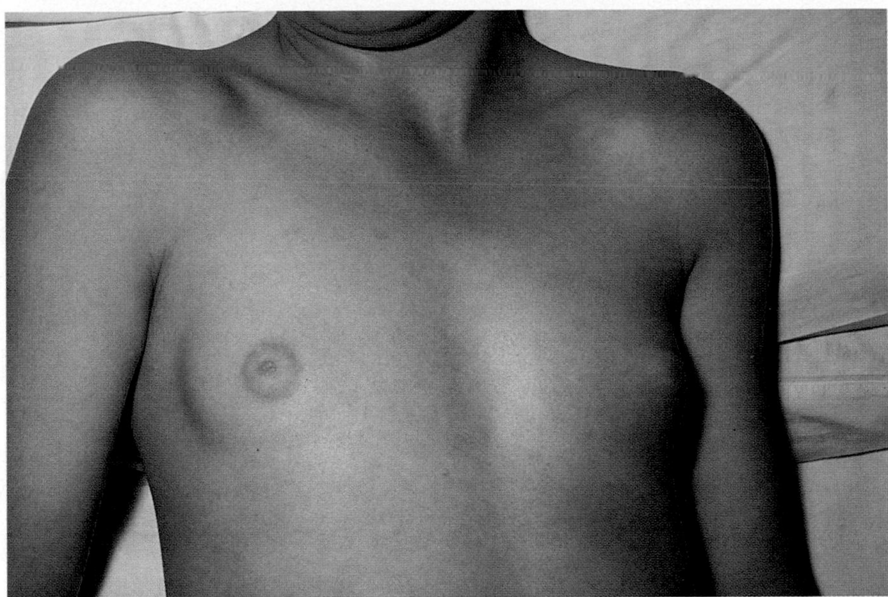

Plate 7.1 Post-pubertal (idiopathic) gynaecomastia: asymmetrical painless duct tissue hypertrophy: endocrinologically normal. Swelling subsided after 3 years of observation without intervention.

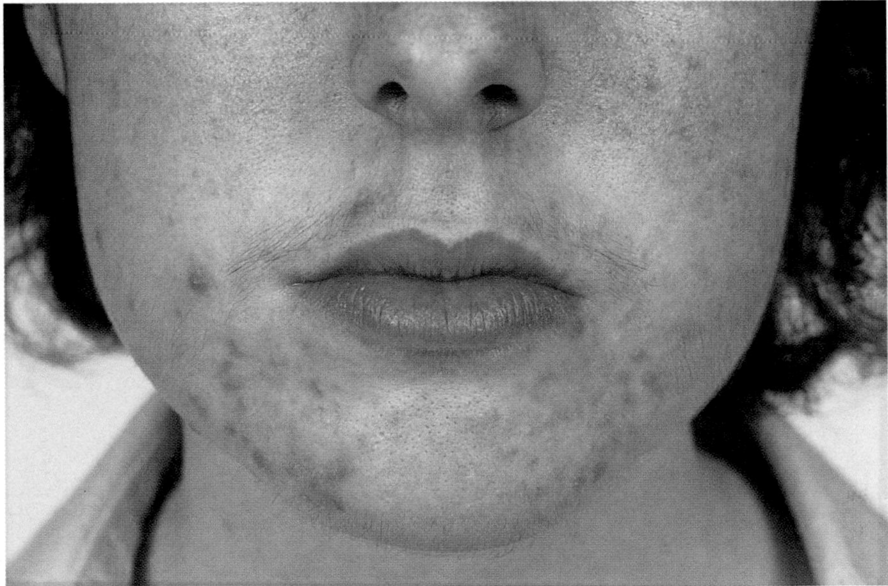

Plate 8.1 Polycystic ovarian disease: hirsutism and acne. Patient presented with infertility despite regular menstrual cycles; investigation confirmed frequent anovulatory cycles; pregnancy followed fourth course of clomiphene.

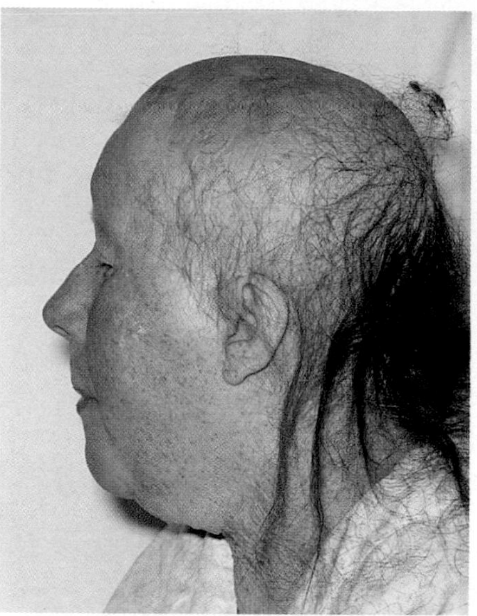

Plate 9.1 Gross hypothyroidism in an elderly female: alopecia and loss of normal facial contours. Patient presented with depression and personality disorder first identified during long-term (institutional) psychiatric care.

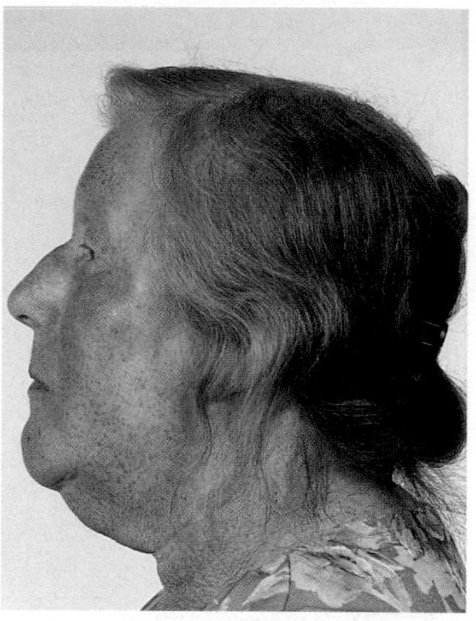

Plate 9.2 Same patient as 9.1 eight months after commencing thyroxine replacement: restoration of hair growth and facial contours. Marked improvement in psychiatric state allowing discharge from hospital into community.

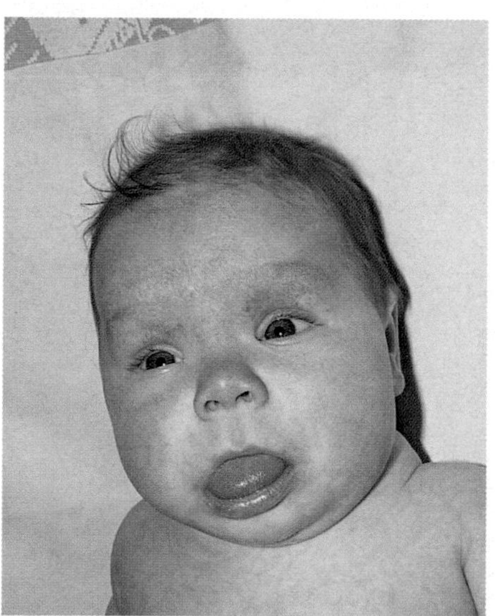

Plate 9.3 Congenital hypothyroidism: bloated facial appearance and large tongue. Routinely identified on neonatal heel-prick serum TSH. Hypothyroidism corrected promptly with thyroxine: normal subsequent growth and intellectual development.

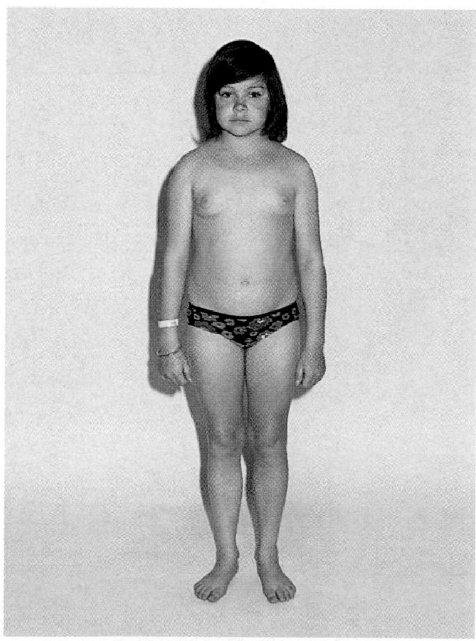

Plate 9.4 Juvenile hypothyroidism in a 16-year old girl: short stature (7 cm below 3rd centile), dull facial features and delayed puberty. Patient presented with poor growth and learning difficulties. Thyroxine restored growth velocity and academic performance.

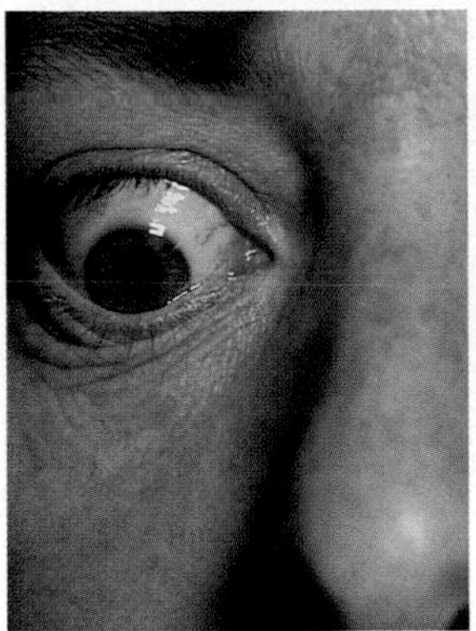

Plate 9.5 Lid lag and retraction in Graves' hyperthyroidism: no evidence of true infiltrative ophthalmopathy.

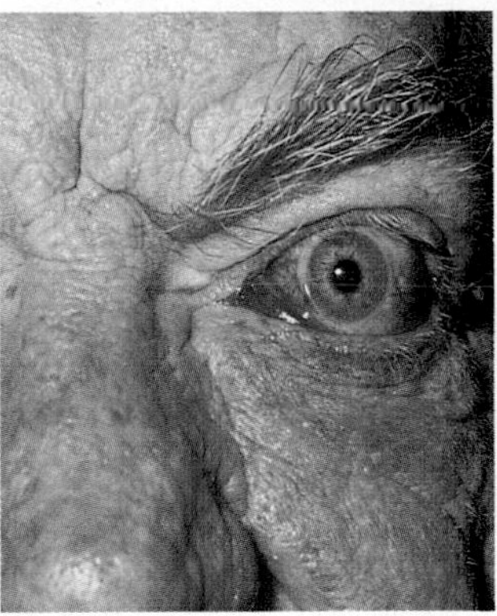

Plate 9.6 Conjunctival oedema (chemosis) and injection masquerading as 'conjunctivitis' in early Graves' ophthalmopathy.

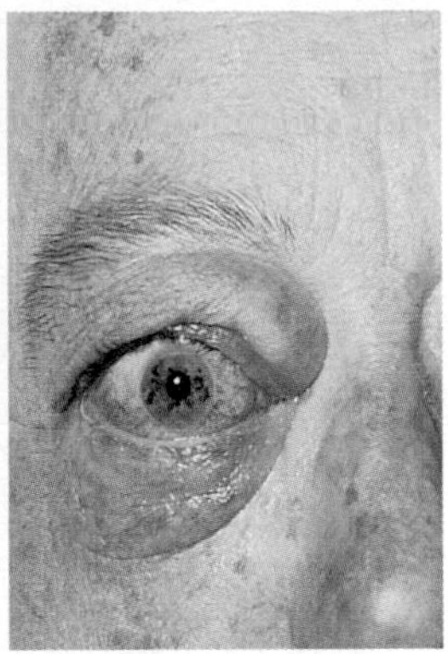

Plate 9.7 Marked chemosis, injection and periorbital oedema in severe Graves' ophthalmopathy: patient required steroid therapy.

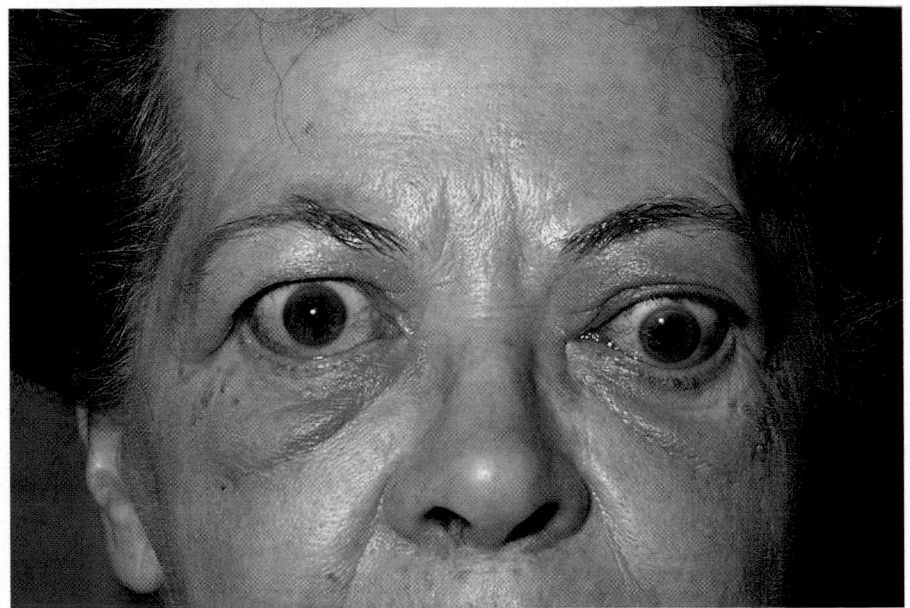

Plate 9.8 Graves' ophthalmopathy with marked conjunctival injection, periorbital oedema and extra-ocular muscle involvement: patient had continuous diplopia and required corrective muscle surgery.

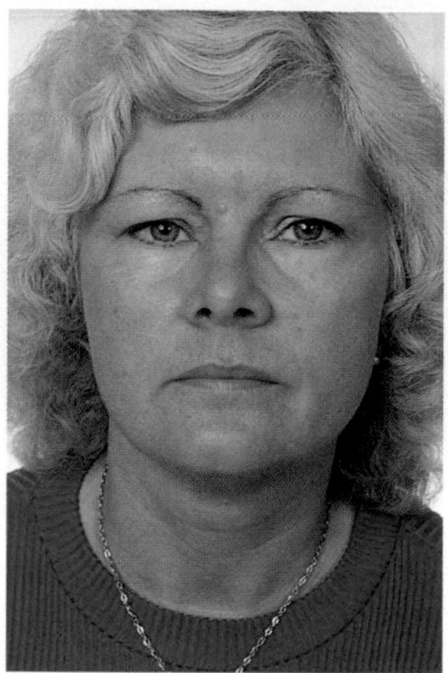

Plate 9.9 Primary (autoimmune) hypothyroidism: no abnormal clinical features. Patient presented only with increasing fatigue. Low free T4, raised serum TSH and high thyroid microsomal (peroxidase) antibody titre.

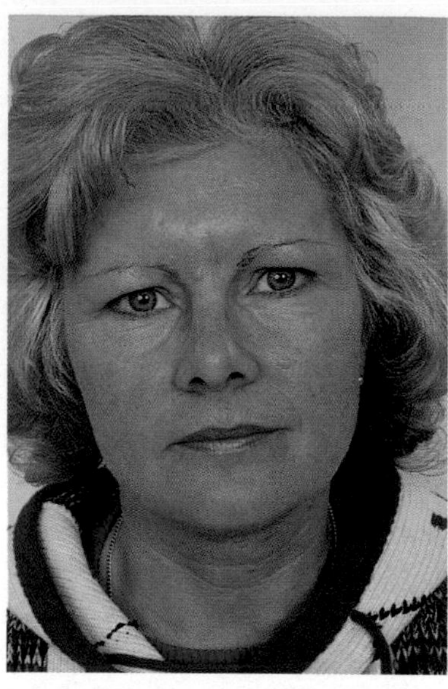

Plate 9.10 Same patient as in 9.9, six months after commencing thyroxine replacement. Fatigue totally reversed. In retrospect, patient did manifest minor facial changes prior to treatment.

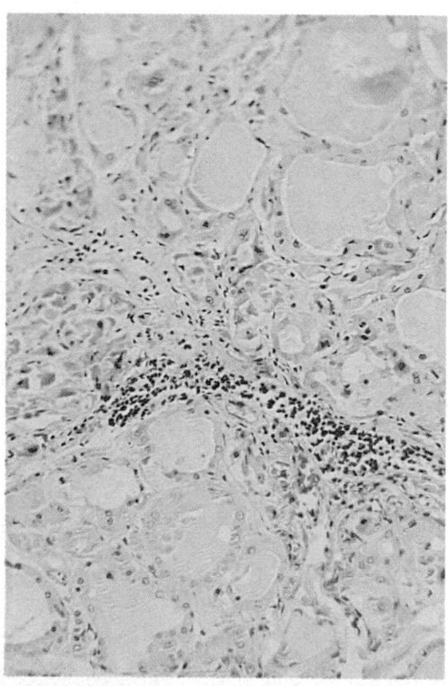

Plate 9.11 Histology of thyroid in surgically treated Graves' disease. Note hallmark of auto-immune disease: a dense lymphocytic infiltrate. Similar changes may be seen in other organ specific immune disorders e.g. adrenal, parathyroid, gonads.

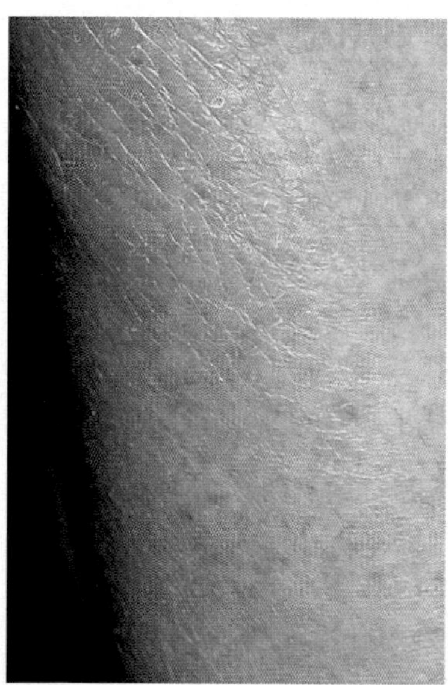

Plate 9.12 Pretibial myxoedema (infiltrative dermopathy): red, indurated thickening on both shins. Patient also had thyroid ophthalmopathy.

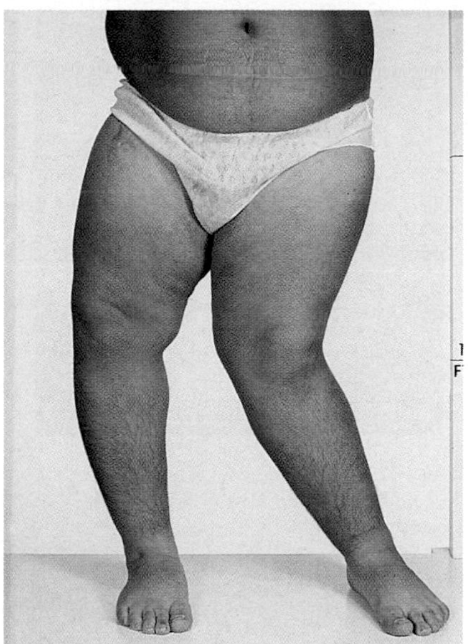

Plate 10.1 Vitamin-D resistant (hypophosphataemic) rickets: 'windswept' knees appearance due to combined genu valgum and varum deformity. Patient treated with high dose vitamin D and phosphate, but deformity persisted.

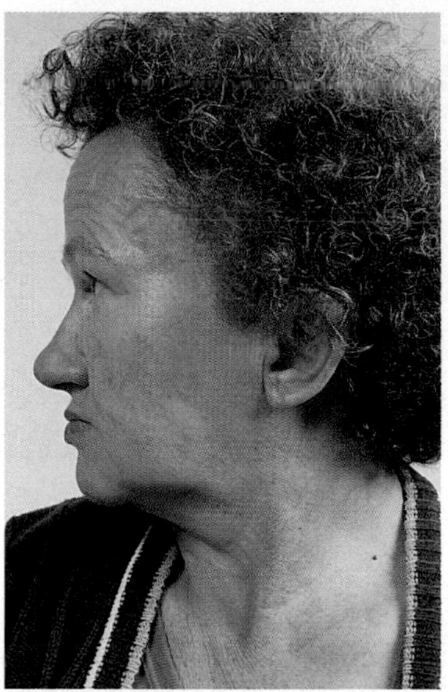

Plate 10.2 Paget's disease of bone: asymptomatic prominent frontal bones, but polyostotic involvement of pelvis and femora responsible for extensive lower limb girdle pain.

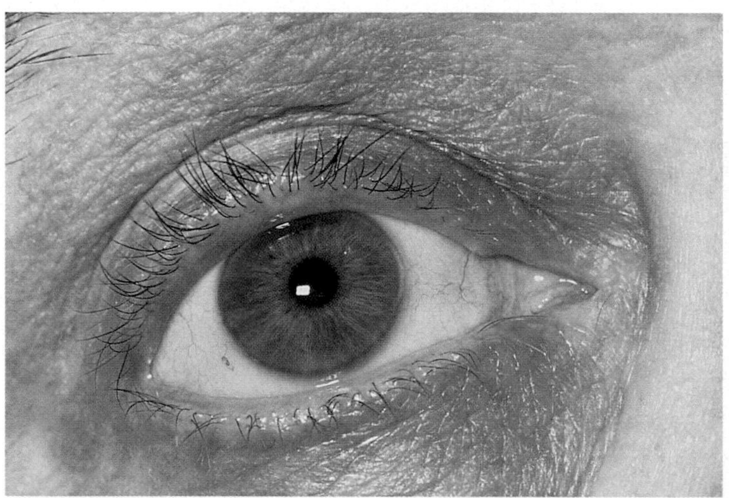

Plate 10.3 Band keratopathy (corneal calcification) in primary hyperparathyroidism: crescentic white band on nasal aspect of cornea. Tympanic membrane calcification also identified. Patient presented with malaise and polyuria: serum calcium 3.4 mmol/l.

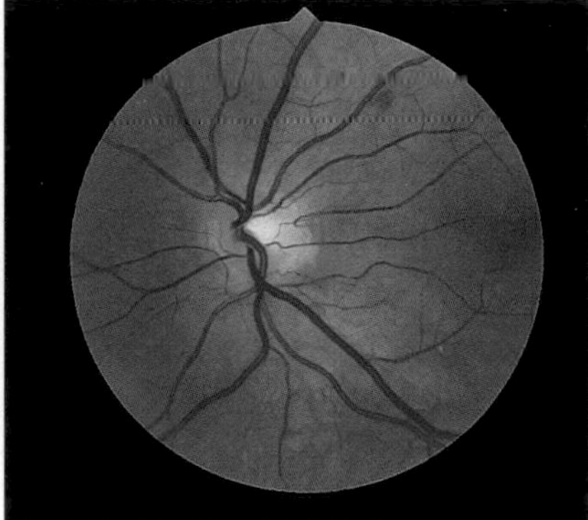

Plate 11.1 Background retinopathy: blot haemorrhage in right superior sector; single dot haemorrhage ('microaneurysm') in left inferior sector of field. No visual impairment

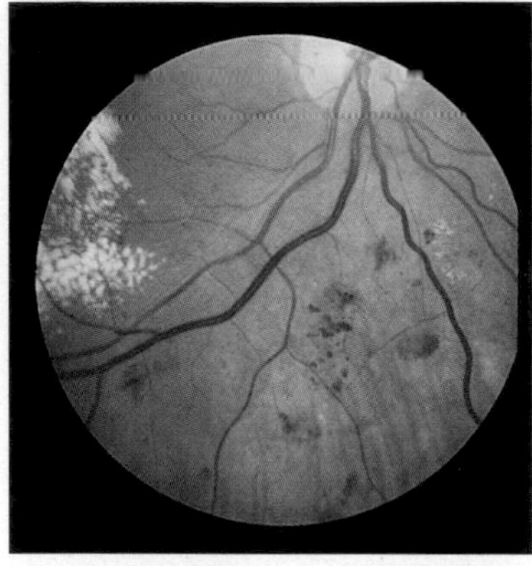

Plate 11.2 Advanced background retinopathy: dot and blot haemorrhages and macular exudate: no visual impairment.

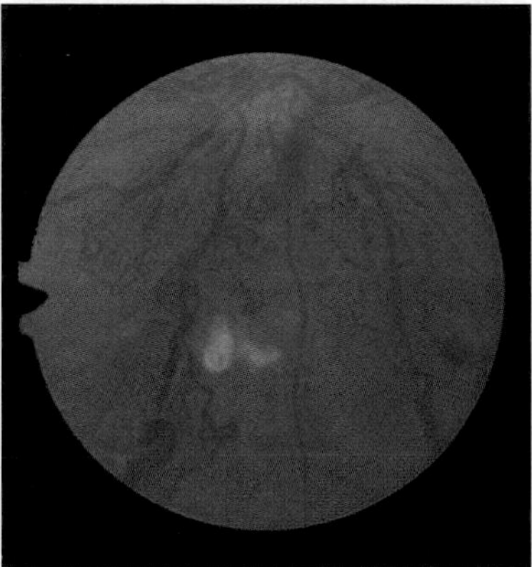

Plate 11.3 Proliferative retinopathy: venular dilatation and new vessel formation: no visual impairment.

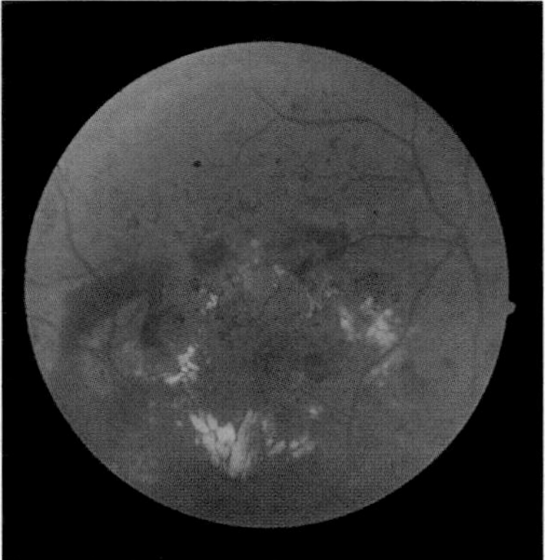

Plate 11.4 Proliferative retinopathy: extensive pre-retinal haemorrhage and exudate. Visual acuity reduced due to scotoma and vitreous haze.

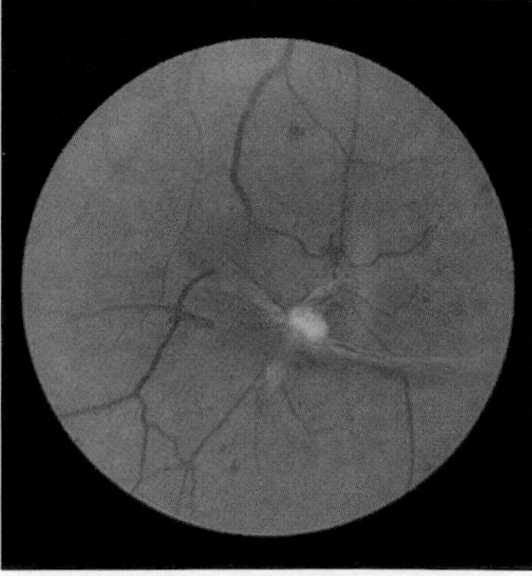

Plate 11.5 Retinitis proliferans: fibrous band at site of previous pre-retinal haemorrhage. Retinal detachment followed one year later.

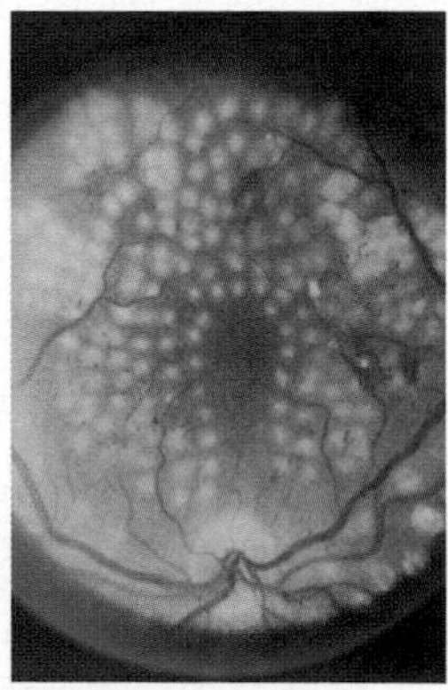

Plate 11.6 End-result of grid pattern laser therapy of extensive retinopathy: despite apparent damage, patient retained visual acuity 6/12, due to sparing of macula.

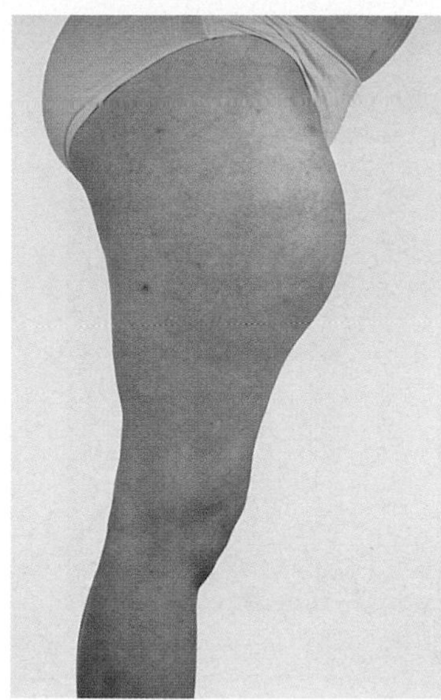

Plate 11.7 Lipohypertrophy due to repeated self-injection of insulin into same area of thigh. Partial resolution followed adoption of an injection-site rotation plan.

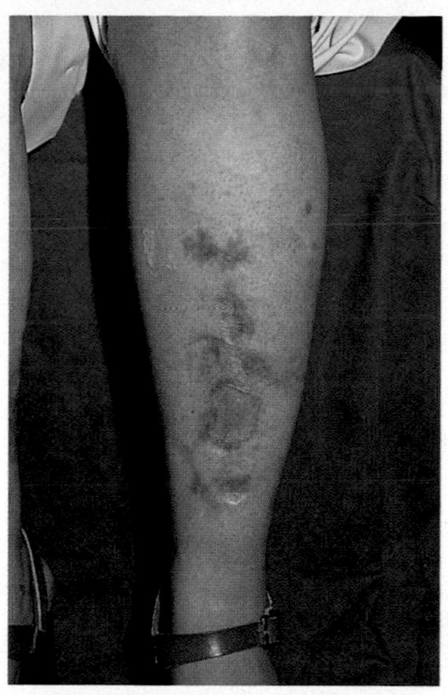

Plate 11.8 Necrobiosis lipoidica diabeticorum: disorder began three years earlier with single, then multiple lesions similar to proximal red patch. Trauma resulted in indolent ulceration with depressed 'tissue-paper' scars (seen distally).

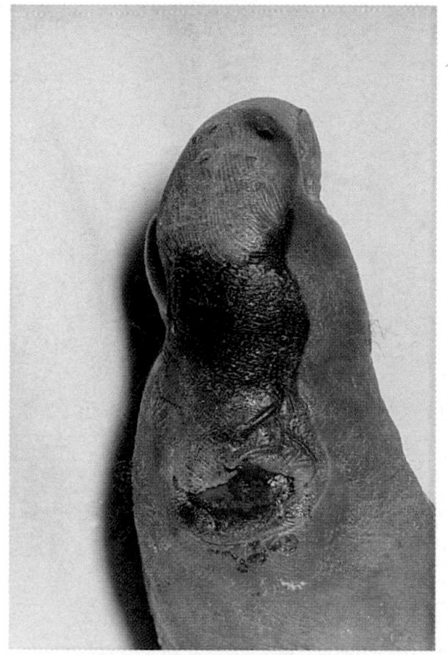

Plate 11.9 Ulcer in an arteriopathic neuropathic diabetic foot following use of (unrecognized) excessively tight new shoes: rapid progression to gangrene of big toe, ultimately requiring forefoot amputation.

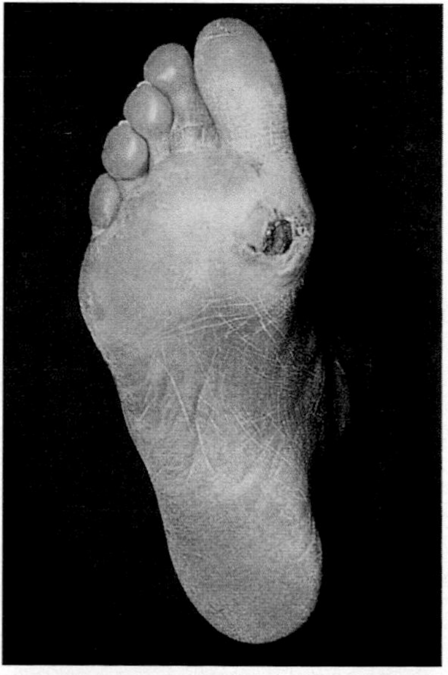

Plate 11.10 Neuropathic (painless) ulcer in typical position over first metatarsal head. Healing was eventually achieved by plaster cast immobilization/protection over a four-month period.

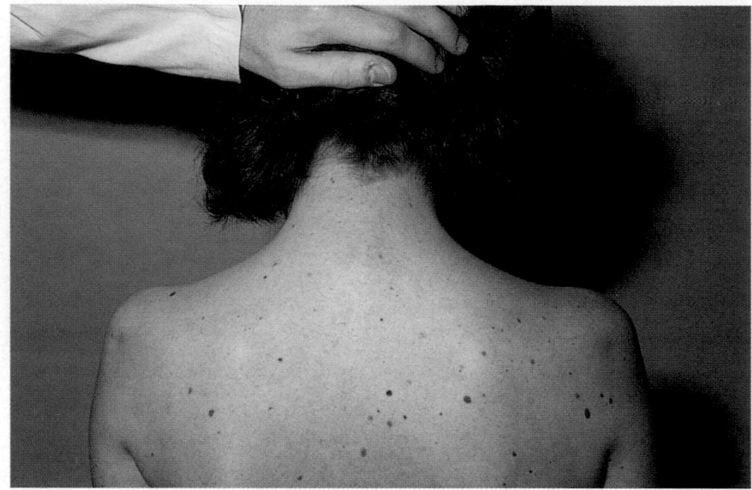

Plate 13.1 Gonadal dysgenesis (Turner's syndrome), karyotype 46-XO: webbed neck and multiple pigmented moles. Patient presented with primary amenorrhoea and short stature.

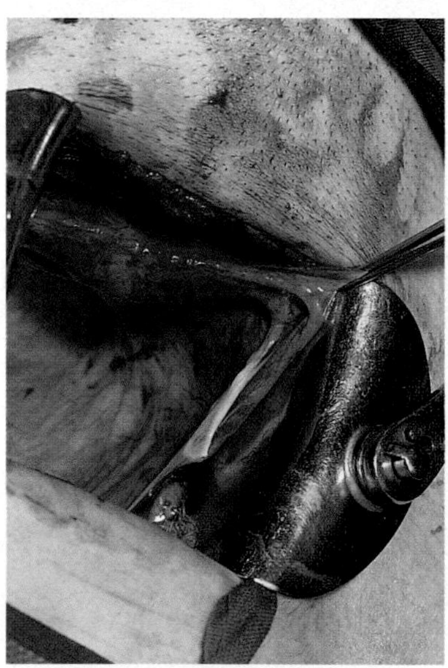

Plate 13.2 Laparotomy in patient shown above: note small uterus and (white) fibrous gonadal streak. No ovarian tissue identified on histology.

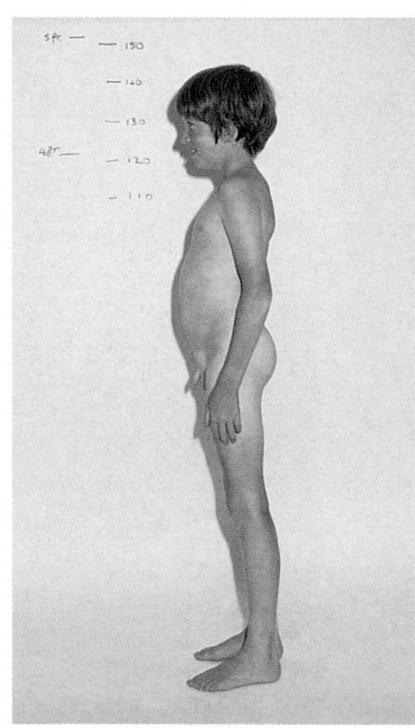

Plate 13.3 Simple delayed puberty in a boy age 17: presented with short stature and absent secondary sexual characteristics. Treated with 4 month course of testosterone which initiated growth and sexual maturation.

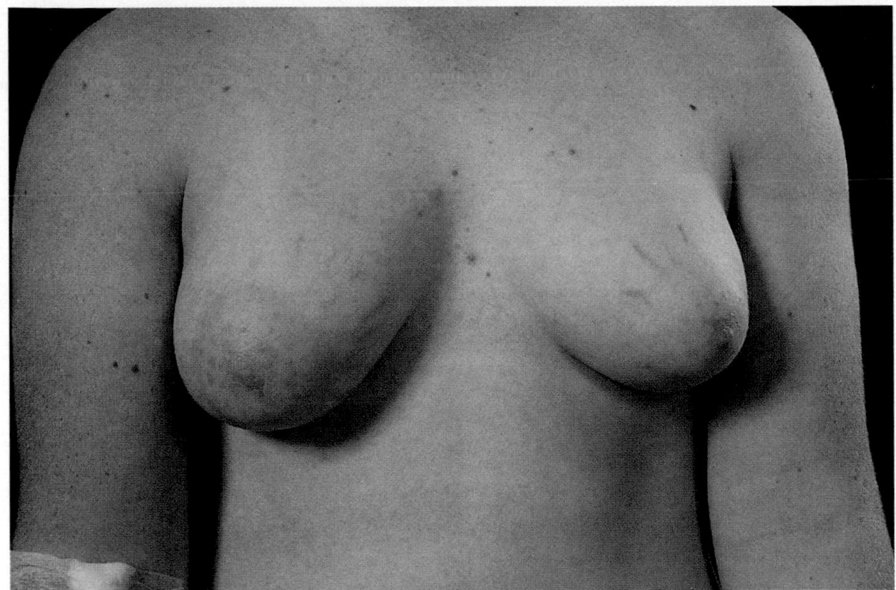

Plate 13.4 Precocious puberty in a nine-year old girl. Hypothalamic tumour (presumed hamartoma) identified on MRI scanning.

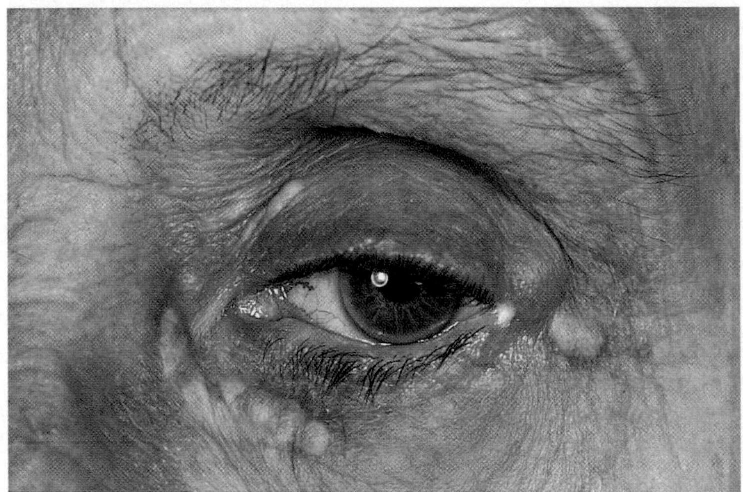

Plate 14.1 Xanthelasmata and marked corneal arcus in familial hypercholesterolaemia. Patient presented with myocardial infarction age 55.

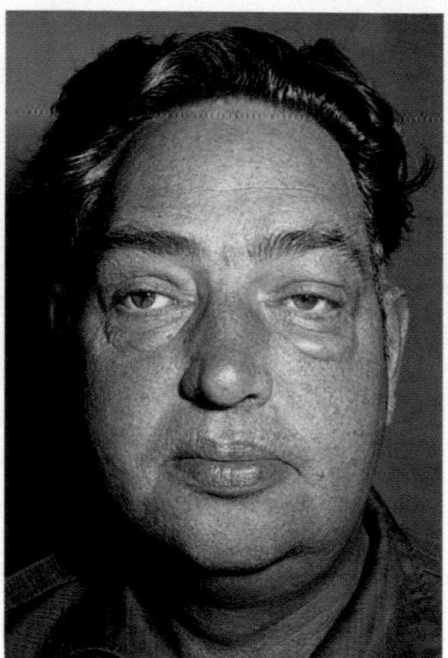

Plate 15.1 Ectopic ACTH syndrome: facial obesity and oedema: patient presented with weakness (due to hypokalaemia) and thyroid mass. At surgery medullary thyroid carcinoma confirmed.

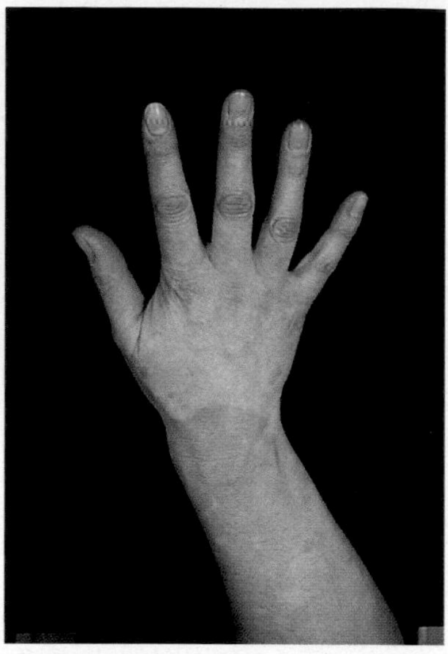

Plate 16.1 Vitiligo of hand: further areas of depigmentation were present on legs and neck. Patient presented with classical Addison's disease, and found to have co-existent asymptomatic hypothyroidism. Patient's sister had Hashimoto's disease.

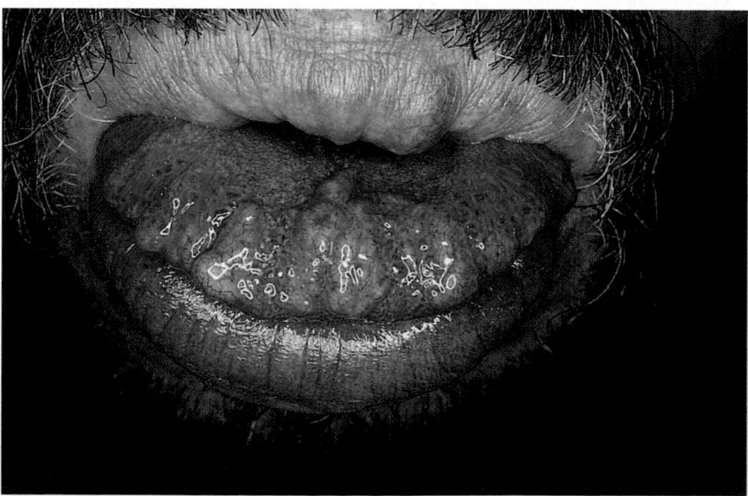

Plate 16.2 Multiple mucosal neuromas in the MEN-2 syndrome: patient presented with hypertension shown to be due phaeochromocytoma. Serum calcitonin raised: thyroidectomy revealed multifocal medullary thyroid carcinoma.

back inhibition. The HCG molecular structure is in fact remarkably similar to LH, and its binds to the luteal LH receptors.

The secretion of HCG begins soon after fertilization and its concentration in the maternal circulation reaches a peak about 50–60 days after the last menstrual bleed. The plasma concentration then falls quite sharply to reach a new level which remains relatively constant until the end of pregnancy. A second, smaller increase is observed between weeks 28–36 of pregnancy (see Fig. 8.9).

It is generally accepted that HCG is luteotrophic during the first weeks of pregnancy and its main role is to maintain the activity of the corpus luteum until the fetoplacental unit becomes endocrinologically autonomous — some 6–7 weeks after fertilization. It also appears to be a potent stimulator of placental progesterone synthesis.

Since HCG can be detected in the blood long after the fetoplacental unit has assumed the role of oestrogen and progesterone synthesis, it is likely that it has other functions. One possibility is that it stimulates the fetal production of dehydroepiandrosterone which can then be converted to oestrogens by the placenta. In the male fetus, HCG stimulates the interstitial cells of Leydig which then begin to secrete testosterone. The small quantities of testosterone produced at this stage stimulate the development of the male sex organs.

Because HCG is only produced by a developing trophoblast, the measurement of its concentration in the maternal blood is used to monitor the health of the trophoblast. In addition, the detection of HCG in the urine forms the basis of the pregnancy test which becomes positive approximately 28 days after conception. The development of a radioimmunoassay to detect the presence of an HCG subunit

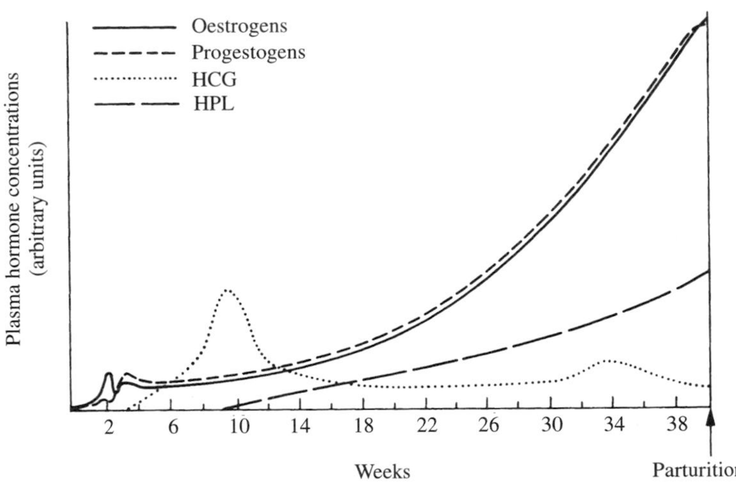

Fig. 8.9. The pattern of changes in maternal plasma hormone concentrations which might be expected during pregnancy. (HCG, human chorionic gonadotrophin; HPL, human placental lactogen, somatomammotrophin.)

in maternal serum now provides a diagnosis of pregnancy even before the first missed period.

Human placental lactogen (HPL)

As HCG production declines after 50–60 days, the syncytiotrophoblast (placenta) begins to secrete another hormone called human placental lactogen (HPL) in increasing quantities. The level of HPL in maternal blood increases steadily throughout the pregnancy, and flattens off towards term. The hormone is a protein consisting of 191 amino acids and is structurally similar to the two adenohypophysial hormones, somatotrophin and prolactin. Its activity resembles that of prolactin; it has very little somatotrophin-like activity.

The precise role of HPL in pregnancy is not yet appreciated. However, it does have several different actions which include lactogenic and growth-promoting effects. Mammotrophic and luteotrophic properties have also been described. In addition, HPL has a lipolytic action and could thus provide an alternative source of energy to glycogenolysis in the mother. The anti-insulin effect of HPL may be responsible for the 'diabetogenic' changes of pregnancy.

Since its production appears to be related to placental (and fetal) weight its concentration in maternal blood serves as a valuable indicator of fetal well-being. Decreasing levels of HPL during early pregnancy suggest that abortion may be inevitable, or if occurring later may indicate placental insufficiency.

Progesterone

The plasma concentration of progesterone rises steadily throughout pregnancy, reaching peak concentrations of approximately 500 nmol/l just before the beginning of labour. The source of progesterone is initially the maintained corpus luteum, but the placenta gradually takes over as principal production site. The placental progesterone can only use cholesterol as the substrate, and not acetate. The cholesterol is usually derived from the maternal circulation. The mechanisms involved in the control of placental progesterone secretion have not yet been determined (but see HCG above). Placental progesterone enters both maternal and fetal circulations, but its function in the fetus is unclear.

The principal urinary excretory product is pregnanediol, but measurement of its concentration during pregnancy serves as an indicator of placental function only to a limited extent since normal levels can vary enormously.

Oestrogens

During pregnancy, the fetoplacental unit becomes the primary source of the steadily increasing plasma oestrogen concentration. Both fetal and maternal adrenals synthesize dehydroepiandrosterone sulphate (DHEAS) and this precursor is deconjugated and aromatized to oestrogens by the placenta. Approximately half of the DHEAS is derived from the fetal adrenals. However, the principal oestrogen produced by the placenta is oestriol with only relatively small quantities of 17β-oestradiol and oestrone being produced. The placental synthesis of oestriol

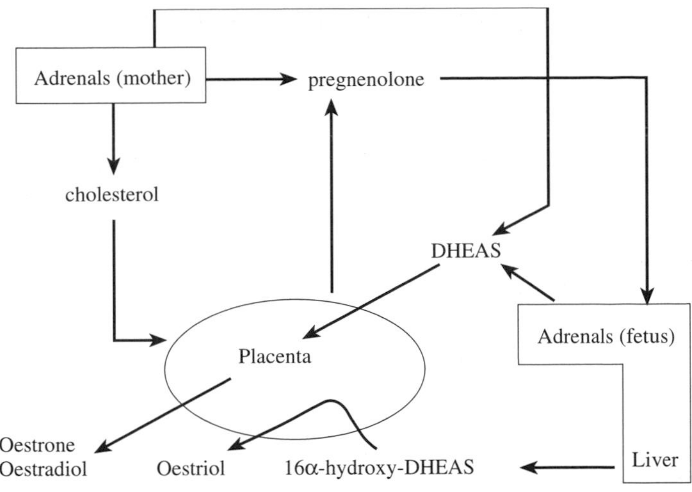

Fig. 8.10. The synthesis of oestrogens by the fetoplacental unit

requires the precursor 16α-hydroxy-DHEA-sulphate which is derived solely from the fetus, while oestradiol and oestrone production depend equally on fetal and maternal DHEAS (Fig. 8.10).

During late pregnancy, the maternal plasma concentration of oestriol is of the order of 400 nmol/l (110 ng/ml) and 17β-oestradiol is approximately 50 nmol/l (15 ng/ml). The measurement of daily urinary oestrogen excretion is used to assess fetoplacental function throughout pregnancy. When fetal function is adversely affected there is a greater fall in oestriol excretion than in total oestrogen excretion.

Maternal hormones

During pregnancy, the adenohypophysis is enlarged and the secretions of corticotrophin, thyrotrophin, and somatotrophin are increased. As indicated earlier, gonadotrophin secretion is inhibited throughout pregnancy.

Adrenal corticosteroid production increases steadily to reach peak levels at parturition. Since plasma protein synthesis is increased during pregnancy it was originally believed that the increase in total cortisol levels resulted from the increase in protein-bound hormone. However, it now appears that the free cortisol component actually increases threefold in late pregnancy. The physiological effects of increased cortisol production during pregnancy remain obscure. Aldosterone production is increased, and this, together with the renal effects of oestrogens and progesterone, causes increased sodium reabsorption from the renal nephron, and hence induces expansion of the extracellular fluid volume.

The thyroid gland may enlarge by approximately 50 per cent during pregnancy as a result of increased thyrotrophin production but only the total thyroxine and triiodothyronine concentrations are raised due to increased protein binding, and hyperthyroidism does not occur.

The parathyroids also often increase in size and activity, possibly induced by the increasing requirement for calcium by the growing fetus. Increased quantities of parathormone are believed to be secreted in order to maintain the maternal calcium level by mobilizing bone calcium, enhancing the absorption of calcium from the gastrointestinal tract (through its action on vitamin D metabolism) and decreasing its renal excretion (see Chapter 10).

Finally, a polypeptide called relaxin isolated from the corpora lutea of ovaries causes the relaxation of the ligaments of the symphysis pubis (also induced by oestrogens and progesterone), a softening of the cervix at the time of delivery, and inhibits uterine motility. Whether these possible effects of relaxin are essential for the passage of the fetus at parturition is still debatable.

Parturition

Parturition is the process by which the fetus is expelled from the uterus at term. Expulsion of the fetus requires both a relaxation of the cervix as well as co-ordinated contractions of the myometrium. The trigger which initiates the process of parturition is still unclear. However, there is evidence in various species, such as the goat and sheep, to suggest that a key factor is the maturation of the fetal hypothalamo–adenohypophysial-adrenal axis resulting in the increased production of adrenal cortisol. In humans, too, there is evidence for an increase in the fetal production of cortisol before parturition. The cortisol may play a crucial role in stimulating enzymes necessary for diverting the conversion of androgen precursors from progesterone to oestrogen. This could be a local event limited to the fetoplacental unit, so that the detection of changes in the ratio of progesterone to oestrogen in the general circulation of the mother might not be possible.

The myometrium

During pregnancy, the mass of the uterine muscle (the myometrium) increases markedly due to an increase in the size of the muscle fibres. The muscle fibres are interconnected by gap junctions and function as a syncytium, so that the flow of electrical current spreads rapidly from cell to cell and allows for a co-ordinated muscular contraction. The contractile process requires the movement of calcium ions from extracellular fluid and/or intracellular storage sites into the cytoplasm where they can bind to the troponin proteins associated with the contractile myosin. The binding of Ca^{2+} to the troponin molecule allows actin proteins to react with the myosin, and as a result of the activation process, a contraction of muscle can develop. Relaxation of the muscle is produced by re-uptake of Ca^{2+} by the intracellular storage sites. The contractile process is influenced greatly by various hormones which will now be briefly considered (Fig. 8.11).

Oestrogens and progestogens

Progesterone is associated with the hyperpolarization of the uterine myometrium, while an oestrogen-dominated uterus shows spontaneous pacemaker potentials and

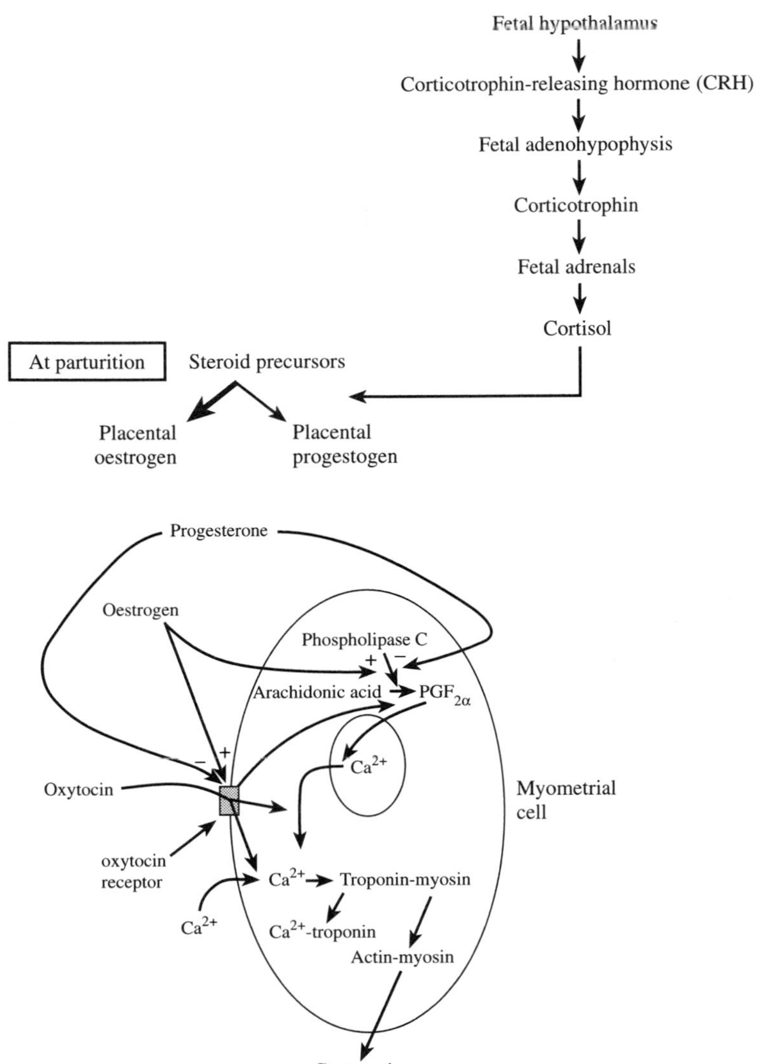

Fig. 8.11. Diagram showing how hormones can increase intracellular Ca^{2+} in myometrial cells during parturition.

cell membrane depolarization. When potentials exceed threshold a burst of spike potentials is propagated across the muscle and this leads to a muscular contraction. Furthermore, oestrogens stimulate the synthesis of oxytocin receptors and intracellular prostaglandins while progesterone inhibits these processes. Oxytocin increases the intracellular concentration of calcium ions through a membrane-mediated effect and by mobilizing intracellular calcium, while prostaglandin increases the movement of calcium from intracellular stores into the cytoplasm (see below). In contrast, progesterone exerts the opposite effects. Thus, an oestrogen-dominated myometrium would be more susceptible to contraction than a progesterone-dominated uterus.

Just before term, the oestrogen to progesterone ratio is often such that the uterus is oestrogen-dominated. Indeed, the increased secretion of placental oestrogens (relative to progesterone), which may initiate parturition, could be produced as a result of increased fetal cortisol synthesis from its progesterone precursor, at least in some species. However, there is little evidence for an increased oestrogen to progesterone ratio just before parturition in women, according to measurements made in blood samples, although such a change need only be local to the myometrium for it to be effective.

Prostaglandins

Prostaglandins (PG) are now believed to play a crucial role in the process of parturition. Recent studies have indicated that $PGF_{2\alpha}$ concentrations in amniotic fluid increase prior to parturition and then continue to rise during the actual birth. The precise cause for the increased production of this prostaglandin has not yet been established. However, as mentioned above, there is evidence to suggest that oestrogens stimulate, and progesterone inhibits, PGF_2 release in the uterus. In addition, oxytocin stimulates uterine PGF_2 release directly.

The prostaglandins are believed to stimulate uterine contractility by increasing the release of Ca^{2+} from the intracellular binding sites.

Oxytocin

Oxytocin is released in pulses from the neurohypophysis during parturition probably as a result of the neuroendocrine reflex initiated by uterine stretch receptors. Oxytocin then stimulates Ca^{2+} influx into uterine muscle as well as decreasing the excitation threshold of the muscle cells.

It is important to remember that oxytocin tends to be effective in an oestrogen-dominated uterus, such as is often the case during labour. In some species, oestradiol stimulates the synthesis of endometrial oxytocin receptors while progesterone has an opposite effect. Therefore, part of the action of the sex steroids on PGF_2 may be mediated by changes in oxytocin receptor numbers.

Oxytocin is also released through the mediation of a neurogenic reflex as the cervix is stretched when the fetus is pushed downwards by the uterine contractions. In addition, as the cervix dilates it may elicit uterine contractions directly, either through a nervous or myogenic reflex.

The cervix

The cervix is prepared for the delivery of the fetus by a process which involves the 'softening' of the tissue due to a decrease in collagen content and their linkage by glycosaminoglycans. Prostaglandins increase the distensibility of the cervix and this is probably one of their important actions prior to, and during, parturition.

The possible role of the polypeptide relaxin in the softening process of the cervix remains speculative since its production by the corpus luteum is maximal during the first trimester after which it decreases, and removal of the corpus luteum of pregnancy after the seventh week of gestation does not appear to be detrimental to the process of parturition.

Lactation

The production of milk is the chief function of the breasts. In the female the breasts develop at puberty, but normally only become functional at parturition. Various hormones are involved in developing and maintaining the breasts, including the gonadal oestrogen and progesterone hormones, and adenohypophysial somatotrophin and prolactin. As described previously, oestrogen stimulates the development of the duct system in the breast while progesterone stimulates growth of the alveoli. However, somatotrophin and adrenocorticosteroids also appear to be necessary for the full development of the ductile system, and prolactin is required for the complete development of the alveolar lobules. During pregnancy, oestrogen, progesterone, and HPL are produced by the placenta in large quantities and it is chiefly in response to these hormones that the breasts develop fully at this stage. Delivery of the child results in an immediate decrease in progesterone levels following the loss of the placenta; the oestrogen concentration also decreases, but less dramatically. This withdrawal of placental hormones results in hormonal domination of the breasts by prolactin which, in the presence of insulin, adrenal corticosteroids, and thyroid hormones, initiates the secretion of milk into the duct system. Release of prolactin is believed to be due at least partly to an inhibition of the release of the hypothalamic inhibitory factor dopamine. Milk will not necessarily flow out of the ducts to the nipple unless suckling takes place. If this occurs, the tactile stimulation of the nipple results in a neuroendocrine reflex release of the neurohypophysial hormone oxytocin which stimulates contraction of the myoepithelial cells surrounding the alveoli, and the smooth muscle of the ductile system. Milk is forced into the main ducts of the breast which ultimately connect to the nipple so that milk ejection can take place (Fig. 8.12).

The plasma basal concentrations of prolactin decrease after birth. However, suckling stimulates the release not only of oxytocin but also of prolactin. Hence, neuroendocrine reflexes are responsible for the secretion of both hormones; an ideal situation, in that the secretion and expulsion of milk from the lactating breasts occur together.

The menopause

As the ovaries begin to run out of ova, plasma inhibin and oestrogen levels begin to fall and (because of a reduced negative feedback) the plasma LH, and particularly FSH, levels begin to rise; consequently, menstrual cycles become more irregular. A perimenopausal condition arises in the early stages of the climacteric (the period of increasingly irregular cycles) when LH and FSH levels are at the upper level of the normal range. Interestingly, it is the plasma FSH concentration which shows the more marked increase perimenopausally, presumably because of the loss of the negative feedback effect of inhibin specifically on this gonadotrophin. It is possible that the accelerated loss of ova in the pre- or perimenopausal

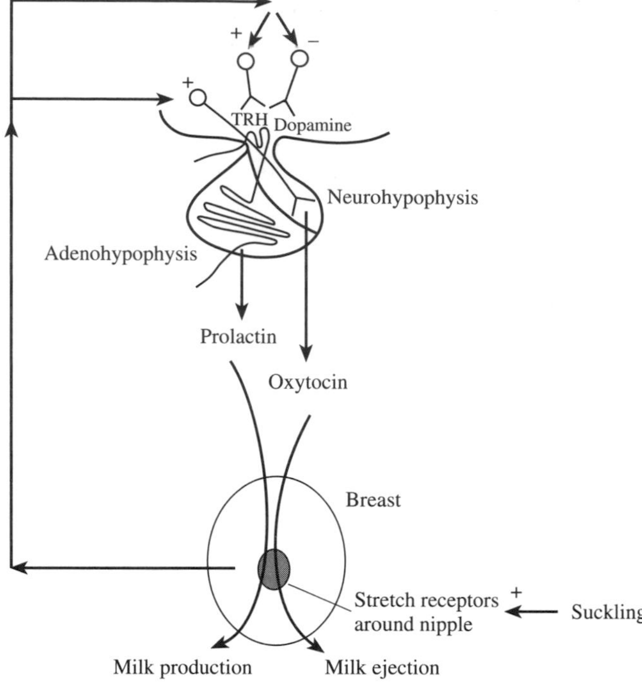

Fig. 8.12. The hormonal control of milk production and ejection during lactation.

phase is linked directly to the raised FSH concentration which stimulates increased numbers of ova to enter ovarian cycles. The menopause itself is the time when the cycles cease completely. At this stage, there are no more ova to ripen, gonadal steroid levels in the plasma are reduced and consequently gonadotrophin levels are raised. With the decrease in ovarian oestrogens, symptoms are associated with the loss of maintenance effects on the reproductive tract and other tissues, an increase in osteoporesis (increased incidence of fractures) and an increased incidence of atherosclerosis and cardiovascular disease. The roles of oestrogen in bone metabolism and cardiovascular regulation are unclear, but certainly oestrogen-replacement therapy is beneficial in many women (see clinical section). Another common problem of the menopause in many women is the 'hot flush' which often occurs at night. The aetiology of this particular symptom is unknown, although it does appear to be related to the hypothalamic production of GnRH.

CLINICAL DISORDERS

Ovulation and the failure to ovulate

The most common endocrine disorders in the female are disturbances of the menstrual cycle. Bearing in mind the broad range of normality, whether such a disturbance is pathological may be difficult to determine. The range extends from a regular cycle of between 25 and 29 days to infrequent or reduced menstrual loss every few weeks or months (oligomenorrhoea). The effect of emotional factors on this rhythm is well recognized, and will be dealt with later. Relative or absolute infertility is commonly but not invariably associated with oligo- or a-menorrhoea. This section will deal with identification of ovulation and subsequently with the causes of anovulation.

Investigations

It is impossible to be certain purely on clinical grounds that ovulation is occurring. The only absolute proof of ovulation is pregnancy, but there are other observations and routine investigations which may help in assessment. These observations and investigations are as follows:

1. *The menstrual cycle.* A regular cycle and dysmenorrhoea suggest, but do not prove, that ovulation is occurring. Conversely, the woman with amenorrhoea is unlikely to be ovulating, although should this occur and fertilization be successful, it can cause considerable confusion in calculating the length of gestation. Sometimes women notice lower abdominal pain for a brief period at ovulation (*Mittleschmerz*).

2. *Basal temperature chart.* The body temperature dips during the follicular phase, and then rises at the time of ovulation. This rise is a direct effect of progesterone. The temperature change can be used to time ovulation, both in those who want to conceive and in those who do not.

3. *Measurement* of *progesterone levels.* A serum progesterone level of 20 nmol/l or more, 7 days before menstruation (i.e. 7 days after ovulation) usually indicates the formation of a corpus luteum, although the normal luteal phase range is 5–60 nmol/l.

Twenty-four hour urinary pregnanediol excretion is also increased, an end-product of progesterone metabolism which is easily measured. The serum progesterone level is nevertheless the most useful test.

4. *Vaginal smears.* This is easily obtained even in a virgin and on cytological examination may reveal characteristic cellular changes in the presence of luteal phase progesterone levels. In addition, the following vaginal smear characteristics are of interest rather than necessarily of diagnostic value.

(a) *Spinnbarkheit.* The effect of rising oestrogen levels up to the ovulatory peak is to thin out cervical mucus. At the time of ovulation a drop of mucus can be placed on a microscope slide, a second slide placed on top of it and the two slides then separated. Well-oestrogenized mucus will form a thread of 7–8 cm before breaking. After ovulation, the effect of progesterone reduces the length of the thread to a centimetre or two.

(b) *Ferning.* On the same principle, well-oestrogenized cervical mucus, when allowed to dry on a slide and examined under the microscope shows a typical 'fern leaf' pattern. This also disappears after ovulation due to the effect of progesterone.

5. *Visualization of the corpus luteum* by laparoscopy is good evidence for ovulation having occurred.

6. *Endometrial biopsy*. Histological examination of the endometrium will show secretory changes in the second half of the cycle if ovulation has occurred.

Failure of ovulation may present as 'primary' or 'secondary' amenorrhoea. Although this is the conventional classification it may be confusing because 'primary' and 'secondary' are terms used differently in other spheres of endocrinology. In the context of amenorrhoea, 'primary' refers to the situation where no menstruation has previously occurred, while 'secondary' refers to the loss of periods after previously normal or (often) irregular cycles.

Primary amenorrhoea

The onset of menarche, which can vary, is controlled by the hypothalamic–adenohypophysial axis. The majority of girls in developed countries have their first period between the ages of 10 and 16, and more than 50 per cent will be menstruating by the age of 13. The age of onset of the menarche has been falling over the past 100 years but is now flattening out. It is reasonable to delay investigating primary amenorrhoea until the age of 17 years, unless secondary sex characteristics have developed (i.e. there is a disparity between physical development and the onset of menstruation) or there are other physical signs or symptoms which suggest chromosomal or hormonal abnormalities.

Causes

Cryptomenorrhoea

This term means 'hidden menstruation' and is not true amenorrhoea, as the uterus does in effect shed its endometrium. The menstrual loss is unable to escape due to a transverse septum in the vagina or complete vaginal atresia. The diagnosis is made from a history of cyclical lower abdominal pain with 'menstrual symptoms'. A transverse septum is treated simply by a cruciate incision which allows free drainage. The complete absence of a vagina is a much more difficult problem and plastic surgery is necessary in order to 'construct' one. Occasionally, the only defect is a failure of utero-vaginal continuity when once again plastic surgery is employed to form a connecting channel. There is no endocrine abnormality present.

Delayed menarche

Primary amenorrhoea may be due to an idiopathic and essentially physiological delay in the onset of menstruation: history often reveals that the patient's mother had a similar problem. This diagnosis is usually made after other causes have been excluded, and often retrospectively. Curiously, the associated short stature so often seen in males with delayed puberty (small delay syndrome) is less frequently seen in females. Investigations reveal serum oestrogen, LH, and FSH to all be low. Although the condition is by definition self-limiting, a short course of oestrogen, pulsatile GnRH, or gonadotrophin is sometimes used to accelerate development and to initiate menstruation. Providing the treatment course is kept to 4 months or less, it is without adverse effect: in particular, there is then no risk of the accelerated epiphyseal fusion which could lead to an impairment of final adult stature.

Chromosomal disorders: Turner's syndrome (see Plates 13.1 and 13.2)
Chromosomal abnormalities can be expected in one-third of girls with primary amenorrhoea by the age of 18. Chromosomal analysis is therefore an essential investigation. The most common abnormality is gonadal dysgenesis (Turner's syndrome) due to loss of an X chromosome during meiosis, resulting in a 45 XO karyotype. The other features of the classical syndrome (marked short stature, ptosis, excess of cutaneous moles, wide carrying angle, webbed neck, and in 30 per cent of cases, either horseshoe kidney and/or coarctation of the aorta) make it likely that the diagnosis will have been made before primary amenorrhoea becomes the significant complaint. However, there may be few or none of these other clinical signs in patients with mosaic forms of gonadal dysgenesis, such as XO/XX, where amenorrhoea and short stature may be the only features.

Patients with gonadal dysgenesis have fibrous 'streak' ovaries and do not usually ovulate (XO/XX mosaics may have a unilateral gonad and ovulate occasionally, while XO/XY mosaics may have unilateral or bilateral ovo-testes with features of masculinization). All cases have poorly developed secondary sex characteristics due to the low level of oestrogens: LH and FSH levels are as expected, markedly raised due to reduced oestrogen feedback.

Menstruation, some growth in stature, and development of secondary sex characteristics can be stimulated by cyclical oestrogen therapy. After a few months, progestogen is added cyclically, in order to regularize the menstrual cycle, and more importantly to reduce the significant risk of endometrial carcinoma when 'unopposed' oestrogen is used. However, despite oestrogen replacement, stature remains very small due to the growth-determining effect of the short arm of the missing X chromosome, and mature height above 57 inches (145 cm) is unusual. The anabolic steroid, oxandrolone, has been used with some success in an attempt to stimulate growth without prematurely stimulating epiphyseal fusion. Human growth hormone has also been used successfully, using doses higher than physiological replacement, and with ultimate mature height some 4–5 cm greater than would otherwise have been the case. There is a significant risk of malignant transformation (gonadoblastoma) in the ovo-testis of XO/XY mosaic forms of Turner's syndrome, so that in these cases, gonadectomy is always performed prophylactically.

The development of egg donation/*in vitro* fertilization techniques has made it possible for patients with gonadal dysgenesis to conceive.

Congenital adrenal hyperplasia
It is possible for a patient with mild forms of late-presenting congenital adrenal hyperplasia to actually present with primary amenorrhoea; there is usually associated hirsutism and accompanying signs of virilism (see Chapter 5).

Primary hypothalamic pituitary disease
Patients with hypogonadotrophic hypogonadism rarely present as primary amenorrhoea, except in the eating disorders mentioned later. However, the occasional non-functioning pituitary adenoma or craniopharyngioma may present at quite a young age.

Testicular feminization
Patients in this category are genetically male but have a complete or partial androgen receptor defect. So-called complete forms are phenotypically (physically) female with normal breast development, a normal or small introitus and a clitoris which is in fact a micropenis with associated hypospadias. Cases may only be discovered when they present with infertility! Incomplete forms representing partial androgen insensitivity also occur, particularly in childhood, and in the context of investigation of the diagnostic dilemma of intersex. Chromosome analysis reveals an XY karyotype: testosterone and FSH levels are usually within normal male ranges, and serum LH often raised.

The testes may be abdominal or inguinal, and because of the malignant potential of ectopic testes, orchidectomy is usually performed if the testes can be located (which is not always possible). Treatment in the complete form may not be necessary, while in the incomplete form, management depends on many factors, including the extent of psychosocial and sexual adjustment and the extent of anatomical abnormality. Extensive genital reconstruction is often necessary, and psychosexual support and counselling mandatory.

Other causes
Many of the causes of secondary amenorrhoea detailed below, such as panhypopituitarism, prolactinoma, and the polycystic ovarian syndrome may rarely be responsible also for primary amenorrhoea.

Secondary amenorrhoea (where menstruation has previously occurred)

Causes

Benign androgen excess: polycystic ovarian disease (see Plate 8.1)
The Stein–Leventhal syndrome was first described in 1935. The originally description included obesity, hirsutism, infertility, polycystic ovaries, and oligomenorrhoea, although it is now recognized that women with polycystic ovary syndrome (PCOD) may show no abnormal clinical features at all, or at most have oligo–or amenorrhea. In fact, PCOD is the most common cause of secondary amenorrhoea, and in population studies, characteristic ultrasound features are seen in 10 per cent of the female population.

Clinical Features The typical range of clinical features of these patients depends to some extent on the degree of testosterone and other androgen elevation. They include infertility, oligo- or amenorrhoea, acne, frontal (male pattern) balding, and varying degrees of hirsutism. The distribution of pathological hair is highly variable, most commonly affecting upper lip, chin, and sideburn areas, as well as lower abdomen and medial aspects of thighs. Obesity increases the likelihood of menstrual irregularity, and by lowering sex-hormone-binding globulin (SHBG), obesity also increases free testosterone activity and hence hirsutism. As mentioned above patients may show no clinical abnormality whatsoever.

Pathophysiology While it is accepted that the normal ovaries secrete testosterone, together with the less active androstenedione and dehydroepiandrosterone, the quantities secreted are insufficient to induce hirsutism. The adrenal cortex is normally the main source of androgens in the female. However, in PCOD, androgen secretion is of ovarian as well as adrenal origin. In addition, the activity of the skin enzyme 5α-reductase which is responsible for dihydrotestosterone (DHT) synthesis may vary between individuals, and therefore condition the cutaneous response to a given level of circulating androgen.

Most patients with PCOD have raised levels of testosterone and androstenedione, and SHBG is usually decreased even without obesity, resulting in an increased free (biologically active) fraction, often referred to as the free androgen index (testosterone:SHBG ratio). When these simple analyses are performed, the entity of true 'idiopathic' hirsutism is seen to be very rare.

Although the precise role of the adrenal gland in this syndrome is uncertain, the results of adrenal and ovarian stimulation (ACTH and/or gonadotrophin) or suppression (dexamethasone and/or oestradiol) tests indicate that the adrenals in some patients make a significant contribution. Accordingly, it has been assumed that in many cases, hyperandrogenism reflects a generalized disorder of steroid-producing tissue. Nevertheless, the precise aetiology of the endocrine changes is unknown, and hypothalamic as well as primary steroid abnormalities have been postulated, and supported by research findings. It is possible that a wide variety of genetic and conceivably environmental triggers may be responsible for the diversity of both clinical and biochemical features. The characteristic ultrasound appearance of peripherally situated ovarian cysts within enlarged ovaries is now the single most important diagnostic finding. (see Fig. 8.13.)

It has been shown that most patients with PCOD manifest insulin resistance: for a given glucose level, insulin levels are abnormally elevated. This is a phenomenon which also occurs in obesity alone, and is therefore more striking still when obesity and PCOD coexist. The reason for this association is unclear: some evidence supports a primary role for hyperinsulism in the genesis of the hyperandrogenaemia, perhaps acting through somatomedins. Glucose intolerance or even overt diabetes (of the non-insulin-dependent type) is therefore common in PCOD, especially if obese. Since insulin resistance is known to be associated both with hyperlipidaemia and early onset atherosclerosis, particularly of the coronary vessels, PCOD may prove to have significant long-term morbidity and mortality implications.

A particularly striking degree of insulin resistance is seen in the HAIR-AN syndrome, so-called because of the association of hyperandrogenism with insulin resistance, and the rare condition of *acanthosis nigricans.* This latter condition

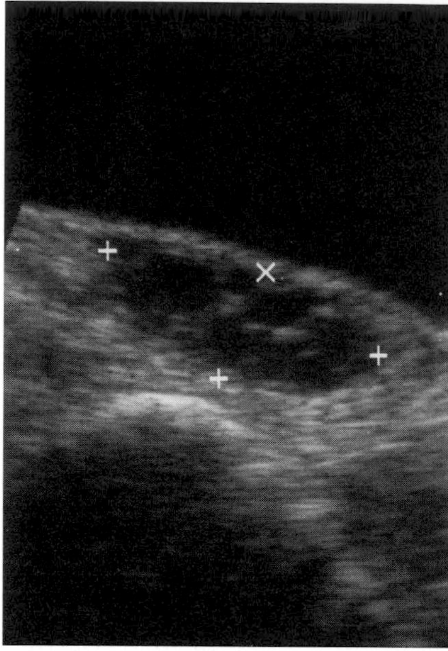

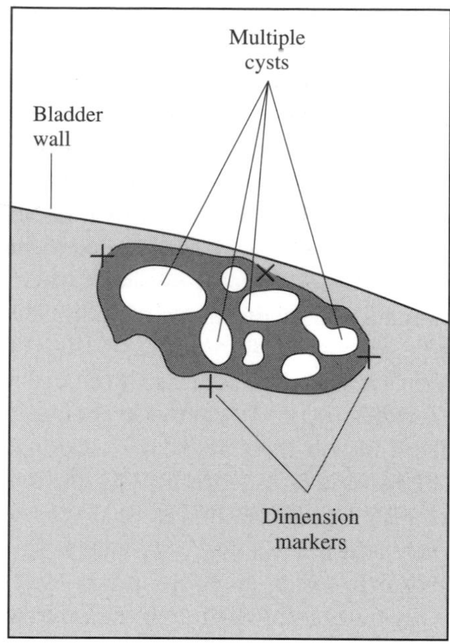

Fig. 8.13. Pelvic ultrasound of a patient with polycystic, peripherally situated cysts in enlarged ovaries.

manifests itself as hyperplastic, ridged, and darkened skin seen most frequently in axillary folds and in the neck.

Differential diagnosis Hirsutism may be due to other factors, and these must be considered in the initial approach to diagnosis (see Table 8.1).

The differential diagnosis of hirsutism is not always easy. True virilism, as manifest by voice deepening, muscular hypertrophy, breast atrophy, or clitoral enlargement immediately excludes PCOD, and focuses attention on all the other pathological processes listed in Table 8.1. The precise diagnostic tests required are dealt with elsewhere, under the titles of the respective conditions.

Table 8.1. The major causes of hirsutism

Ovarian:
- Benign androgen excess (including the polycystic ovary syndrome, PCOD)
- Ovarian masculinizing tumours (hilus cell, arrhenoblastoma, gynandroblastoma)

Adrenal:
- Androgen-producing adenoma or carcinoma
- Cushing's disease or syndrome
- Congenital adrenal hyperplasia

Other:
- Oral contraceptives with androgenic progestogen, phenytoin
- Hyperprolactinaemia

Management The treatment of PCOD is complex. Simple cosmetic depilatory creams and waxes satisfy many patients and electrolysis (in expert hands) is of value with more sparse, darker hairs. However, in all cases a detailed social history is essential, since a number of patients have major psychosocial problems which render comparatively minor hirsutism a major problem of stigma and self-consciousness. In these cases, the management of the whole patient is of greater significance than that of the hirsutism.

In some patients with more severe degrees of hirsutism affecting the face, the peri-areolar and intermammary areas, the lower back and the sideburn area, simple cosmetic approaches, including shaving, are rarely acceptable. It has been shown that the administration of oestrogens can suppress androgen production through a combination of LH suppression, increase of SHBG concentration, and down-regulation of androgen receptors. Over a period of 6–12 months, oestrogens can produce some clinical improvement but never complete control of hirsutism: this period of treatment is necessary for the hair cycle to be restored from terminal hair production towards a more normal vellus hair pattern. It is important to use a form of contraceptive pill which includes a progestogen which is non-androgenic (e.g. desogestrel or cyproterone).

Additional benefits may result from the use of corticosteroids which suppress the adrenal component. However, the potential disadvantages of necessarily long-term therapy often outweigh the benefits and this form of therapy is not frequently used.

Using comparatively high dosage, the drugs cyproterone (50–100 mg daily) and spironolactone (100–200 mg daily) have been shown to possess peripheral anti-androgenic effects. Used with or without oestrogen, they represent appropriate drugs for more severe cases. Other approaches may prove to be valuable. Drugs which inhibit cutaneous 5α-reductase, such as finasteride, may prove very valuable. A direct approach to reversing hyperinsulinaemia has also been proposed, and drugs for achieving this are still under development.

Partial or wedge resection of the ovary has been used for many years to induce ovulation, a procedure which resulted from a 60-year-old observation that ovarian biopsy sometimes induced a temporary restoration of menstrual cycles. Other surgical procedures, capable of being performed laparoscopically, are being assessed. However, anovulation eventually recurs in most patients after these interventions. The anti-oestrogen clomiphene, acting by blocking oestrogen feedback to the pituitary (and thereby causing an LH surge) is often successful. Other approaches involve suppressing endogenous LH and FSH by high-dose GnRH agonists, such as buserelin, followed by pulsatile pump-delivered LH administration. However, some patients sadly remain entirely refractory to treatment.

Premature menopause: primary ovarian failure

The menopause occurs in 90 per cent of women between the ages of 48 and 52, although continued secretion of oestrogen may occur for a further 3–5 years. In some women, menopause occurs up to 25 years earlier than this, providing typical 'hot flushes' and other symptoms, noted later in this chapter, as part of the menopausal syndrome. As in the normal menopause, oestrogen levels are low, and LH and FSH elevated. Aetiology is now identified in most instances as a destructive auto-immune process, forming part of the auto-immune endocrinopathy syndrome which also includes pernicious anaemia, hyperthyroidism, Hashimoto's disease, and Addison's disease; see Chapter 16).

Infertility in this condition is obviously irreversible, but oestrogen deficiency should be treated by oestrogen/progestogen replacement to avoid the complications of accelerated osteoporosis and premature atherosclerotic coronary artery disease and stroke.

Hypothalamic or pituitary tumours: prolactinoma

Any tumour of the hypothalamus or of the adenohypophysis may interfere with GnRH or LH/FSH release, and hence ovulation and menstruation are inhibited. Prolactinomas are the most common, sometimes but not invariably associated with galactorrhoea. Rather than tumour tissue physically interfering with cellular function and hormone release, raised prolactin directly inhibits LH and FSH release by a negative feedback loop. Measurement of serum prolactin is accordingly a routine investigation of all patients with any disturbance of ovulation (see Chapter 4). Treatment is very simple, involving the use of one of the many available dopamine agonists, either ergot- or non-ergot-related.

Hyperthyroidism

Amenorrhoea is a common and reversible feature of hyperthyroidism. Oligomenorroea and infertility are also seen. The mechanism is unclear but may reflect the reduction of free oestrogen and androgen induced by an increase in SHBG.

Post-pill amenorrhoea

Approximately 10 per cent of women ceasing oral contraceptives have subsequent irregular or absent menstruation. Some cases are found to have underlying benign androgen excess, others have hyperprolactinaemia. It does not represent a separate entity, and does not appear to be a direct consequence of prolonged hormonal contraception.

Chronic hypothalamic anovulation and anorexia nervosa (see also Chapter 4)

Endocrinologically, these conditions form a continuum. In the former, anxiety and stress (sometimes quite subtle and inapparent) result in inhibition of cerebral–hypothalamic pathways. This is probably an atavistic response to stress and threat which is common within the animal kingdom. In girls, the social trigger of a change of school is not unusual, and indeed amenorrhoea of this type may also be primary. The phenomenon is almost always reversible by reassurance, discussion, and occasionally psychotherapy.

In anorexia (and bulimia) nervosa, a more severe psychiatric disturbance is present associated with marked weight loss due to anorexia, hyperactivity, and often self-induced vomiting and purgation. At a body weight of less than 40 kg or a body mass index (BMI) of approximately 15, amenorrhoea is almost invariable. As anticipated, serum oestrogen, LH, and FSH are all also low in this condition.

Premenstrual tension

This term is used to denote a very variable and complex group of symptoms occurring, as its name implies, at some time during the 10–14 days before menstruation. Fluid retention is often a part of this syndrome and may contribute to other symptoms listed below. There is some evidence to suggest abnormal sensitivity to oestrogen (since anti-oestrogens often abolish the symptoms) or progesterone deficiency. However, it must be emphasized that there may be a considerable emotional component in this condition, and objective measurement of body water compartments may be normal.

Clinical features

The symptoms include a sensation of lower abdominal discomfort, distension, nausea, breast discomfort, and a general 'bloated feeling'. There may be increased frequency of micturition, change of bowel habit, an increase or decrease in acne, and a darkening of the skin under the eyes. There is often quite severe depression and reduction of libido.

Treatment

Treatment includes oral contraceptives in some patients, anti-oestrogens, such as tamoxifen, in others. Progesterone or a related progestogen may be given in the second half of the cycle. Norethisterone 5 mg, a nortestosterone derivative, is given by mouth from the first day that symptoms appear until the onset of menstruation, or as a 400 mg progesterone suppository. In cases of marked fluid retention, diuretics, such as thiazides, are often a valuable addition to therapy. The dopamine agonist, bromocryptine, has been shown to provide benefit in some cases, even in the absence of hyperprolactinaemia. Alternative medicine in the form of acupuncture and hypnosis helps some patients.

The menopause

By definition, menopause is the stage in a woman's life when ovulation, and hence menstruation ceases, usually preceded by a fall in circulating oestrogen. However, the systemic changes associated with the menopause may occur before, or months or years after cessation of menstruation. The menopause may also be associated with psychological consequences: the belief that there is a loss of physical attraction and of 'unwantedness'. At the same time, children are usually at an age when they are seeking their own self-expression outside the home, and the woman feels that she has lost her maternal role. These more social factors cannot be divorced from other psychological changes such as depression, irritability, and lassitude which may be oestrogen-dependent. The woman's reaction to the menopause may in addition be influenced by religious factors. These psychological effects and the social background have to be considered when assessing the significance of the hormonal changes.

The low oestradiol level is responsible for the atrophy of the breasts, labia, uterus, and vaginal epithelium; the associated dryness of the vagina renders this organ more susceptible to infection and results in discomfort during intercourse (dyspareunia). The low oestrogen level of the hormone may contribute to uterine prolapse and susceptibility to bladder infections. The fall of oestrogen levels is partly responsible for a rise in the plasma cholesterol concentration, which contributes to the markedly increased incidence of cardiovascular and cerebrovascular disease. The precise mechanism of menopausal flushes is not certain. Some evidence supports a relationship to pulsatility of LH and FSH and may involve release of prostaglandins. Osteoporosis (see Chapter 10) is accelerated by low oestradiol levels seen in postmenopausal women, and most particularly in premature menopause.

Treatment

It is generally agreed that hormonal replacement therapy (HRT) is justified if typical oestrogen-dependent symptoms are causing distress. Treatment is also mandatory in premature menopause, whether natural or iatrogenic, since both atherosclerotic events and osteoporosis are strikingly less frequent in treated cases.

Nevertheless, there is a gradual progression towards a philosophy of routine oestrogen replacement. Thus, it has been calculated that a 30 per cent reduction in hip and other fractures would result from routine oestrogen replacement, together with a 30–50 per cent reduction in the incidence of myocardial infarction and stroke. Providing that progestogens are co-administered in non-hysterectomized women, the incidence of uterine carcinoma is not increased, and the comparitively small increase in breast tumour incidence is probably insignificant. However, to be effective, oestrogens probably need to be given at least until the age of 70: current data suggest that many patients are, in practice, reluctant to commit themselves in this way and default from therapy.

A more selective approach to HRT may be an attractive alternative. Thus, patients with abnormally low bone density at menopause or with a family history of osteoporosis, and those with either hyperlipidaemia or strong family history of atherosclerosis might be those most benefited by HRT (and also those most motivated to continue treatment for the requisite period).

Oestrogens may be replaced orally using a variety of formulations, including conjugated equine oestrogens and oestradiol. They may also be given by transcutaneous patches (which avoid first pass hepatic metabolism now thought to be metabolically disadvantageous), or by implantation of oestrogen (and sometimes additional androgen) pellets.

A progestogen need only be given with an intact uterus, since there is an increased risk of endometrial carcinoma if unopposed oestrogen is used. A compound with both androgenic and oestrogenic action (tibolone) has been evaluated, and has the advantage of minimizing the ongoing periodic menstrual loss which is not appreciated by the postmenopausal woman. Whether it has all the benefits of other forms of HRT remains to be proven. Similarly, continuous oestrogen and continuous progestogen are being introduced into clinical practice: this formulation also results in little or no 'breakthrough' bleeding.

The immediate benefits of oestrogen replacement are undoubted when severe menopausal symptoms are due to oestrogen deficiency; the benefits are more variable where there is marked emotional overlay. If the major problem is vaginal, an oestrogen cream is of value.

The problem of female infertility

It is clear that by inhibiting regular ovulation, every condition mentioned in this chapter can cause either sub- or infertility. In the systematic evaluation of female infertility (which is outside the scope of this book), confirmation of regular ovulation is the first step. Any defect in ovulation must then be explained, using the approaches mentioned above. Nevertheless, in many instances, female infertility is due to non-endocrine factors, only a few of which are readily amenable to intervention and correction: the reader is referred to gynaecological texts for further discussion on these situations. Finally, some form of egg donation is proving to be the desired approach in many instances.

FURTHER READING

PHYSIOLOGY

Evans, W.S., Sollenberger, M.J., Booth, R.A., jun., Rogol, A.D., Urban, R.J., Carlsen, E.C., *et al.* (1992). Contemparary aspects of discrete peak-detection algorithms. II. The paradigm of the luteinizing hormone pulse signal in women. *Endocrine Reviews,* **13**, 81–104.

Handwerger, S. (1991). The physiology of placental lactogen in human pregnancy. *Endocrine Reviews,* **12**, 329–36.

Johnson, M.M. and Eveitt, B.J. (1995). *Essential reproduction* (Fourth edition). Blackwell Science.

Norman, R.J. and Brannstrom, M. (1994). White cells and the ovary — incidental invaders or essential effectors? *Journal of Endocrinology*, **140**, 333–6.

Richardson, S.J. (1993). The biological basis of the menopause. In *Baillière's clinical endocrinology and metabolism.* Vol. 7, The menopause,. pp. 1–16. Ballière Tindall, London.

Turner, R.T., Riggs, B.L., and Spelsberg, T.C. (1994). Skeletal effects of estrogen. *Endocrine Reviews,* **15**, 275–95.

CLINICAL

Belchetz, P.E. (1994). Hormonal treatment of the postmenopausal woman. *Lancet,* **330**, 1062–71.

Derksen, J., Nagesser, S.K., Meinders, A.A., *et al.* (1994). Identification of virilizing adrenal tumours in hirsute women. *New England Journal of Medicine*, **331**, 968–73.

Dunaif, A., Green, G., Phelps, R.G., *et al.* (1991). Acanthosis nigricans, insulin action and hyperandrogenism: clinical, histological and biochemical findings. *Journal of Clinical Endocrinology and Metabolism,* **73**, 590–5.

Healy, D.L., Trounson, A.O., and Andersen, A.N. (1994). Female infertility: causes and treatment. *Lancet*, **343**, 1539–44.

Jeffcoate, W. (1993). The treatment of women with hirsutism. Clinical Endocrinology, **39**, 143–50.

Penzias, J., Allan, A.S., and de Cherney, A.H. (1994). Advances in clinical *in vitro* fertilization. *Journal of Clinical Endocrinology and Metabolism*, **78**, 503–8.

Randall, V.A. (1994). Androgens and human hair growth. Clinical Endocrinology, **40**, 439–58.

Rodin, A., Thakkar, H, Taylor, N., and Clayton, R. (1994). Hyperandrogenism in polycystic ovary syndrome. *New England Journal of Medicine,* **330**, 460–5.

Saenger, P. (1993). Current status of diagnosis and therapy in Turner's syndrome. *Journal of Clinical Endocrinology and Metabolism*, **77**, 297–301.

9

The thyroid

PHYSIOLOGY

The thyroid gland, so named by Thomas Wharton in 1656, was at that time believed to have nothing more than the cosmetic role of making the neck more shapely. We now appreciate that this important endocrine gland secretes two hormones which have various general effects on metabolism and which are particularly important for normal growth and development. These hormones are iodinated molecules called iodothyronines; they are triiodothyronine (T_3) and tetraiodothyronine (T_4, also known as thyroxine).

Another hormone called thyrocalcitonin (or simply calcitonin, CT) is produced by thyroid parafollicular cells, and is involved in the regulation of calcium metabolism. Detailed consideration of calcitonin is therefore included in Chapter 10.

Development, anatomy, and histology

The thyroid gland develops as a diverticulum in the middle of the floor of the primitive pharynx. The diverticulum becomes bilobed, is diplaced caudally, and eventually fuses with part of the fourth pharyngeal pouch. It is attached to the floor of the pharynx at this stage by the thyroglossal duct which normally disappears by the second month after conception. Only the foramen caecum, at the junction between the anterior two-thirds and the posterior one-third of the developing tongue, remains at its point or origin. The ultimobranchial body from the fifth pouch becomes incorporated into the developing thyroid, and it is thought that it is the source of the parafollicular cells.

The fully developed thyroid is a highly vascular bilobed gland, the two lobes being connected together by a thin band of tissue called the isthmus. It is one of the largest of the endocrine glands in the body, and weighs approximately 20 grams. It lies over the ventral aspect of the trachea to which it is attached by connective tissue. Each lobe of the thyroid receives arterial blood from two sources: the superior thyroid arteries (which arise from the external carotids); and the interior thyroid arteries (from the subclavian arteries). Autonomic nerve fibres (cholinergic and adrenergic) enter the thyroid from the laryngeal nerves.

Under the microscope, thyroid tissue is composed of numerous follicles. Each follicle consists of a central colloid-filled cavity lined by follicular cells. Other cells, called parafollicular cells, are dispersed between the follicles. Enhanced thyroid activity over a prolonged period is usually accompanied by a decrease in colloid (reduced follicular volume) and a hypertrophy and increase in number of the follicular cells, which become columnar and may proliferate into the colloid. Decreased thyroid activity is associated with a flattening of the follicular cells.

The follicular cell cytoplasm contains a microtubular network, and microvilli containing canaliculi project from the apical membrane into the colloid. The follicular cells also have a prominent endoplasmic reticulum. Lysosomes and mitochondria are scattered throughout the cytoplasm.

The iodothyronine hormones (T_3 and T_4)

Synthesis, storage, and release

The synthesis of tri- and tetraiodothyronine involves iodine which is normally ingested in the form of iodides in the diet. The follicular cells concentrate iodide by means of an active pump mechanism closely related to the Na^+K^+-ATPase system in the basal membrane, so that the intracellular iodide concentration is usually 25–50 times greater than the plasma concentration. This process is sometimes called 'iodide trapping'. The thyroid iodine content is normally around 600 μg/g tissue.

Once inside the cell, iodide is rapidly oxidized to a more reactive form (which remains undefined) in the presence of peroxidase enzyme which is located mainly near the apical membrane. The reactive iodine is promptly 'organified' by binding to amino acids and other intracellular units. Most of the reactive iodine is organified by linking to tyrosine amino acids incorporated into thyroproteins as tyrosyl groups. These are important components of a specific thyroidal protein molecule synthesized by the follicular cells, called thyroglobulin. Initially, the various tyrosyl groups are iodinated in one or two possible positions forming mono- and diiodotyrosyl units on the thyroglobulin molecule (see Fig. 9.1). An internal coupling reaction between the various iodinated tyrosyls then occurs as the thyroglobulin undergoes structural alteration. As a result of this coupling reaction some tri- and tetraiodinated thyronine groups are formed, still incorporated within the thyroglobulin protein. These reactions occur mainly at the follicular cell–colloid interface prior to the secretion of the thyroglobulin into the colloid. This protein containing the iodothyronines is then stored in the follicles as a colloid.

The activity of the iodide pump, the organification of the reactive iodine, the synthesis of thyroglobulin, and the coupling reaction are all stimulated by the adenohypophysial hormone, thyrotrophin (also known as thyroid-stimulating hormone, TSH).

When the follicular cells are stimulated by thyrotrophin, colloid is taken into the cells by endocytosis. The intracellular microtubular network may be involved in this process. Once within the cells the colloid droplets fuse with lysosomes containing protease enzymes, which migrate rapidly towards the site of endocytosis. Consequently, the thyroglobulin molecules are degraded and the iodinated units enter the cytoplasm. Mono- and diiodotyrosines are rapidly deiodinated by cytoplasmic dehalogenases and the tyrosyl and iodide residues can then be re-utilized in new thyroglobulin synthesis. Tri- and tetraiodothyronines are released into the

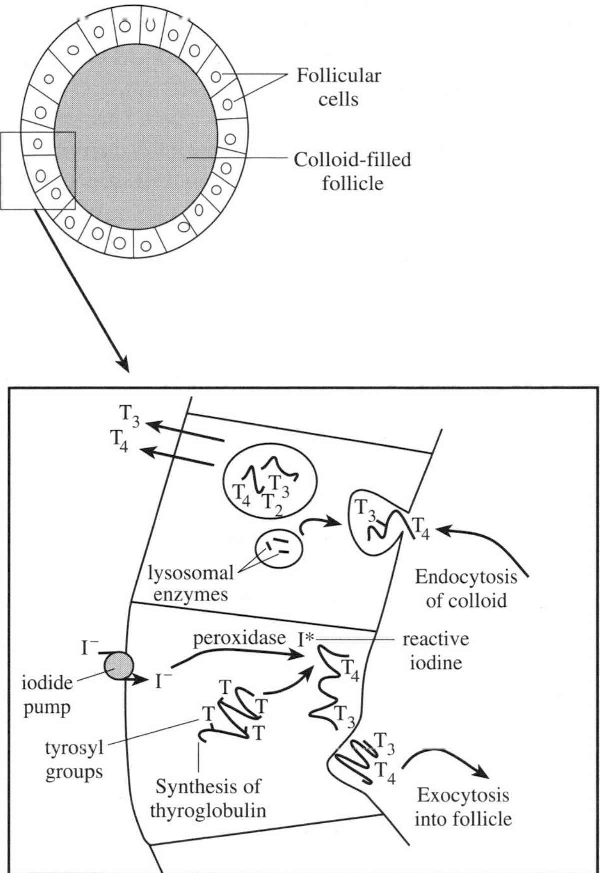

Fig. 9.1. Mechanisms involved in the synthesis of thyroglobulin.

general circulation (see Fig. 9.1). These various processes are stimulated by thyrotrophin.

The main iodothyronine produced by the thyroid gland is thyroxine (T_4). The average T_3 and T_4 concentrations in the thyroid are approximately 0.02 and 0.3 μmol/g, respectively (15 and 200 μg/g), while the plasma concentrations of the two iodothyronines are of the order of 1.4–3.0 nmol/l and 60–160 nmol/l respectively. Plasma concentrations reach a peak soon after birth (probably associated with the surge in thyrotrophin which follows delivery, and which may be induced partly by the sudden decrease in the environmental temperature) but decrease within the first few years to levels which remain relatively unchanged thereafter. Although thyroid disease is more prevalent in women than men, the plasma iodothyronine levels, their production and metabolism are generally similar in both sexes under normal circumstances (but cf. pregnancy, p. 185).

Transport of T_3 and T_4

Once T_3 and T_4 have entered the general circulation they are transported mostly bound to plasma proteins. The T_4 molecule has a high affinity for a glycosylated globulin previously named thyroxine-binding globulin but now more appropriately called thyronine-binding globulin (TBG). It is also transported bound to a pre-albumin (thyroxine binding prealbumin, TBPA) while small quantities are bound to the albumin fraction. Of the total T_4 in the blood over 75 per cent binds to TBG and between 15–20 per cent to the TBPA with less than 0.05 per cent being present unbound (free). T_3 is predominantly transported bound to TBG while very little binds to albumin and practically none to the TBPA. Because of the slightly lower affinity of T_3 for the plasma proteins, the percentage of this hormone present unbound in the plasma is quite high (approximately 0.5 per cent) relative to T_4. The difference between the free components of T_3 and T_4 in the blood probably accounts for at least part of the disparate activities of the two hormones. Therefore T_4 (more avidly bound to plasma proteins) has a longer biological half-life ($t^{1/2}$, approximately 7–9 days) and a longer latent period (approximately 72 hours) than T_3 which has a $t^{1/2}$ of 2 days and a latent period of 12 hours.

Oestrogens decrease the hepatic clearance, and increase the synthesis, of TBG and consequently are associated with an increased circulating pool of iodothyronines (e.g. in pregnancy).

Peripheral conversions

The iodothyronines cross target cell membranes with relative ease. At least part of this transport into some target cells appears to be carrier-mediated. The carriers for T_3 and T_4 are saturable, require ATP, and appear to be influenced by the extracellular Na^+ concentration.

T_4 can be deiodinated to various alternative iodinated forms. By far the most important of these is the conversion of T_4 to the more active T_3. It has been estimated that the normal thyroid gland only contributes some 20 per cent of the extrathyroidal pool of T_3, with the remainder being produced by monodeiodination of the outer tyrosyl groups of T_4 to T_3 by peripheral tissues. This is now believed to be an important mechanism for cellular regulation of the amount of active hormone in the immediate environment since T_3 is more potent than T_4 on a molar basis. Various deiodinases have now been characterized, one (type 1) being active in converting T_4 to T_3 providing the latter molecule to the plasma, while another (type 2) provides T_3 for intracellular use. However, while this cellular conversion mechanism indicates that T_4 is a prohormone (i.e. circulating precursor molecule) it must be emphasized that T_4 is also a hormone in its own right since it produces specific effects and probably has its own specific target receptors.

In addition to the cellular conversion of T_4 to the more potent T_3 there is now evidence for another conversion of T_4 by the same peripheral tissues, with a possible physiological role. This second conversion mechanism is also a deiodination of the T_4 molecule but the iodide removed in this instance is from the inner tyrosyl unit. The resulting metabolite is called reverse T_3. However, this alternative tri-iodothyronine molecule is biologically inactive. Recent estimates suggest that less than 3 per cent of the rT_3 present in the circulation is actually formed within the

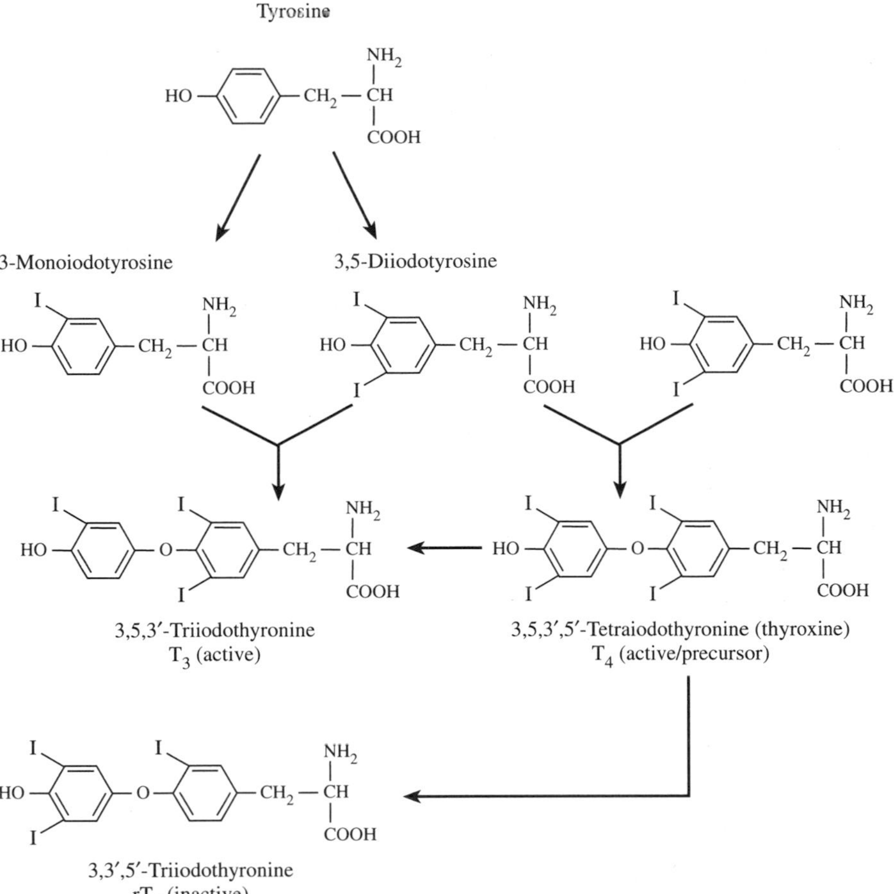

Fig. 9.2. Diagram showing the peripheral conversion of thyroxine (T_4) from the thyroid to the biologically active triiodothyronine (T_3) and the biologically inert reverse triiodothyronine (rT_3).

thyroid gland, the remainder being produced by peripheral tissues conversion. The normal plasma rT_3 concentration has been estimated to be approximately 0.3 nmol/l. Therefore it now seem likely that the peripheral tissues can regulate directly how much active thyroid hormone is present in the immediately vicinity by increasing or decreasing T_4 conversion to either active T_3 or inactive rT_3 (Fig. 9.2). The precise regulators of this switching system have not been determined although nutritional status may be a major factor. Thus, caloric restriction results in preferential reverse-T_3 synthesis, suggesting that the conversion mechanism functions as an energy conservation system.

Actions

Both thyroid hormones T_3 and T_4 are associated with the same general effects on cellular metabolism and activity. The most documented effect is the increase in basal metabolic rate (BMR) which they induce in many tissues. The increase in BMR is associated with an increased oxygen consumption and an increased production of heat (calorigenic effect).

The effects of T_3 and T_4 on metabolism in responsive tissues involve carbohydrates, fats and proteins, and they are at least partly related to the important influence that these hormones have on the processes of growth and development. Other effects of iodothyronines may be indirect and related to important interactions between these hormones and others, such as the catecholamines.

Maternal iodothyronines can cross the placenta, but only in limited quantities; consequently, fetal T_3 and T_4 are vital for stimulating normal growth and development *in utero*.

Metabolic effects

Basal metabolic rate

After the long latent period, thyroxine (and triiodothyronine) increase the basal metabolic activity of most cells in the body, the most notable exceptions being the cells of the brain, spleen, and testes. The BMR can increase by as much as 100 per cent in the presence of excess hormones, or decrease by much as 50–60 per cent in severe hypothyroidism. Associated with the increased BMR is an increase in the number and size of mitochondria and a rise in the intracellular concentrations of many enzymes (e.g. of the respiratory chain). In addition, the iodothyronines increase Na^+K^+-ATPase activity, and an enhanced Na^+ and K^+ transport across the cell membrane is an important component of the hormone-induced increase in energy expenditure.

In the presence of raised iodothyronine levels, the increased BMR is accompanied by a slight rise in body temperature and a lower tolerance of heat as the body's heat-dissipating mechanisms are stimulated. Not surprisingly, when there is a decrease in circulating iodothyronines there is a decreased tolerance of the cold.

Carbohydrate metabolism

All aspects of carbohydrate metabolism are increased by T_3 and T_4 directly (e.g. due to stimulation of enzyme systems), and indirectly by potentiation of the effects of other hormones. There is an increase in the rate of absorption of glucose by the intestinal tract, an increased uptake of glucose by peripheral cells, such as muscle and adipose tissue, and enhanced glycolysis and gluconeogenesis as well as glycogenolysis. However, insulin-induced glycogenesis is also increased. Some of these effects are probably at least partly due to potentiation of the actions of other hormones, such as the catecholamines and insulin. Furthermore, many of the effects of iodothyronines on carbohydrate metabolism appear to be dose-dependent, accounting for the biphasic actions often reported.

Fat metabolism

As result of the generalized increase in cellular metabolic activity, the iodothyronines stimulate lipolysis in adipose tissue and other cells, which tends to increase the plasma free fatty acid concentration. However, they also stimulate the cellular oxidation of these fatty acids. Therefore, while these hormones stimulate the synthesis, mobilization, and degradation of lipids, the latter effect is usually the more prominent when raised iodothyronine levels are present resulting in general depletion of the body's stores of fat, a fall in body weight and a decrease in circulating lipid concentrations (e.g. triglycerides, cholesterol, phospholipids). On the other hand, there may be an increase in the plasma concentrations of cholesterol and other lipids, and an increased body weight, when thyroid hormone levels are depressed.

Part of the effect of T_3 and T_4 on fat metabolism is due to the potentiation of catecholamine activity which causes increased lipolysis via the adenyl cyclase–cyclic AMP second messenger system.

Protein metabolism

The effects of iodothyronines on protein metabolism are of particular importance to growth and development and are clearly illustrated by the clinical condition of hypothyroidism in the child. In this situation, physical growth is severely affected and the child is stunted, often despite normal plasma somatotrophin concentrations. Hyperthyroidism in the child is associated with initial accelerated growth, but the epiphyses of the long bones fuse at an earlier age and final height attained may again be reduced.

In general, both protein anabolism and catabolism are stimulated by the thyroid hormones, but an excess of the circulating iodothyronines induces a greater protein degradation than synthesis. This results in a net protein deficit which is manifest by decreased muscle mass and weakness and a fall in body weight. On the other hand, decreased hormone levels are usually associated with a small positive nitrogen (i.e. protein) balance because, again, protein degradation is influenced more than protein synthesis. In this case there is consequently a decreased turnover of protein and other materials in addition to a decrease in protein synthesis. Therefore, in both hypothyroidism and hyperthyroidism, growth, development, and the maintenance of structural and other tissues are usually impaired. One consequence of increased protein catabolism when T_3 and T_4 levels are raised is that there is an increased presentation of amino acids to the liver resulting in a substrate-induced increase in gluconeogenesis.

The point to note is that the thyroid hormones play an extremely important role in normal growth, maintenance, and development of tissues, in addition to the effects of other growth-promoting hormones such as somatotrophin and insulin. Indeed, iodothyronines influence many aspects of the somatotrophin-somatomedin axis (see Chapter 4). For example, hypothyroidism is associated with a decreased sensitivity of pituitary somatotrophe cells to stimuli such as hypoglycaemia, and decreased hepatic production of IGF-I and its principal plasma binding protein, IGFBP3.

Vitamin metabolism

One consequence of the general metabolic effects of the thyroid hormones is the increased requirement for vitamins which play an essential role as coenzymes. A vitamin deficiency can therefore accompany hyperthyroid activity despite a stimulated appetite, unless adequate additional sources are made available. One particular role for the iodothyronines is the direct stimulation of vitamin A synthesis from carotenes in the liver. Hypothyroidism is sometimes associated with a raised plasma carotene concentration which, if sufficiently high, can produce a yellowish tinge to the skin similar to that seen in jaundice.

Effects on bone

Bone metabolism, both resorption and synthesis, is stimulated by the iodothyronines, the former being affected to the greater extent. Thus, in the presence of excess T_3 or T_4 there is an increased demineralization of the bone associated with an increased risk of fractures, hypercalcaemia, and loss of calcium and phosphorus in the urine and faeces. In addition, there is an increased turnover of the protein (collagen) matrix.

Cardiovascular consequences of thyroid activity

As a result of the raised BMR there is an increased oxygen requirement by the tissues and an increased production of heat. These factors are partly responsible for the increase in cardiac output, and the increased blood flow to the surface vessels to allow for increased loss of heat from the skin. In addition to these influences on the cardiovascular system, the thyroid hormones may have a direct action on the heart as well as by potentiating the chronotropic and inotropic effects of circulating catecholamines. The force of contraction of the heart muscle is influenced by the thyroid hormones directly, but the effect can vary. Slight increases in plasma hormone levels increase the force of contraction, but large excesses chronically appear to decrease the strength of the heart beats probably due to the increased protein catabolism in this tissue.

The interaction between iodothyronines and catecholamines is incompletely understood, but catecholamine beta blocker drugs can reduce the tachycardia and other signs of excess iodothyronines in thyrotoxicosis. One explanation may be that iodothyronines stimulate the synthesis of β-receptors, for instance in cardiac muscle.

Effects on the central nervous system

The iodothyronines are vital not only for physical growth but also for mental development. In the absence of these hormones form birth to puberty, the child remains mentally, as well as physically, retarded (cretinism) due to poor development of cellular processes, hypoplasia of cortical neurones, and delayed myelination of nerve fibres. If the deficiency is not corrected within a few weeks of birth irreversible damage occurs. In the adult, hypothyroidism is characterized by poor mentation, poor memory, and lack of initiative. Psychological changes may also occur. The reflex relaxation time also is often delayed.

The effect of the thyroid hormones on the central nervous system (e.g. cortical arousal, stimulation of the reticular formation) are believed to be due, at least partly, to a potentiation of catecholamine activity.

Mechanisms of action

The iodothyronines can penetrate the plasma membranes of target cells with relative ease, at least partly by way of active transport processes, and specific intracellular receptors have been identified. For instance, two genes coding for iodothyronine receptors (thyroid receptors, TR) have been identified in the human. Both of the resulting receptor proteins have a 10-fold greater affinity for T_3 than for T_4, and have been shown to be expressed in all T_3-sensitive tissues. Thus, the expression of both receptors is found in many tissues, but the ratio of the two can vary. Inheritance of general resistance to thyroid hormones (a cause of hypothyroidism) has been linked genetically to one of the receptor (TR-β) genes, and various mutations have now been identified. These are associated with varying defects in iodothyronine-receptor binding. The T_3-receptor complex probably binds to specific sequences along nuclear DNA in a dimeric form, altering the rate of transcription of these genes into mRNA and subsequent new protein synthesis. A nuclear mechanism of action would explain the long latency before physiological effects are induced.

At present, various other possible, non-nuclear, mechanisms are still under investigation.

One mechanism previously ascribed to thyroxine consisted of an 'uncoupling' of oxidative phosphorylation in mitochondria, whereby some of the energy produced by oxidation is lost at heat. To produce the same quantity of ATP, increased metabolism (and therefore raised oxygen consumption) would be required. However, extremely high (toxic) concentrations of the iodothyronines are required to produce this effect which cannot be related to some of the other known actions of the hormones, and this mechanism is now considered to be physiologically inappropriate.

The two additional mechanisms of action which are currently being studied are: (1) a direct stimulation of the mitochondria (which increase in size and number and have an increased content and activity of various enzymes, e.g. of the respiratory chain) increasing mitochondrial protein synthesis; and (2) a direct effect on plasma membrane transport mechanisms (e.g. for amino acids), probably following an initial increase in cAMP generation, although the stimulation of membrane-bound ATPase is also likely (Fig. 9.3). In addition, some of the potentiating effects of the iodothyronines on other hormone activities may be related to the intracellular cAMP system.

Although no single unifying mechanism of action for the thyroidal iodothyronines has yet been identified, the direct stimulation of nuclear transcription processes resulting in increased intracellular protein synthesis is almost certainly the most likely to be important.

Thyrotrophin receptors

It is important to emphasize the prime importance of the thyrotrophin receptor to thyroid disease since it is subject to considerable influence by a variety of antibodies.

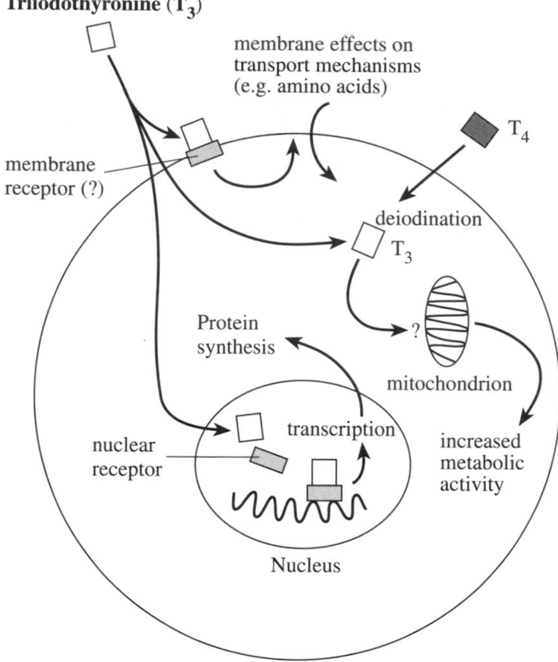

Fig. 9.3. Mechanisms of action of triiodothyronine (T_3).

Control of release

The adenohypophysial hormone thyrotrophin regulates most aspects of iodothyronine synthesis and release from the thyroid. It stimulates iodide uptake from the plasma by the follicular cells, either by stimulating iodide 'pump' (trapping) activity or by increasing the number of 'pumps' on the basal membrane. It also stimulates peroxidase activity and the iodination of the tyrosyl groups on thyroglobulin, and influences the coupling reaction so that formation of iodothyronines on the protein molecule is increased. Thyrotrophin also stimulates the synthesis of thyroglobulin by increasing the rate of incorporation of thyroidal amino acids. The uptake of colloid by endocytosis, the fusion of colloid droplets with lysosomes, and the degradation of thyroglobulin resulting in liberation of T_3 and T_4 into the blood, are also events which are stimulated by the adenohypophysial hormone. Thyrotrophin's actions are mediated by stimulation of membrane-bound adenyl cyclase and subsequent cAMP generation.

Finally, thyrotrophin exerts a tonic maintenance effect on the thyroid and its blood supply. In the presence of excessive quantities of thyrotrophin, the size and number of follicular cells increase, and with prolonged stimulation there is increased vascularity and eventual hypertrophy of the gland.

Thyrotrophin release is controlled mainly by the hypothalamic tripeptide thyrotrophin-releasing hormone (TRH) which reaches the adenohypophysial thyro-

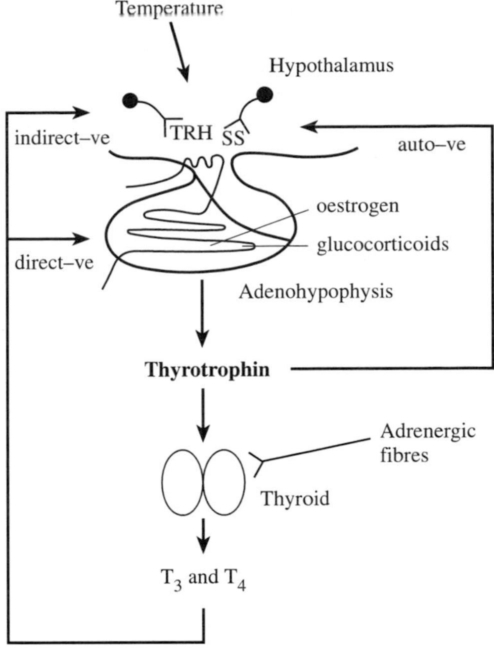

Fig. 9.4. Diagram showing some on the factors involved in the control of thyroxine (T_4) and triiodothyronine (T_3) production from the thyroid gland. (TRH, thyrotrophin-releasing hormone; SS, somatostatin.)

trophe cells by the local portal blood system (see Chapter 2). Another hypothalamic neuropeptide, somatostatin, also influences thyrotrophin release; it has an inhibitory effect on the thyrotrophe cells. The circulating free T_3 and T_4 concentrations also have a controlling influence on thyrotrophin release by exerting direct and indirect negative feedback effects at the adenohypophysial and hypothalamic levels respectively (see Fig. 9.4). Oestrogens appear to increase thyrotrophe responsiveness to TRH, perhaps by stimulating the synthesis of TRH receptors, this being the one clear sexually dimorphic response relating to the thyroid–gonadal axis.

Glucocorticoids from the adrenal cortex inhibit thyrotrophin release from the adenohypophysis, but only when they are present in the circulation in excessive quantities such as in Cushing's syndrome. Pharmacological amounts of glucocorticoids also appear to reduce thyrotrophe responsiveness to TRH, and this is seen in patients with Cushing's syndrome.

Environmental temperature has long been known to influence T_3 and T_4 production. Within 24 hours of being in a cold environment there is usually an increase in plasma T_4 concentration, reaching a maximum in a few days. The plasma thyrotrophin concentration, on the other hand, does not appear to increase at least during short-term exposure to cold.

The autonomic innervation to the thyroid has also been considered as having some influence on hormone function of the gland, partly by varying the blood flow to the tissue. An adrenergic fibre network directly innervates the basement membranes of the follicles. Catecholamines, like thyrotrophin, appear to stimulate aspects of thyroid function (e.g. increased colloid uptake) via the adenyl cyclase–cAMP system. However, adrenergic antagonists only inhibit the effects of catecholamines. Another molecule, vasoactive intestinal peptide (VIP) is released from autonomic (non-sympathetic) nerve terminals. This peptide can also stimulate thyroidal blood flow and hence could influence iodothyronine secretion.

Goitre and goitrogens

Any enlargement of the thyroid is called a goitre and substances which induce goitre formation are called goitrogens. For example, certain monovalent ions interfere with thyroid iodide uptake and can therefore, in certain circumstances, cause decreased T_3 and T_4 production. Ions such as thiocyanate and perchlorate decrease iodide uptake by competitive inhibition and, as a consequence of reduced T_3 and T_4 secretion, cause an increased release of thyrotrophin (by reduced negative feedback) which then stimulates the thyroid. Some goitrogens occur naturally, and can be found in certain vegetables (e.g. thiocyanates in cabbage).

Goitre may also be a consequence of reduced iodide content of the diet, and hence of iodide uptake. In certain areas of the world where there is reduced iodide in the soil and hence in vegetable products, a deficiency of this ion can result in the formation of so-called endemic goitre. However, iodine is now added to table salt or given by depot injection in many countries, and this cause of goitre is now less common.

Large quantities of iodide also exert numerous poorly understood, but clinically useful, inhibitory influences on the thyroid gland. The best recognized, though ill-understood, phenomenon is the Wolff–Chaikoff effect representing an inhibition of organification of trapped iodide by excess iodide (or iodine) administration. In addition, iodide in pharmacological dosage induces a marked inhibition of thyroidal release of T_3 and T_4 which is of singular therapeutic value in the management of gross hyperthyroid states such as thyroid crisis (storm).

CLINICAL DISORDERS

Introduction

Thyroid hyperfunction and hypofunction share a prevalence of approximately 2 per cent of the adult population. Together with diabetes mellitus (2–5 per cent of the adult population) these are among the most common endocrine disorders encountered. In addition, a number of thyroid disorders are not associated with abnormal hormone secretory function, and will be considered separately.

All types of thyroid pathology may be subtle in their initial clinical presentation. Bearing in mind their frequency in the community and the wide variation in their mode of presentation, a high index of suspicion is required to make an early diagnosis, particularly in the presence of other medical disorders with which thyroid disease is often associated, or with which it may be confused. Much thyroid dysfunction is based on auto-immune pathology: as indicated later in this chapter, variation in thyroid function occurs spontaneously across the full range from hypo- to hyperfunction: the factors which determine these spontaneous fluctuations remain largely unknown.

Excess

Graves' disease

The description of this disorder, which gains its eponym from the Irish physician who first described it, is also attributed to the physicians Basedow and Parry. It affects approximately 1:100 of the adult population, as ascertained from cross-sectional population studies. Hyperthyroidism is the principal, but not exclusive manifestation of this disorder, which can induce symptoms and signs in virtually every organ system.

Aetiology

Although it was initially conceived that excessive native pituitary thyrotrophin (TSH) was the aetiological factor, it is now clear that physiological TSH secretion is invariably suppressed by the excessive T_4 and T_3 secretion found in hyperthyroid Graves' disease (nevertheless rare cases of hyperthyroidism have been described where a TSH-producing pituitary adenoma has been responsible for a hyperthyroid state). The responsible thyroid stimulating protein in Graves' disease has been characterized as a 7-S IgG class immunoglobulin arising from the lymphocytes within as well as outside the thyroid gland. This stimulator (TSAB) is a unique antibody to the thyroidal TSH receptor. It is produced by an abnormal clone of B-cells, and associated with an abnormal ratio of CD4 (helper) to CD8 (suppressor) cells. The characteristic, but not invariable ocular involvement of Graves' disease is mediated by one or more distinct but still poorly characterized orbital-stimulating immunoglobulins. By a still unidentified mechanism, these result in the characteristic oedema and mucinous infiltration of retro-orbital fat and extra-ocular muscles. Similarly, the cutaneous condition of pretibial myxoedema (more correctly, infiltrative Graves' dermopathy) is due to mucinous infiltration of the dermal and subdermal layers, although the responsible inducing agent has not yet been isolated.

Sometimes, Graves' hyperthyroidism appear to follow an episode of subacute thyroiditis of presumed viral origin, suggesting that viral-induced antigen presentation or release from thyrocytes may be the precipitating step in some cases, followed by an abnormal immunological response. Some cases follow the administration of iodine or iodide. This is a common ingredient of multivitamin and anticough medication as well as being present in the contrast media used in radiological imaging. It is now known that iodide not only acts as a facilitatory substrate, but also possesses specific immunostimulatory activity: in individuals with the thyroid auto-immune hallmark (positive thyroid microsomal antibody, TMA: more correctly now referred to as peroxidase antibody, TPO), iodide administration has also been shown to increase TPO antibody titre.

Where population-based prophylactic iodide administration has been used with a view to prevention of endemic goitre, an increased prevalence of hyperthyroidism has been documented: this phenomenon is referred to as the Jod–Basedow phenomenon. A similar iodide-precipitated syndrome is frequently seen following the administration of the iodine-rich anti-arrythmic drug, amiodarone. In this latter case, although the typical clinical picture of hyperthyroidism may occur, bizarre disturbance of thyroid function tests (e.g. high circulating thyroid hormone levels with paradoxically normal TSH) is also common. This is not an iodide effect, and is due to receptor blocking effects of the amiodarone molecule, and inhibition of peripheral T_4 to T_3 conversion. Despite the clearly important role of iodide, in most cases of Graves' disease it is not possible to identify the primary trigger factor.

Graves' disease may be associated with other auto-immune disorders of the thyogastric group, including pernicious anaemia, Addison's disease, hypoparathyroidism, premature ovarian failure, insulin-dependent diabetes mellitus, and the obscure focal depigmentation disorder, vitiligo. These disorders share a common association with the histocompatibility antigens HLA-B8 and DR 3 and 4 and DQ, and are further discussed in Chapter 16. Furthermore, auto-immune thyroid disease embraces a spectrum from Graves' disease through Hashimoto's disease to 'idiopathic' primary hypothyroidism. Individual patients may pass spontaneously through these functional extremes over a period of weeks, months, or years. Furthermore, any thyroid functional status may be associated with the characteristic ophthalmopathy. It is common to find different forms of these and other types of thyrogastric immune disorders in different members of the same family as well as within individuals: coexistence of up to five of the above group in a single patient has been described.

Clinical features

Although it may be seen at any age, this form of hyperthyroidism is most common in young to middle-aged females: the female preponderance (approximately 3:1), which is seen in all auto-immune thyroid disorders remains unexplained. The signs and symptoms can be subdivided into three groups: (1) those associated directly with thyroid hormone excess; (2) those due to potentiation of sympathetic action; and (3) those due to extrathyroidal actions of related immunoglobulins.

Thyroid hormone hypersecretion

These actions may be very subtle, comprising only weight loss and heat intolerance due to hypermetabolism: in fact the disorder may be totally asymptomatic in the earliest phases. Patients tend to be physically and mentally hyperactive and there may be both a skeletal and cardiac myopathy, giving rise to tiredness, weakness, and breathlessness. Both supraventricular arrhythmias (usually atrial fibrillation) and precipitation of cardiac failure may be seen, more particularly in older patients. Osteoporosis may occur (due to increased bone turnover and preferential resorption) and amenorrhoea (due partly to gonadotrophin suppression) may be present. A diffuse goitre with overlying bruit (due to increased thyroid vascularity) is found in about two-thirds of cases.

Thyroid crisis (thyrotoxic storm) is seen in very severe cases, often precipitated by additional physical, surgical, or infective stress. Circulating thyroid hormone levels are not invariably higher than in patients without this dramatic presentation, and many of the clinical features are due to sympathetic components (see below): untreated, the mortality of such thyroid crises exceeds 80 per cent.

Sympathetic potentiation

Although circulating catecholamine levels are normal or even reduced, both T_3 and T_4 potentiate sympathetic receptor effects so that many features of hyperthyroidism mimic those seen in patients with simple anxiety states or with adrenal medullary tumours (phaeochromocytoma).

Tachycardia, sweating, and tremor together with intestinal hypermotility (inducing diarrhoea) are the principal autonomic features, and some of the manifest anxiety is probably based on a direct sympathetic effects on brain neuronal activity. The ocular signs of lid lag and retraction which give rise to the characteristic wide-eyed look of hyperthyroid patients are also mediated by the increased sympathetic tone of Mueller's muscle (levator palpebrae superiorus). (see Plate 9.5) There is also a major component of autonomic hyperfunction in patients with thyroid crisis, which is highly relevant to the therapy used in this fortunately uncommon problem which is dealt with later in this chapter.

Extrathyroid manifestations (see Plates 9.6–9.8 and 9.12)

The ophthalmopathy, dermopathy, or acropachy which come into this classification are found in more than 50 per cent of all patients with Graves' disease and are not attributable to T_4 and T_3 excess. As indicated earlier, these features are produced by abnormal circulating antibodies to incompletely identified antigens in the target tissue concerned.

Thyroid ophthalmopathy is represented by various degrees of swelling of peri-orbital and retro-orbital tissues (including the conjunctivae and extraocular muscles). Such eye disease (either unilateral or bilateral) may be the only or the initial manifestation of Graves' disease, then leading to the term 'ophthalmic or euthyroid Graves' disease'. The clinical course of thyroid ophthalmopathy is largely unaffected by treatment of the associated thyroid dysfunction, although there is data to suggest that incidental hypothyroidism occurring in the course of treatment of the hyperthyroid state may induce or aggravate eye changes. Ophthalmopathy tends to progress in the first few weeks or months following diagnosis, then stabilizes and undergoes very slow, but rarely complete regression over a period of years.

Patients show measurable degrees of ocular protrusion (proptosis or exophthalmos) due to increased volume and oedema of retro-orbital fat. In more severe cases muscle infiltration and ultimately fibrosis occurs, effectively shortening extraocular muscles and resulting in double vision (diplopia). A similar process in the levator palpebrae superiorus (together with the proptosis) is responsible for the persistent upper lid retraction often seen in this condition. Diplopia is usually

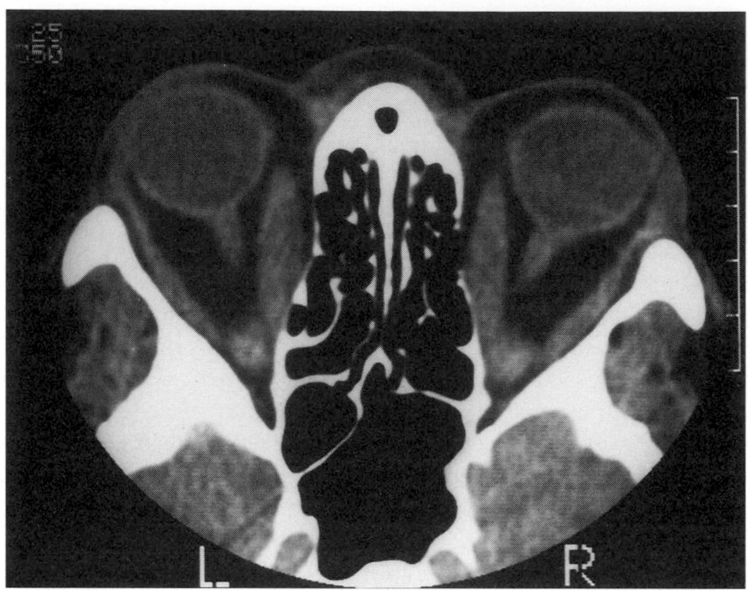

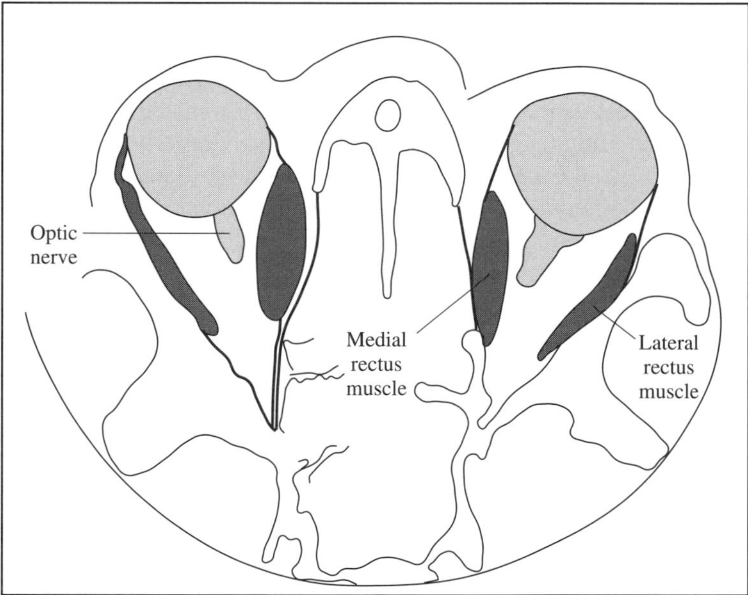

Fig. 9.5. Orbital CT scan of patient with thyroid ophthalmopathy: note dominant involvement (thickening) of the medial rectus muscle.

maximal during lateral and upward gaze because of dominant involvement of the medial rectus and inferior oblique muscles. Even more severe degrees of proptosis are associated with exposure keratitis (due to corneal exposure), optic neuritis (due to tension on the optic nerve), and retinal vascular insufficiency (due to combined tension and pressure on the retinal artery): singly or together these may, in untreated cases, result in blindness.

The related conditions of an intracutaneous infiltration commonly seen on the shins (pretibial myxoedema or infiltrative dermopathy) and a pseudo-clubbing of the nails (thyroid acropachy) with or without recession of the nail bed (onycholysis) are seen less commonly and are purely of aesthetic importance. Splenomegaly and lymphadenopathy are sometimes present, reflecting the lymphoproliferative immunological basis of Graves' disease. Uncommonly, this lymphoproliferative process extends to the development of lymphoma within the thyroid. This condition should always be suspected in a patient with a personal or family history of autoimmune thyroid disease in the presence of a firm goitre which is increasing in size.

Investigations

1. In classical cases, both serum free T_3 and T_4 concentrations are elevated at diagnosis. However, mild or early cases, particularly patients living in areas of iodine deficiency, may show only an elevation of serum free T_3 due to preferential synthesis of the iodine-poor T_3 molecule (T_3-toxicosis). Serum TSH concentrations are invariably suppressed below the normal range.

2. Isotopic uptake of tracer doses of radioactive iodine or technetium (whose thyroid trapping is similarly thyroid–stimulator-dependent) is increased: this is an essential test, since it allows clear differentiation of Graves' disease from subacute thyroiditis and thyrotoxicosis factitia (where uptake is suppressed), and from toxic nodular goitre (where uptake is either raised or normal). A simultaneous thyroid scintiscan image will show the characteristic diffuse goitre in Graves' disease (see Fig. 9.6) in contrast to the multifocal pattern of nodular goitre or the single focus of a hyperfunctioning solitary nodule or adenoma.

3. Thyroid antibodies directed against microsomal thyroid cell antigens are present in approximately 90 per cent of cases (as compared with about 10 per cent of the 'normal' population), and can therefore provide help in differential diagnosis of the thyrotoxic state. Similarly, TSAB can be directly assayed by a number of bio- and immuno-assay techniques, and represent the biological and immunological hallmark of the disorder in most, but not all cases.

4. Prior to the availability of highly sensitive TSH assays, the TRH stimulation test was sometimes employed, relying on the fact that supraphysiological levels of thyroid hormones induce a suppression of the normal TSH response to TRH by direct pituitary feedback. This test may be viewed as an alternative *in vivo* assay of circulating serum-free T_3 and T_4 levels, but is in practice only rarely required bearing in mind the diagnostic value of a suppressed serum TSH level.

5. In suspected ophthalmopathy a CT scan readily quantifies the degree of extraocular muscle involvement, and is useful in the differential diagnosis of proptosis, particularly in its occasional unilateral form. Hess charting of eye

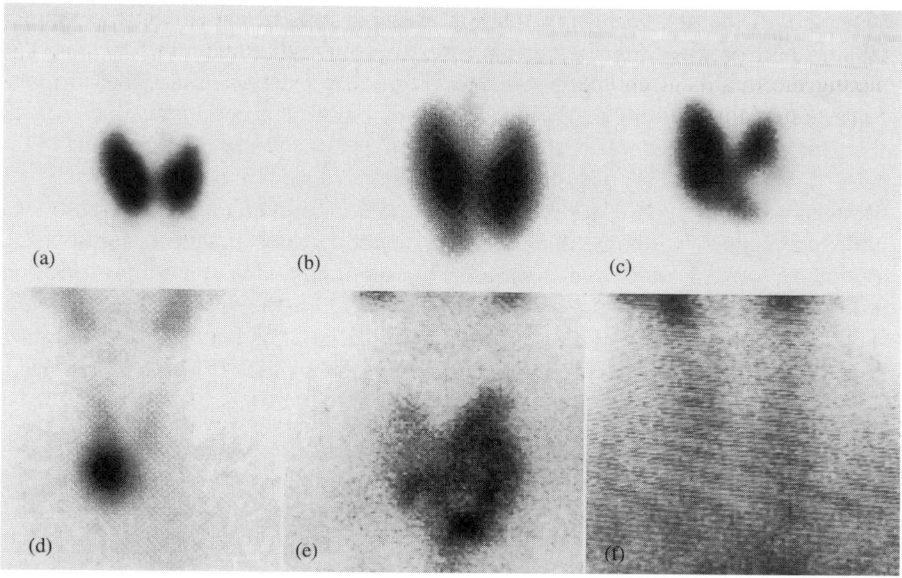

Fig. 9.6. Representative thyroid isotope scans: patients were given pertechnetate (Tc-99m) and scanned with a gamma camera: (a) normal scan; (b) Graves' disease; (c) 'cold' nodule; (d) 'hot' (autonomous) nodule; (e) multinodular goitre; (f) the suppressed image of subacute thyroiditis: an identical pattern is seen in thyrotoxicosis factitia.

movements, measurement of visual acuity, and intraocular pressure changes on upgaze are additional methods of documenting progress of infiltrative eye disease. CT-demonstrable extraocular muscle thickening may be seen in up to 80 per cent of patients with Graves' hyperthyroidism, even in the absence of obvious eye involvement.

Treatment

No form of therapy for Graves' disease is ideal, and life-long follow-up is essential in every case, for reasons which will be made clear. Initial management consists of the optional administration of β-adrenergic blocking agents, either propranolol 120–160 mg a day, or a more cardioselective agent, such as nadolol, if indicated. The tremor, tachycardia, and anxiety elements respond within hours. Although these drugs have been found to have minor inhibitory effects on peripheral tissue conversion of T_4 to T_3, their use does not interfere with subsequent investigation, so that symptomatic treatment need not be delayed until biochemical and isotopic confirmation of the clinical diagnosis.

It is interesting that the disorder has been shown to be self-limiting in approximately 20–30 per cent of cases, although this expectant approach is not a viable management option: such an event may take years to occur, and in most instances represents waning levels of TSAB. In some instances, it has been shown to be due to the development of TSH receptor-blocking antibodies. There is also evidence of cyclicity in the activity of the disease, even involving spontaneous transitions between hypothyroid and hyperthyroid states. The following treatment alternatives exist, and there are very few absolute indications for any one approach. Increasingly, after detailed discussion, patients' own preferences are considered in making the treatment choice. In practice, it often proves necessary to use more than one modality.

Antithyroid drugs

The major (thiocarbamide) group of drugs act by inhibiting two major steps in thyroid biosynthesis: the organification and coupling of iodide and tyrosines. It has also been shown that some members of the group (methimazole and carbimazole) have a direct action on the immunological process itself. This pharmacological attribute probably explains the higher eventual remission rates than would be expected simply by the administration of a drug which (temporarily) affects hormone biosynthesis. On the other hand, propylthiouracil, in addition to its biosynthetic blocking effects has a further effect in blocking peripheral tissue thyroxine deiodination to triiodothyronine. This attribute makes it the drug of choice in more severe forms of hyperthyroidism. The lower transplacental secretion and breast milk excretion of propylthiouracil also makes it a preferred drug in pregnancy, if high dosage of antithyroid drugs proves to be necessary. Potassium perchlorate is used rarely as an antithyroid drug. It acts by blocking iodide trapping.

Carbimazole or methimazole (20–40 mg daily) or propylthiouracil (200–400 mg daily), together with tapazole (principally used in the United States) are the only drugs in common use. Six- or eight-hourly dosage is desirable in the early stages of treatment in view of the short half-life of these drugs imposed by hypermetabolism. Once euthyroidism is achieved, the dose may be either titrated against circulating T_3 and T_4 levels, or more simply a block-replace regime can be used, employing the higher doses mentioned above, together with physiological replacement of T_4 (100–150 μg) daily. Single daily dosage is usually possible once euthyroidism is achieved, thereby improving patient compliance. Drug therapy is usually continued for 12 to 24 months: in general, the longer duration of therapy, the better the chances of 'remission'. Normalization of isotope trapping by the thyroid, as assessed by thyroidal technetium uptake measurements performed at intervals during therapy, or the more direct but related measurement of TSAB, are relative indications of potential remission, especially if taken together with reduction of goitre size: the above findings have been used with some success as a guide to when therapy should be terminated.

Relapse occurs in some 50 per cent of cases, requiring a second or even third course of therapy. Alternatively, surgery or radioactive iodine therapy can be used in the treatment of such relapses. Drug side-effects of skin rash and migratory joint pains occurs in approximately 5 per cent of patients, and are sometimes eliminated by changing to an alternative thiocarbamide drug. Agranulocytosis, which is usually reversible when the drug is ceased, is seen in approximately 1 case in 500 in patients given thiocarbamides, although much more frequently and less reversibly with potassium perchlorate (explaining the far lower usage of this drug). Patients need to be accordingly forewarned that the development of the clinical hallmark of agranulocytosis, a severe sore throat, requires immediate clinical assessment.

Subtotal thyroidectomy

Surgery is only indicated with larger goitres causing superior mediastinal compression, or in some patients relapsing after antithyroid drugs. The risk of persistent hyperthyroidism after surgery is as high as 20 per cent (depending on the experience of the operator), with an incidence of hypothyroidism up to 60 per cent if the surgeon strives to avoid the risk of recurrence by a more radical approach. The potential surgical complication risks of hypoparathyroidism and recurrent laryngeal nerve palsy should be rare events: thyroidectomy should only be performed by those surgeons with established expertise. Pre-operatively, patients must be rendered euthyroid either with antithyroid drugs or with 10 days' of iodine loading (Lugol's iodine 0.5–1.0 ml daily), although it has been shown that full beta-adrenergic blockade alone may safely be used for pre-operative management, where urgency demands it.

Radioactive iodine

Radioactive iodine (^{131}I) is the treatment of choice in most patients above the age of 40 and is being increasingly used in younger patients, particularly those with intolerance to, or relapse following antithyroid drugs. It has been shown that older patients with Graves' disease have a higher relapse rate following antithyroid drugs, so that a more definitive approach to treatment is logical. Traditionally, a 3–5 millicurie (mCi); (110–180 megabecquerel, mBq) dose was used, given by mouth. Euthyroidism developed over a period of months, rather than weeks, sometimes requiring additional temporary antithyroid drug therapy: non-response was treated by repeat doses, required in up to 50 per cent of cases. In addition, the overall incidence of treatment-induced hypothyroidism was approximately 10 per cent in the first year, increasing at the rate of 2–3 per cent per annum.

Both the slow response as well as the delayed hypothyroidism (requiring very careful patient follow-up) has prompted the adoption of a more definitive ablative regime using 15–20 mCi (550–730 mBq) doses. With this approach, the patient is often rendered euthyroid in 4–6 weeks, thyroid replacement can usually be initiated at that time without necessarily awaiting the development of hypothyroidism, and then continued on a life-long basis. Subsequent management is then that outlined under the section on hypothyroidism. Some patients are curiously radioresistant and require up to 50 mCi (1800 mBq) to achieve euthyroidism. Possible carcinogenic, teratogenic, and leukaemogenic effects of radioiodine therapy have been carefully excluded over more than 40 years of carefully monitored usage world-wide. Providing it is not given during pregnancy (which should not be allowed to occur within 3 months of radioiodine), there is no longer any contraindication to its use except in young children, in whom natural caution still dictates an avoidance of unnecessary radiation exposure. Children also need to be kept out of contact with radioiodine-receiving patients for approximately 10 days.

Treatment of extrathyroidal manifestations

Minor eye involvement requires no therapy, although dryness and irritation (due to corneal and conjunctival exposure) respond to the instillation of artificial tears (e.g.

hypromellose drops). In some cases, diuretics will reduce minor degrees of peri-orbital oedema and discomfort.

Progressive extraocular muscle involvement and peri-orbital oedema are indications for the use of systemic corticosteroids (prednisolone 40 to 80 mg daily); even retrobulbar administration of steroids has been employed with benefit. Other types of immunosuppressive regimens have been tried, alone or together with corticosteroids but not with uniform success. Orbital irradiation is sometimes used to supplement corticosteroids. Its precise action is not known, but is often effective, and reduces the need for extended courses of corticosteroids. None of these approaches are indicated in established, stable or non-progressive cases. More severe degrees of proptosis which induce visual loss are an indication for high-dose steroid as a matter of urgency. If unsuccessful, this is followed within 48 hours by surgical orbital decompression, usually by a transantral approach often performed by a joint ENT and ophthalmic surgical team approach.

Infiltrative dermopathy sometimes responds to topical steroid (fluocinolone) administration under occlusive dressings, but a total remission is unusual.

Other forms of hyperthyroidism

Nodular toxic goitre

This disorder is usually found in an older population than Graves' disease. There are probably multiple interactive causes. Periods of thyroid involution and regeneration, perhaps contributed to by episodic iodine deficiency and repletion may be relevant: over a period of time, this may result in autonomous foci, one or more of which may subsequently become hyperfunctioning. Thyroid antibodies are present in approximately 25 per cent of cases with corresponding intrathyroidal lymphocytic aggregations seen in surgically removed glands. This finding supports an autoimmune component in some cases.

Clinical features

The lack of extrathyroidal (especially eye) signs in this type of hyperthyroidism may result in the diagnosis being missed or delayed. Otherwise, the clinical features are those of Graves' disease. A readily palpable nodular thyroid gland is usually palpable, and the goitre is sometimes retrosternal, and of sufficient size to induce upper mediastinal compression. Clinical presentation is frequently with atrial fibrillation, with or without cardiac failure: since patients are often elderly, coronary ischaemia probably plays a contributory role in many cases. Since this disorder is eminently treatable, it should be at least considered in every elderly patient with cardiac failure: over the age of 60, the prevalence of hyperthyroidism in women is as high as 5 per cent.

Investigations

1. Free T_3 and T_4 levels are elevated and serum TSH levels suppressed.
2. Isotope uptake by the thyroid is not invariably increased, but the scan demonstrates multifocal areas of increased and decreased activity (see Fig. 9.6).

Treatment

Radioiodine is almost uniformly safe and effective. Larger doses of 15–20 mCi (550–730 mBq) are used since the multinodular toxic gland is more radioresistant, and multiple further doses are sometimes required. The intention is to ablate hyperfunctioning areas, allowing previously suppressed areas to recover function. Accordingly, post-therapy hypothyroidism only occurs in about 5 per cent of cases. Surgery is reserved for large goitres which are either causing mediastinal compression or are cosmetically unacceptable. Antithyroid drugs may be used, as in Graves' disease: however, relapse following discontinuation is almost invariable, even after prolonged courses of treatment, and more definitive, destructive therapy as outlined above is the normal choice.

Autonomous hyperfunctioning nodule

An apparently single hyperfunctioning nodule may be either part of a multinodular gland (where the remaining thyroid tissue is functionally inactive) or a true thyroid adenoma: in the latter case it is sometimes referred to as Plummers' disease.

Clinical features

The clinical picture is similar to that seen in multinodular toxic goitre, but normally only a solitary nodule is palpable in the thyroid: even this may not be apparent on routine examination, since the lesion may be partly or wholly retrosternal in location.

Investigations

Biochemical investigations confirm hyperthyroidism as above, and isotope scan shows a solitary hyperfunctioning area with no uptake within the remaining thyroid gland (see Fig. 9.6).

Treatment

Cases respond equally well to surgical excision or radioiodine ablation. With the latter approach, large doses of 12–15 mCi (440–550 mBq) selectively ablate the nodule without affecting the remaining thyroid, which is not iodine-avid because of negative feedback TSH suppression. Part or all of this previously inactive thyroid tissue regains function once the autonomous nodule is rendered inactive. This 'recruitability' can be assessed prior to ablative therapy by repeating an isotope scan after thyrotrophin priming (10 units intramuscularly daily for 3 days).

Subacute thyroiditis (De Quervain's disease)

This is an important differential diagnosis to consider in every hyperthyroid patient. Only in some cases is there clinical or serological evidence for a viral aetiology.

Clinical features

Patients often but not invariably present with a sore throat, occasionally incorrectly diagnosed as a 'simple' sore throat (pharyngitis) and with variable severity of thyrotoxic features (due to inflammation-induced hormonal discharge). Pain may radiate to the ears. During the acute phase, the thyroid is uniformly enlarged and often quite tender, with fever in some cases. Following the hyperthyroid phase (lasting 1–3 weeks) approximately 50 per cent of patients pass into a hypothyroid phase (due to defective thyroid hormone synthesis) which lasts 1–3 months. Euthyroidism is almost always re-established in due course. Nevertheless, occasional cases appear to progress to Graves' disease, while in others (approximately 5 per cent) hypothyroidism is permanent.

Investigation

1. During the acute phase, serum-free T_3 and T_4 concentrations are elevated, later becoming subnormal with elevated serum TSH in those patients who enter a hypothyroid phase.

2. Thyroid isotope uptake and scan show complete or almost complete suppression of the thyroid image, providing the differential diagnosis from Graves' disease.

3. Thyroid antibodies are present in less than 10 per cent of cases, and usually not to a very high titre.

Treatment

Since the disorder runs a self-limiting course, therapy is often unnecessary. However, the initial pain often responds well to aspirin in high (4–6 g daily) dosage. Occasionally, because of the severity of thyroid pain and tenderness, prednisolone 20 to 40 mg daily is needed, given in gradually reducing doses over a 2–3 month period. Excessively rapid reduction in steroid dosage is often associated with a flare-up of the disorder.

Beta-adrenergic blocking drugs reduce the catecholamine-related clinical features, but antithyroid drugs are universally ineffective in this condition, since enhanced biosynthesis is not the primary cause of the thyroid hyperfunction. Symptomatic hypothyroidism occurring in the recovery phase requires treatment with thyroxine, but usually not beyond 3–4 months.

Thyrotoxicosis factitia (thyrotoxicosis medicamentosa)

Self-administration of thyroid hormones for 'kicks' is not uncommon, pharmacists and nurses being occupationally exposed. The clinical features are those which one would expect, but with an impalpable thyroid gland. Investigations confirm elevated serum-free T_3 and T_4 levels, but isotope uptake and scan show a totally suppressed image and thyroid antibodies are consistently negative. Although the approach to treatment appears obvious, it is often difficult to achieve an admission of self-administration, and underlying psychiatric problems require careful evaluation.

Post-partum thyroid dysfunction: PPTD

This common disorder is being increasingly recognized, and affects approximately 6 per cent of all women during the postpartum period. It occurs almost exclusively

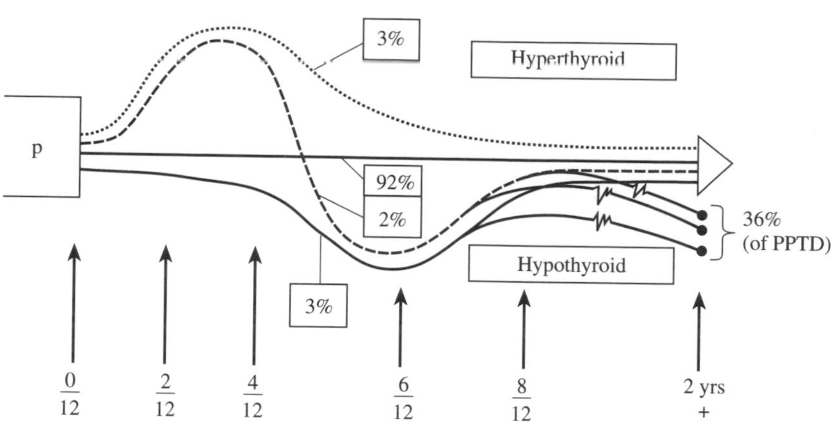

Fig. 9.7. The natural history of postpartum thyroid dysfunction (thyroiditis). (PPT, postpartum thyroid.)

within the pool of women who enter pregnancy with positive thyroid antimicrosomal antibody (TPO) titres (i.e. 12 per cent of all women). Accordingly, 50 per cent of initially TPO antibody-positive women will develop the syndrome, although not necessarily with symptoms. A hyperthyroid phase (at approximately 3 months postpartum) and/or a hypothyroid phase (at approximately 4–6 months postpartum) may be clinically or subclinically (biochemically) evident, and symptoms may be incorrectly attributed to postnatal depression and anxiety. Almost certainly, PPTD is triggered by a reversal of the previous immunotolerant state of pregnancy. (see Fig. 9.7.)

Conventional biochemical criteria are used for diagnosis (see also hypothyroidism, p. 228). Isotope uptake studies (if feasible in non-lactating women) reveal suppressed thyroidal uptake. An important differential diagnosis is postpartum Graves' disease 'relapse', occurring either in a patient with a previous episode of Graves' disease, or as an initial presentation: in this group, thyroidal isotope uptake will, as expected, be increased.

Treatment of the hyperthyroid phase is limited to the use of beta-adrenergic blockers, since the hyperthyroidism is due to release of preformed hormone: as in subacute thyroiditis, antithyroid drugs have no effect. Thyroxine replacement in the hypothyroid phase is logical.

The implications of this disorder include the almost invariable recurrence of the syndrome in subsequent pregnancies, and the later development of permanent hypothyroidism in perhaps 30–50 per cent of cases. Accordingly, repeat thyroid function screening at 3–5-year intervals might represent an appropriate follow-up policy in this high-risk group of patients. It has also been proposed that routine thyroid antibody screening should be performed in all antenatal registrants, in order to identify those at risk for subsequent specific postnatal 'tracking'.

Ectopic (tumour-associated) hyperthyroidism (see Chapter 15)

Hyperthyroidism during pregnancy

Hyperthyroidism occurring during pregnancy may be missed, since hypermetabolism is a common accompaniment of normal pregnancy. Conversely, when measurement of circulating total (rather than serum-free) T_4 and T_3 is performed for diagnostic screening, a false suggestion of hyperthyroidism is raised, since thyronine-binding proteins are increased by the elevated plasma oestrogens of normal pregnancy. In fact, Graves' disease presenting for the first time in pregnancy is uncommon, because of the immunotolerant state characterized by pregnancy: during pregnancy, pre-existing Graves' disease may undergo an apparent partial or complete remission, only to recur quite dramatically postpartum.

The usual diagnostic criteria are used, as outlined above. Isotope uptake tests are avoided in pregnancy because of possible teratogenic effects of irradiation.

Once diagnosed, antithyroid drugs are used in titration dosage, aiming to minimize the dosage necessary to normalize serum-free T_3 and T_4 levels. Under-dosage results in an increased incidence of miscarriage and premature labour; over-dosage results in excessive transplacental passage of antithyroid drugs, producing intrauterine and neonatal goitre and hypothyroidism. This cannot be prevented by concurrent T_3 or T_4 administration, since there is only limited permeability of the placenta to these hormones.

Many patients can be ultimately controlled during pregnancy with 5–10 mg of carbimazole (or equivalents) daily. Some physicians prefer to use propylthiouracil specifically in pregnancy, since transplacental passage is lower, coupled to reduced secretion rate in breast milk. This latter attribute may be of importance where higher dosage of drugs is necessary, and which would otherwise risk the development of neonatal goitre.

Neonatal hyperthyroidism

This condition is due to transplacental passage of thyroid-stimulating immunoglobulins. It may therefore be seen in offspring of women with Graves' disease even if in remission, since thyroid-stimulating immunoglobulins may continue to be elevated. The infant shows many of the features of adult Graves' disease, including proptosis, but the condition is transient and subsides completely within 4–6 weeks without therapy. Considering the frequency with which pregnancy complicates current or previous Graves' disease, the comparative rarity of this disorder remains unexplained.

Thyrotoxic crisis

This condition is uncommon, and as indicated earlier, clinical features are dominated by the sympathomimetic effects of hyperthyroidism. Patients often present critically ill with hyperthermia, confusion, and cardiac irregularities. More commonly, a clinically unrecognized or partially treated degree of hyperthyroidism is precipitated into crisis by trauma, surgery, infection, or radioiodine therapy (which can produce radiation thyroiditis). Occasionally, it is still seen in incorrectly prepared patients undergoing thyroidectomy.

Treatment must often be initiated prior to biochemical confirmation. Because the major features are due to excessive β-adrenergic activity, intravenous propranolol 1 to 2 mg is given, and repeated half-hourly as necessary so as to maintain a ventricular rate of 80 to 100. Reduction of thyroid hypersecretion must be concurrent. In less severe cases, propylthiouracil 200 mg is given every 4 hours, by nasogastric tube if necessary, utilizing the fact that in contrast to carbimazole, this drug additionally inhibits peripheral T_4 to T_3 conversion, which may be of crucial benefit in such ill patients.

More severe cases are treated with intravenous sodium iodide, 1 gram every 8 hours for three doses. Iodide is the only drug capable of producing an almost instantaneous suppression of thyroidal hormone release as well as inhibiting organification of iodine by the Wolff–Chaikoff effect. There is no evidence of any beneficial effect of glucocorticoids, although these are still sometimes given to patients in dosage of 300 mg of intravenous cortisol infused over a 24-hour period. The untreated mortality approaches 100 per cent. but careful and early treatment should be almost universally effective.

Deficiency

Primary hypothyroidism: Hashimoto's disease

This common disorder affects approximately 1 per cent of the adult population. Subclinical cases of biochemically confirmed hypothyroidism are being increasingly documented, sometimes raising the question of large-scale population screening as a means of identifying early cases. The prevalence is highest in elderly females, but may occur at any age and in either sex.

Aetiology (see Plate 9.11)

As with Graves' disease, most cases of primary hypothyroidism represent a component of the thyrogastric autoimmune group of disorders, and probably represent the end result of a cell-mediated destructive immune response directed against the thyroid follicular cell. However, in some cases, a TSH receptor-blocking antibody can be identified. Accordingly, hypothyroidism need not always be considered a permanent condition. It is insidious in onset, and may sometimes represent a transition from 'burnt out' Graves' disease. Goitre is usually not present in these cases, but is by definition a feature of Hashimoto's disease.

Uncommonly, hypothyroidism may be due to a severe defect in thyroid hormone biosynthesis, either inherited or resulting from the additional effect of iodine and other goitrogens. This will be discussed later in the chapter.

Clinical features (see Plates 9.1, 9.2, 9.10, 9.11)

Generalized tiredness and lethargy are the most common features, although there may be no symptoms or signs whatsoever. Classical cases show the following features:

1. In the cardiovascular system there is bradycardia, occasionally gross congestive cardiomyopathy, or pericardial effusion. The ECG is characteristically low voltage in type.

2. Neuromuscular symptoms, such as weakness, muscle cramps (pseudo-claudication), and a cerebellar ataxia are occasionally complicated by psychiatric features including depression or organic psychosis.

3. The skin is dry and flaky and there may be anaemia of varying morphology. Alopecia (hair loss) is common, the voice is deep and husky and there is usually some weight gain, although the concept that many cases of simple obesity are due to thyroid hypofunction has been shown to be totally incorrect. In severe cases, there may be evidence of serous effusions, in pericardial or peritoneal cavities, and occasionally in the form of a scrotal hydrocoele.

4. Females may show heavy periods (menorrhagia) and be infertile, and impotence and lack of libido is common in males.

The thyroid gland is mostly impalpable: if present, a goitre suggests the diagnosis either of Hashimoto's disease or biosynthetic block. In addition to the features listed above, delay in reflex relaxation time is common, best identified in biceps or Achilles reflex.

Investigation

1. Serum-free T_4 (but often not free T_3) concentrations are subnormal, and are accompanied by an elevated serum TSH due to negative feedback effect. Early cases may show only an elevation of serum TSH with normal free hormone levels: it is questionable whether any of such patients' symptoms can be attributed to their thyroid status.

2. Thyroid antibodies, both to thyroglobulin and microsomal antigen (thyroid peroxidase, TPO) are positive in the majority of cases, and usually in even higher titres (exceeding 1:6400) in Hashimoto's disease.

3. Thyroid isotope uptake, although reduced, is rarely necessary for confirmation, although in hypothyroidism due to biosynthetic defect, and in approximately 50 per cent of Hashimoto's disease cases, thyroidal iodide trapping is increased and accordingly isotope uptake is paradoxically elevated.

4. Secondary features, such as a mild normocytic or macrocytic anaemia and variable degrees of hypercholesterolaemia, are often present, the latter finding probably representing the basis of the increased prevalence of atherosclerosis found in this disorder.

5. Diagnostic confusion may arise where the conventional measurement of total serum T_4 is used as the initial diagnostic test: a low measured total serum T_4 may

be due to reduced thyronine-binding proteins as found in hypoproteinaemic patients or with congenital or drug-induced reduction in thyroid-binding prealbumin (TBPA) or globulin (TBG). Confusion may also arise in sick patients who are in fact euthyroid, but who show low serum T_4 and/or T_3 levels partly due to the binding phenomena mentioned above. Even free hormone levels may be reduced in certain instances (such as chronic renal failure and anorexia nervosa) due to associated (functional) hypothalamic-based hypopituitarism. The precise cause of, and rationale for treatment of this so-called 'sick-euthyroid' syndrome has still not been clearly established, although most studies show little benefit from correcting under-function in these disease-associated disturbances of thyroid function. Perhaps they are best regarded as functional adaptations to a disease state.

6. It is essential to exclude hypothyroidism due to hypopituitarism or hypothalamic disease, where serum TSH is in the measurable normal or low range and may therefore cause confusion with the various forms of sick euthyroid syndrome.

Treatment

Thyroxine is more appropriate than T_3 because of its longer half-life, providing stable circulating hormone levels throughout the 24-hour period following once-daily administration. Even multiple daily doses of T_3 produce widely fluctuating serum T_3 levels, and except for short treatment periods, is considered unsatisfactory. Similarly, T_4/T_3 mixtures have no advantage over T_4 alone, since T_4 is deiodinated in peripheral tissues: as a consequence of this, in athyroid patients on normal replacement doses of T_4, serum-free T_3 is almost invariably within the normal range.

Thyroxine replacement requirement in the hypothyroid patient is mostly between 50 and 200 μg daily, given as a single daily dose. Treatment is usually more gradually introduced in patients over age 60, and a 25 μg daily dose is a safer initiating dose in those with known ischaemic heart disease (in whom treatment can otherwise precipitate angina, myocardial infarction, or cardiac failure). In the occasional patient with severe cardiac ischaemia or failure, it may be safer not to treat the hypothyroidism unless symptoms are disabling.

Except in this latter group of patients, it is logical to titrate the thyroxine dose until serum-free T_4 and TSH concentrations are normalized. Dosage increments should not be made until 4 weeks on the previous dose have elapsed to allow for equilibration with serum-binding proteins. As indicated earlier, serum-free T_3 will ultimately rise into the normal range due to peripheral conversion from administered T_4.

Over-replacement with thyroxine carries a number of potential problems. Precipitation of cardiac failure in elderly patients with pre-existing cardiac disease is occasionally seen. More contentiously, it has been shown that bone mineral density falls more rapidly in over-replaced patients (see osteoporosis, Chapter 10). It has therefore become accepted wisdom to ensure that in long term replacement, suppression of serum TSH below the normal range is avoided.

Reinforcement of the need for life-long replacement is essential: a significant number of patients discontinue therapy or default from follow-up, making some form of computerized recall highly desirable. There is controversy about the wisdom of treating patients with solitary elevations of serum TSH (but normal circulating free thyroid hormones). Some of these individuals may demonstrate significant hypercholesterolaemia and accordingly may be at increased risk from premature atherosclerosis. Whether thyroxine therapy reverses this risk still remains to be proven. Current data suggest that the transition rate of such subtle biochemical anomalies to a clinical hypothyroid state occurs at the rate of about 5 per cent per annum.

Special forms of hypothyroidism

Hypothyroid coma

This is uncommon, and represents the most extreme form of hypothyroidism. It may be precipitated by environmental cooling, by anaesthesia, or by a variety of hypnotic and antidepressant drugs. In addition to the classical features (which may have evaded previous diagnosis) there is hypothermia and a variable degree of confusion and depressed state of consciousness. In most cases this is due to a dilutional hyponatraemia (due to a lack of the thyroxine-dependent ability to excrete a water load) and less commonly due to hypoxia and hypercapnia with a resulting respiratory acidosis (due to hypoventilation).

The therapeutic options consist of treating cautiously with small doses of thyroid hormones (usually T_3) or use of a massive administration of parenteral thyroxine. The latter approach is justified by the knowledge that much of the effect of thyroxine is based on peripheral interconversion to T_3, the rate of this transformation being dependent on metabolic rate. Accordingly, recovery from hypothermia and hypometabolism will itself affect the rate of hormone availability. External warming of patients is undesirable, but the infusion of heated parenteral fluids may be of some value, and additional corticosteroid is usually given in the form of a continuous intravenous infusion of cortisol 300–400 mg over 24 hours, since adrenal function may be impaired. Supportive ventilation is often necessary since hypoxia and hypercapnia are frequently encountered. Untreated, the mortality is high and even with treatment a mortality rate of 20–30 per cent is usual.

Neonatal hypothyroidism (see Plate 9.3)

Large-scale screening programmes have suggested that this disorder has a prevalence of between 1 in 3000 and 1 in 5000 deliveries, although there are significant regional differences. It is mostly due to agenesis of the thyroid, although rare cases are due to immunologically based disease similar to the adult form. Since the disorder causes severe mental retardation unless promptly treated, and since it is not always possible to make a clinical diagnosis at birth, universal screening of all neonates is now commonplace. This is normally based on TSH assay of heel prick or cord blood. National programmes have been organized in many countries, and the cost-effectiveness of such schemes is well documented.

Self-limiting neonatal hypothyroidism may also occur as a consequence of drug over-treatment of a thyrotoxic mother or the transplacental passage of TSH-blocking antibodies from mothers who are, or have been hypothyroid.

Juvenile hypothyroidism (see Plate 9.4)

Although clinical features are qualitatively similar to adult hypothyroid patients, in childhood certain features predominate. There is delayed sexual maturation. Mental slowness may be striking but occasionally absent. Retardation of linear growth may be marked, and hypothyroidism must be considered in every child or young adult presenting with short stature. Short lower limbs are occasionally striking, and skeletal age assessment often shows retardation even below that which is expected for the observed height. The cause and diagnostic procedure is identical to adult hypothyroidism.

Treatment is always gratifying, but care must be taken not to replace with excess thyroxine; in infancy and early childhood, this may be associated with premature fusion (synostosis) of cranial bones resulting in mental retardation, or of long bones (resulting in permanent short stature). Accurate titration of thyroxine to maintain serum TSH in the normal reference range is therefore mandatory.

Goitre

Patients may present at any age with a thyroid enlargement. Although there is some obvious overlap, diagnosis and management is most easily divided into generalized and localized thyroid swellings.

Generalized thyroid enlargement

Endemic goitre

Numerically this is the most common cause of goitre in the world, and is encountered in up to 50 per cent of certain ethnic groups such as the New Guinea highlanders and natives of the Himalayas. The common denominator is the low dietary iodine consumption, based on the leaching of soil iodides in mountainous areas. To a lesser extent, this phenomenon is encountered even in minor hilly areas of many countries. In rare instances, genetic inbreeding and the consumption of cabbage-type goitrogens may compound the problem, by inducing defects in thyroid hormone biosynthesis. More severe cases are also hypothyroid, and endemic goitrous cretinism with severe mental retardation may occur in those individuals who are severely iodine-deficient from birth, brain damage resulting in these cases directly from iodine deficiency rather than from the hypothyroid state itself. The control of endemic goitre is one of the major achievements of modern medicine, utilizing the injection of depot iodinated oils in some communities, or the use of iodized salt and bread in others. The organization of such community programmes often presents major logistic difficulties. The occasional consequence of the Jod–Basedow phenomenon (induction of hyperthyroidism by iodide) has been dealt with in an earlier section (p. 216).

Sporadic non-toxic goitre

Diffuse or nodular goitre is common in some countries, and has multiple aetiologies.

'Physiological' goitre Transient thyroid enlargement is sometimes detected in the neonate, in puberty, and in pregnancy. The precise mechanisms are unknown, but may reflect temporary increased hormone demand, possibly superimposed on a mildly abnormal gland (subtle biosynthetic defect or autoimmune component).

Drug-induced goitre Apart from obvious drugs, such as thiocarbamides used in the treatment of Graves' disease, a number of other drugs inhibit thyroid hormone synthesis, negative feedback stimulating TSH and hence follicular cell hypertrophy and hyperplasia in order to restore normal hormone production states.

Lithium carbonate (used in the treatment of depression) blocks dominantly hormone release and organic binding, but also to a lesser extent other stages of synthesis. Up to 20 per cent of patients receiving lithium develop goitres, and a proportion of these develop hypothyroidism. Positive thyroid microsomal antibody titres are a risk factor. Iodides (used in anticough formulations, radiography contrast media, and in many other drug and multivitamin preparations) inhibit hormone release and organification (the so-called Wolff–Chaikoff effect). Vitamin A, phenylbutazone, ρ-aminosalicylic acid, resorcinol, thiocyanates, and other less frequently used drugs can also induce goitre. In all cases, hypothyroidism may also be induced, particularly if patients have an associated mild inherited biosynthetic defect, or underlying previously unrecognized thyroid auto-immune disorder.

Hereditary disorders of thyroid biosynthesis Mild or severe defects of synthesis occur most commonly at the level of organification of iodine with tyrosine, less commonly affecting other stages of biosynthesis. The disorders are usually inherited as autosomal recessive characteristics, expression being incomplete since environmental factors (drugs, iodine deficiency or excess, natural goitrogens) are sometimes needed for the disorder to become clinically apparent. Patients are often quite young at presentation. Negative feedback stimulation induces TSH release and hence goitre formation. Various classical syndromes have been described, including Pendred's syndrome (organification defect with sensorineural deafness). If defects are more severe, hypothyroidism may also be present.

Hashimoto's disease This eponymous diagnosis represents the archetype thyroid autoimmune disease, linked as indicated earlier to specific histocompatibility antigens and found both individually or in familial association with the other organ-specific autoimmune disorders listed in Table 16.2. It refers specifically to the association of hypothyroidism, goitre, and positive TPO antibodies (sometimes in a titre greater than 1:6400).

The classical histological finding of focal and diffuse lymphocytic infiltration and fibrosis is responsible for the goitre which is almost invariably found in these patients. The gland is firm to palpation, but still mobile, the occasional more focal varieties giving rise to confusion with regard to a a differential diagnosis of carcinoma or lymphoma (whose prevalence is greater in patients with auto-immune thyroid disease).

A broader spectrum of Hashimoto's disease is now recognized, with some patients undergoing spontaneous transition between hypothyroid, euthyroid, and hyperthyroid states.

Multinodular goitre This is common in the second half of life, and may represent the end result of one or more of the pathological processes listed above, in addition to iodine deficiency. The nodular pattern is presumably brought about by periodic involution and regeneration of regions of the gland, due to fluctuating environmental changes. The palpatory findings are usually diagnostic, and the goitre may occasionally be large enough to cause major mediastinal compression. Malignant change is often suspected in such glands, but is actually uncommon.

Investigation of goitre

1. Serum-free T_3 and T_4 levels are required to determine whether thyroid function is normal. Serum TSH may occasionally be elevated even with normal serum T_3 and T_4, reflecting the compensatory negative feedback response. Alternatively, the biochemical profile may be that of hyperthyroidism (see earlier), reflecting hyperfunction of autonomous thyroid foci.

2. Thyroid isotope uptake and scan (using either radioiodine or technetium) or thyroid ultrasound is capable of distinguishing diffuse from nodular goitres. Isotope uptake is increased typically in biosynthetic and most drug-induced goitres (except for defects in the iodide trap or with lithium therapy), and in some cases of Hashimoto's disease. It is usually normal or even low in multinodular goitre, with characteristically variable foci of increased and decreased isotope uptake in scintiscans (see Fig. 9.6).

3. Thyroid antibodies to microsomal (thyroid peroxidase) and thyroglobulin antigen are very high in Hashimoto's disease (greater than 1:6400) with occasionally elevated titres in multinodular and in drug-induced goitre. They are by definition absent in biosynthetic goitres.

4. Thyroid aspiration cytology (needle biopsy) may provide diagnostic findings in Hashimoto's disease, or when an autoimmune component is suspected in multinodular goitre.

Treatment

Some diffuse goitres occurring during puberty and pregnancy require no therapy and are self-limiting. When responsible for goitre, drug therapy may require discontinuation, but where continuation is essential (e.g. lithium in depression) supplemental thyroxine will normally induce regression of the goitre. The response of biosynthetic goitre to suppressive T_4 therapy (100–200 μg daily) is variable. Younger patients may expect significant and even total regression, but in later life, for reasons which are unclear, a less complete response is common.

The goitre of Hashimoto's disease responds variably to suppressive thyroxine therapy, and is more likely in younger patients. Thyroxine replacement is often required on the basis of overt or biochemical hypothyroidism. Euthyroid cases with positive antibody status require close observation with annual or biennial thyroid function assessment to identify transition to abnormal functional status.

The response of multinodular goitres to suppression is uniformly poor. Patients in whom there is little disability require only reassurance, but where there is evidence of cervical or mediastinal compression, thyroidectomy is indicated. In such cases, the prevalence both of postoperative hypothyroidism and hypoparathyroidism is high. Haemorrhage or degeneration may occur suddenly into individual thyroid nodules causing acute discomfort and even sudden mediastinal obstruction.

Thyroid hormone resistance syndromes

Thyroid hormone receptors are present on all body tissue cells, and there is evidence of physiological variability in tissue responses to circulating T_3 and T_4. Over and above this, however, a variety of rare syndromes has been described where genetic alteration in the action, transport, or metabolism of thyroid hormones has apparently occurred. Characterization of the defect(s) has been difficult, some researchers showing defective binding of T_3 to nuclear receptors within *in vitro* cell systems such as fibroblasts. Recently, mutations in the thyroid hormone-receptor beta-gene have been identified, and are likely to be responsible for the majority of reported cases.

The clinical syndromes which result from such receptor defects depend on the sites of the lesion. A well-recognized variant is that in which the pituitary receptors alone fail to normally recognize T_3 or T_4. This feedback 'reset' results in a hyperthyroid syndrome with raised T_3 and T_4 levels, a goitre and paradoxically normal or minimally raised serum TSH concentrations. Although there is no ophthalmopathy, this disorder comes into the differential diagnosis of Graves' hyperthyroidism. The only other disorder providing the same spectrum of findings is the equally rare TSH-producing pituitary adenoma.

If T_4 and T_3 insensitivity involve both pituitary and peripheral tissues, the patient is clinically hypothyroid, but in the presence of normal, or even raised T_4, T_3, and TSH levels. It has often been suggested that a proportion of biochemically euthyroid patients with apparently hypothyroid symptoms (especially fatigue) may have such a syndrome, although it is exceedingly difficult to prove: clinically assessable parameters of peripheral thyroid hormone action are limited to basal metabolic rate, ankle reflex relaxation time, cardiac systolic time intervals (measurable by echocardiography), and a few very non-specific enzyme changes. None the less, the existence of such wide and yet apparently physiological differences in thyroid hormone levels within the normal range, plus the fact that individual subjects without thyroid disease 'track' at remarkable constant levels within this range does lend some support for potentially significant individual receptor status. This may have biological (and pathological) conseqences.

A further interesting type of hormone resistance occurs one step earlier in the thyroid–thyrotrophin feedback loop: resistance to the action of thyrotrophin caused by mutations in the thyrotrophin receptor gene(s). These may produce their effects by inactivating either the thyrotrophin receptor itself, or alternatively the G protein (guanine nucleotide-binding) which couples the receptor to adenylate cyclase. In both cases, partial defects result in euthyroidism with raised serum TSH, while complete defects result in classical (but antibody-negative) hypothyroidism. A number of cases of the latter syndrome have been recorded, presenting as both congenital and familial hypothyroidism.

The solitary thyroid nodule

Around 5 per cent of a random Western population harbour a palpable nodule if the neck is carefully examined. The aetiology of these is variable. Malignancy is often suspected, but is rarely found in incidentally discovered nodules. A focally dominant area in a basically multinodular goitre is a common finding when subsequent thyroid isotope or ultrasound scans are performed, but true adenoma, a solitary colloid nodule or a cyst is found in approximately 80 per cent of cases coming to surgery. Haemorrhage into or acute cystic degeneration of such a solitary nodule or multinodular goitre may result in an acute presentation with pain and swelling without preceding history. A similar picture can also be seen with some cases of focal subacute thyroiditis. Clinical features which suggest malignancy are a lack of mobility of the nodule, progressive increase in size over a 3–6 months observation interval, and hoarseness.

Investigation

1. Except with large autonomous hyperfunctioning nodules, serum-free T_3, T_4, and TSH are usually normal.

2. Thyroid (nuclear) isotope scanning may demonstrate a greater than normal uptake in the palpable thyroid tissue (hot nodule) which if large (usually greater than 4 cm diameter) may be associated with other evidence of thyroid hyperfunction. The scan may show that the nodule represents a single palpable feature of a multinodular goitre which is unsuspected clinically. A 'warm' or 'cold' solitary nodule carries a rather greater risk of being neoplastic, yet only 5 per cent of such nodules are actually malignant at operation.

3. Thyroid ultrasound has the ability to delineate cystic from solid tissue at the site of a palpable nodule, but the identification of cystic change does not exclude neoplasm.

4. Thyroid aspiration cytology through a fine needle (FNAB) is a useful and safe procedure and is normally performed on any nodule which is increasing in size or confirmed by scanning to be solitary, whether 'hot' or 'cold'. Smears are usually reported as non-malignant, suspicious, or malignant. False positive and negative reports do occur, but these are rare in the hands of an experienced cytopathologist.

Treatment

Aspiration cytology may result in the removal of a substantial quantity of fluid from a cyst, providing therapy as well as diagnosis. However, re-accumulation occurs in more than 50 per cent of cases and the replacement of this fluid by a sclerosing agent such as tetracycline, may reduce recurrence rate. The decision whether to watch or to operate on patients with solitary nodules is highly individual, but largely dependant on the level of expertise and confidence in aspiration cytology. Only if findings are 'malignant' or 'suspicious' is hemithyroidectomy normally performed.

If investigation reveals that an apparently solitary nodule is actually part of a multinodular goitre, the risk of malignancy falls sharply. However, carcinoma can occur in multinodular goitres, and surgery is justified for any thyroid swelling which is progressively enlarging, irrespective of cytology findings. The follow-up of patients with benign cytology can be a major commitment with a small return. It is often safe to discharge such patients from follow-up procedure, with notification by the patient if any enlargement is noted.

Thyroid carcinoma

Thyroid cancer is not uncommon, and more frequently found in females. Causative factors are hard to identify, although irradiation (therapeutic to children with lymphomas) or accidental (as in the survivors of the Hiroshima and Nagasaki nuclear explosions) is associated with a markedly increased incidence of papillary thyroid tumour formation. There is also a higher incidence of lymphoma in patients with autoimmune thyroid disease. The overall prognosis of thyroid tumours is generally better than with most other cancers.

Clinical features

Most thyroid cancer presents as a neck lump which is apparent to the patient or their friend or relative. Because of their malignant nature, they may not be so mobile in the neck, and can be clinically tethered to deep tissues. Invasive characteristics may result in hoarseness (due to recurrent laryngeal pressure or infiltration) and occasionally dysphagia. Only rarely is carcinoma associated with thyroid dysfunction: occasional cases of metastatic differentiated carcinoma have been reported with hyperthyroidism.

1. Papillary carcinoma is the most common, presenting in children and adults and occasionally first identified from their metastatic potential to regional lymph nodes.

2. Follicular carcinoma is slightly less common, usually found in older age groups and characterized by blood-borne distant metastases to lungs, bone, and other tissues.

3. Anaplastic carcinoma is a more rapidly progressive tumour found rather more commonly in the older age groups and infiltrating locally as well as metastasizing distally.

4. Medullary thyroid carcinoma is the least common type of 'thyroid' tumour, and represents a neoplasm of the parafollicular C cells of embryonic neural crest origin. It may be familial and associated either in the individual or in relatives with

other endocrinopathies, such as hyperparathyroidism and phaeochromocytoma, and with multiple mucocutaneous nodules (see MEN syndromes, Chapter 16). Because the C cell produces calcitonin, plasma assay of the hormone provides a tissue marker for this disorder. The diarrhoea which often accompanies this syndrome is not due to elevation of calcitonin, but to the presumptive cosecretion of another peptide which currently evades identification. Ectopic hormone production is common, usually involving ACTH hypersecretion: the diagnosis of medullary thyroid carcinoma should be considered in every patient presenting with Cushing's disease, since the neck tumour may not be obvious: indeed the C cell tumour may be in the thymus, pancreas, or lung.

5. Thyroid lymphoma is always to be considered in a firm or hard, uniform or nodular thyroid swelling which is increasing in size. There is sometimes a past or family history of autoimmune thyroid disease.

Investigation

The approach previously described for solitary nodules should be followed. Aspiration cytology is often useful but can be occasionally misleading since cytological (and even histological) characterization of the neoplastic from benign follicular morphology can be difficult. Measurement of serum thyroglobulin is a useful guide to the extent of tumour mass in differentiated thyroid tumours. Although it is present in the circulation in many non-malignant thyroid disorders, in these latter cases it can be suppressed by exogenous thyroxine. In contrast, the diffusion of thyroglobulin from malignant thyroid epithelium is non-suppressible.

Treatment

In early cases of papillary or follicular carcinoma, excision by hemithyroidectomy is often curative. Thyroxine is usually given since a proportion of tumours, particularly of the follicular variety are TSH-dependent, and hence it is logical to treat with maximum TSH suppression. Since some tumours are multifocal, many surgeons advocate total thyroidectomy, followed by whole-body radioiodine scanning. Iodine-avid metastases may be identified in this way, and accordingly treated by larger destructive radioiodine doses. The relative virtues of aggressive ablative approaches and more conservative thyroxine suppression regimes continue to be debated, and are difficult to resolve since these tumours behave in a highly individual manner. The overall prognosis in thyroid cancer is surprisingly good, papillary cases showing a survival of approximately 80 per cent at five years, whatever the treatment. Advanced tumours may respond to external megavoltage therapy, or to a variety of cytotoxic agents.

Medullary thyroid carcinoma is often metastatic at diagnosis, and very resistant to any form of intervention. Since this condition may be familial, screening of first-degree relatives using serum calcitonin determinations is logical, but their treatment remains controversial. However, there is an increasing trend towards thyroidectomy in relatives with raised calcitonin levels (See chapter 16).

Lymphoma may be treated by surgery, but is usually quite responsive to chemotherapy or radiotherapy.

FURTHER READING

PHYSIOLOGY

Dumont, J.E., Lamy, F., Roger, P., and Maenhaut, C. (1992). Physiological and pathological regulation of thyroid cell prolifeation and differentiation by thyrotropin and other factors. *Physiol. Rev.*, **72**, 667–98.

Ludgate, M.E. and Vassart, G. (1995). The thyrotrophin receptor as a model to illustrate receptor and receptor antibody diseases. In *Bailliere's clinical endocrinology and metabolism*, Vol. 9 (1). Autoimmune endocrine diseases. Chapter 5, 95–113.

Porterfield, S.P. and Hendrich, C.E. (1993). The role of thyroid hormones in prenatal and neonatal neurological development – current perspectives. *Endocrine Rev.*, **14**, 94–106.

CLINICAL

Bahn, R.S. and Heufelder, A.E. (1993). Pathogenesis of Graves' ophthalmopathy. *New England Journal of Medicine*, **329**, 1468–75.

Bergholm, U., Adami, H.O., Bergstrom, R., *et al.* (1989). Clinical characteristics in sporadic and familial meedullary thyroid carcinoma: a nationwide study of 249 patients in Sweden from 1959 through 1981. *Cancer*, **63**, 1196–1204.

Boyages, S.C. (1993). Iodine deficiency disorders. *Journal of Clinical Endocrinology and Metabolism*, **77**, 587–91.

Burch H.B. and Wartofsky, L. (1993). Life-threatening thyrotoxicosis. *Endocrinology Metabolism Clinics North America*, **22**, 263–77.

Burrow, G.N. (1993). Thyroid function and hyperfunction during gestation. *Endocrine Reviews*, **14**, 194–203.

Docter, J, Krenning, E.P., de Jong, M., *et al.* (1993). The sick euthyroid syndrome: changes in thyroid hormone serum parameters and hormone metabolism. *Clinical Endocrinology*, **39**, 499–518.

Eguchi, K., Matsuoka, N., and Nagataki, S. (1995). Cellular immunity in auto-immune thyroid disease. *Clinical Endocrinology and Metabolism*, **9**, 71–94.

Franklyn, J.A. (1994). The management of hyperthyroidism. *New England Journal of Medicine*, **330**, 1731–8.

Gagel, R.F., Robinson, M.F., Donovan, D.T., *et al.* (1993). Medullary thyroid carcinoma: recent progress. *Journal of Clinical Endocrinology and Metabolism*, **76**, 809–14.

Hall, R., Richards, C.J., and Lazarus, J.H. (1993). The thyroid and pregnancy. *British Journal of Obstetrics and Gynaecology*, **100**, 512–15.

Kerr, D.J, Burt A.D., Boyle, P., *et al.* (1986). Prognostic factors in thyroid cancer. *British Journal of Cancer*, **54**, 475–82.

Mazzaferri, E.L. (1993). Management of a single thyroid nodule. *New England Journal of Medicine*, **328**, 553–9.

Perros, P.E., Crombie, A.L., and Kendall Taylor, P. (1995). Natural history of thyroid-associated ophthalmopathy. *Clinical Endocrinology*, **42**, 45–50.

Sheppard, M.C. and Franklyn, J.A. (1992). Management of the single thyroid nodule. *Clinical Endocrinology*, **37**, 398–401.

Tandon, N. and Weetman A.P. (1994). T-cells and thyroid autoimmunity. *Journal of the Royal College of Physicians*, **28**, 10–18.

Thoresen, S.O., Akslen, L.A., Glattre, E., *et al.* (1989). Survival and prognostic factors in differentiated thyroid carcinoma — a multivariate analysis of 1055 cases. *British Journal of Cancer*, **59**, 231–40.

Toft, A.D. (1994). Thyroxine therapy. *New England Journal of Medicine*, **331**, 174–80.

10

Calcium regulation, bone, and its metabolic disorders

PHYSIOLOGY

Calcium ions play an essential role in numerous physiological functions. For example, they are involved in many intracellular metabolic pathways as co-enzymes and regulators. They influence membrane permeability to sodium ions and therefore are important in determining the degree of neuromuscular excitability. They also take part in the release of neurotransmitters (e.g. acetylcholine at neuromuscular junctions) and are involved in numerous excitation–secretion coupled events in endocrine and exocrine cells. They are a crucial component of the contractile process in muscle fibres. In blood, the calcium ion is an important factor in the cascade mechanism of coagulation. Such examples demonstrate the importance of calcium ions and indicate the necessity for their quite precise regulation in the extracellular fluid.

Over 99 per cent of calcium in the body is found in the bones (approximately 1000 g in the average adult) where it provides strength and rigidity to the skeletal framework. The bones therefore serve as the principal store of calcium in the body, although about 99 per cent of this calcium is found as complex crystals of hydroxyapatite [$Ca_{10}(PO_4)_6(OH)_2 \cdot xH_2O$], which is not readily available for rapid mobilization. However, the remaining 1 per cent is readily exchangeable, is present as calcium phosphate salts, and provides an immediate buffer to sudden changes in the blood calcium concentration with which it is in equilibrium (Fig. 10.1). The normal level of calcium in the plasma is between 2.3 and 2.6 mmol/l with approximately 50 per cent of the calcium free (i.e. unbound, ionized) and the remainder bound either to plasma proteins (about 45 per cent) or associated with anions such as citrate or lactate (5 per cent). The citrate, lactate, and other salts are diffusible through capillary membranes. The bound and ionized calcium components are in dynamic equilibrium with each other.

Apart from the continuous, inevitable loss of calcium from the body (in dead cells, nails, blood, etc.) the pathways by which calcium can enter or leave the extracellular fluid are the gastrointestinal tract and the kidneys, respectively. Therefore, regulation of the plasma calcium ion concentration, not surprisingly, involves these two tissues as well as the principal storage sites (the bones). The control mechanisms are endocrine and consist of: (1) parathormone from the parathyroid glands and (2) the vitamin D_3 (cholecalciferol) metabolites, which act together to raise the concentration of calcium in the blood; while (3) calcitonin from the thyroid parafollicular cells acts to decrease it. Other hormones have been

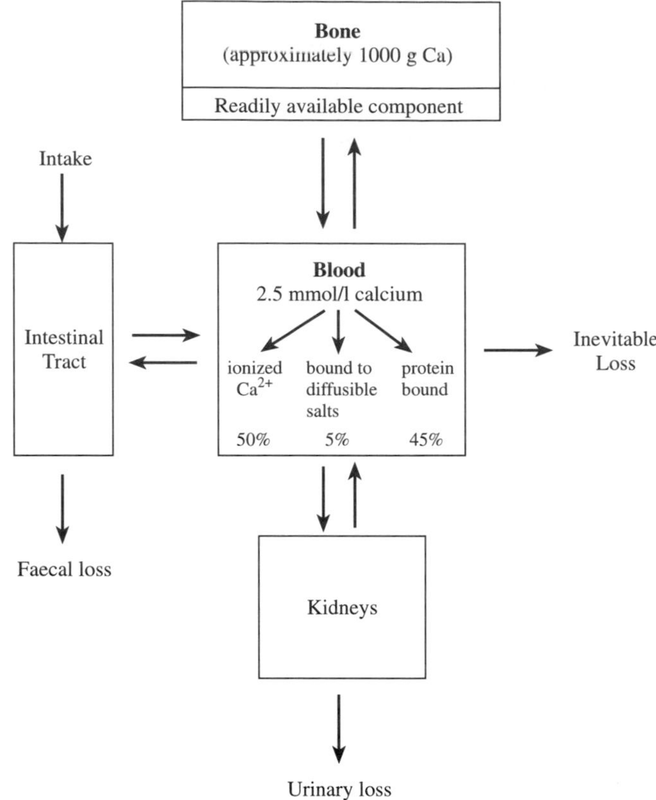

Fig. 10.1 Diagram illustrating the principal organs involved in normal calcium metabolism.

identified recently which can also influence calcium ion regulation, one example being parathormone-related peptide (PTHRP).

The parathyroid glands

Anatomy, histology, and development

The parathyroid glands are derived from the third and fourth branchial pouches. In humans there are usually four glands, one at each of the superior and inferior poles of the two lobes of the thyroid situated close to the posterior surface. However, the number and location of the parathyroids can vary considerably. Each gland is surrounded by a fibrous capsule through which the blood vessels, unmyelinated nerve fibres, and lymphatics penetrate in a distinct stalk. Inside the gland, arterial blood enters a capillary plexus.

There are two principal types of epithelial cell in the gland, the chief and oxyphilic cells. The chief cells are the principal source of parathormone. There are two types of chief cell: 'light' cells which are believed to be inactive and not actually engaged in hormone synthesis; and 'dark' cells which contain some small membrane-bound granules believed to hold the hormone and which are considered to be active. The ratio of active to inactive cells is normally 1 to 3 but this can decrease to 1 to 10 in suppressed glands. The oxyphilic cells appear after puberty and increase in number with age. They are derived from the chief cells and are not usually capable of synthesizing parathormone; their function, if any, is uncertain.

Parathormone (PTH)

Synthesis, storage, and release

Parathormone is a large single-chain polypeptide (approximately 9.5 kDa) consisting of 84 amino acids. The initial precursor molecule called pre-proparathormone, which contains the signal peptide, consists of 115 amino acids. The signal sequence is lost as the molecule enters the endoplasmic reticulum. The remaining proparathormone sequence, a 90-amino acid precursor (approximately 12 kDa), is present only in small concentrations in the glands. It has far less biological (< 0.2 per cent) and immunological activity than PTH which is the major secretion of the parathyroids. Cleavage of the precursor molecule occurs in the Golgi complex, with PTH then packaged into secretory granules prior to the release process.

The NH_2-terminal portion of the PTHRP molecule has some homology with human PTH and can bind to PTH receptors. It was first identified in tumours associated with hypercalcaemia of malignancy. It is immunologically distinct from PTH. A physiological role for PTHRP on calcium transport in the fetus is possible since it has been identified in the placenta. Furthermore, it may stimulate calcium transport into milk as expression of its mRNA in mammary glands has been shown in lactating rats.

Actions of PTH

The actions of parathormone are directed primarily at raising the plasma calcium concentration and also at decreasing the plasma phosphate concentration. These actions occur at the three tissues concerned with calcium metabolism mentioned earlier (see Fig. 10.2).

Bone

The immediate buffering capability of the readily exchangeable calcium phosphate salts in bone is influenced by parathormone, but the hormone's principal effects on this tissue are more related to the longer-term restoration of equilibrium between the extracellular and bone calcium levels. The latter, longer-term, effects of PTH are associated with the increased synthesis of enzymes (e.g. lysosomal enzymes) which induce the breakdown of the bone matrix to release calcium (and phosphate) into the extracellular fluid. The process of bone matrix dissolution which culminates in the release of calcium ions into the blood is called bone resorption.

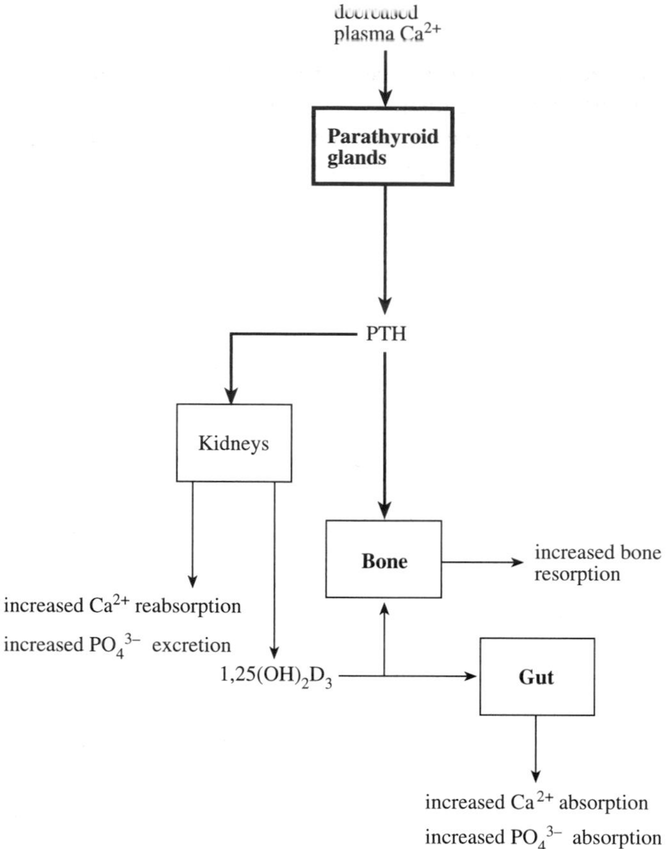

Fig. 10.2 The general actions of parathormone (PTH).

Bone consists essentially of three cell types and a matrix containing the calcium salts. The cells which lay down new bone matrix are called osteoblasts. Once these cells become surrounded by new bone, they convert to osteocytes which have osteolytic activity (bone matrix resorptive activity). The third cell type is the osteoclast which stimulates bone resorption by releasing lysosomal proteolytic enzymes such as collagenase. Parathormone has three separate effects on bone cells:

(1) it stimulates osteoclastic and osteocytic activities;

(2) it increases the osteoclast pool by stimulating the formation of new osteoclasts; and

(3) it induces a (transient) depression of osteoblastic activity.

As a consequence of these actions on bone cells by PTH, the net result is an increased mobilization of calcium and phosphate from the bone matrix.

Kidneys

Historically, the first observed effect of PTH was an increase in renal phosphate excretion. This effect at least partly results from a direct inhibition of phosphate transport in both proximal and distal convoluted tubules. Originally, this renal effect on phosphate was believed to account for the subsequent increase in the plasma calcium concentration since an increased excretion of phosphate alters the equilibrium between the dissociated ions and the readily exchangeable calcium phosphate salts. Thus, a greater dissociation of the salt occurs in order to maintain the equilibrium state and consequently the calcium ion concentration increases.

However, it is now known that PTH also has a direct effect on calcium reabsorption in the kidneys. More than 95 per cent of the filtered calcium load is reabsorbed along the renal nephron by passive and active transport mechanisms in different segments. There is substantial evidence for an inhibition of proximal tubular calcium reabsorption by parathormone, but this hormone also greatly enhances the active transport of this ion out of the distal nephron (distal convoluted tubule and possibly from sections of the collecting duct). The overall effect of PTH on the renal handling of calcium is therefore to decrease the loss of the ion from the body by reducing its urinary excretion.

Parathormone also increases the urinary excretion of sodium, potassium, and bicarbonate ions while decreasing the excretion of magnesium ions. In addition, ammonium and hydrogen ion excretion is reduced. The effect of PTH on sodium and phosphate is probably located at the proximal convoluted tubule along with the block on calcium reabsorption in this segment. Increased presentation of tubular sodium to the distal nephron may then enhance potassium excretion by stimulation of the Na^+–K^+ exchange mechanism in the distal convolution cells.

Another important effect of PTH in the kidneys is the stimulation of 1α-hydroxylase, an enzyme which converts 25-hydroxy-vitamin D_3 (25-hydroxychole-calciferol) to the biologically potent 1,25-dihydroxy-vitamin D_3 metabolite (1,25-dihydroxycholecalciferol). This molecule increases the body calcium stores and raises the plasma calcium ion concentration (see vitamin D_3 metabolites, p. 248).

Gastrointestinal tract

The stimulatory influence of PTH on the absorption of calcium from the upper small intestine is indirect, and is mediated by vitamin D_3 metabolites particularly $1,25(OH)_2D_3$ formed in the kidneys. The possibility that PTH might have a minor, direct, effect on calcium absorption remains controversial. Parathormone also stimulates the absorption of phosphate from the small intestine and again this effect is mediated by the $1,25(OH)_2D_3$ metabolite.

Mechanism of action

Parathormone binds to specific receptors on the plasma membranes of its target cells. In kidney and bone cells, PTH binding to its receptor results in G protein subunit dissociation and catalytic unit activation. The catalytic unit is adenyl cyclase and its stimulation results in the formation of the intracellular second messenger cAMP. The cAMP then activates a protein kinase in the target cell and this in turn probably phosphorylates the various intracellular proteins associated with PTH actions on cellular activity. For example, phosphorylated proteins in the luminal brush borders of renal cells are associated with the inhibition of phosphate reabsorption by these cells. Other proteins phosphorylated by the cAMP-activated protein kinase are the various enzymes which mediate the various transport and bone resorptive actions of PTH. Effects of cAMP in the PTH target cells may include mobilization of intracellular calcium ions in the cytoplasm. However, PTH also appears to stimulate the phosphatidyl inositol and calcium transport pathways in target cells. Activation of these pathways results directly in the movement of calcium ions from extracellular and intracellular sites into the cytoplasm and the consequent activation of proteins. The mitochondria and microsomes are the principal intracellular stores of calcium, and the PTH-induced mechanism(s) of action may then stimulate the net efflux of calcium ions from these stores into the cytoplasm. In addition, there is a movement of calcium ions across the cell membrane into the cytoplasm, and the effect of this can be observed as a transient (paradoxical) decrease in the extracellular calcium concentration. It may be that PTH binds to two different receptors, like other hormones, and induces different effects by activating either intracellular mechanism.

With respect to the actions of PTH on bone, no PTH receptors have (yet) been identified on the main target cells, the osteoclasts. Instead, they have been shown to be present on osteoblasts. Thus, it is likely that in addition to its inhibitory effects on osteoblastic activity PTH also stimulates the synthesis of an osteoclast-stimulating factor (OSF). Increased osteoclastic and osteocytic activity is associated with the increased production of various enzymes, such as acid phosphatase and collagenase, which may act on components of the bone matrix to stimulate calcium mobilization. Increased accumulation of citrate and lactate in the bone matrix has also been associated with PTH activity, and these probably participate in the bone decalcification process (Fig. 10.3).

Control of release

There is an inverse correlation between the plasma calcium concentration in the range 1.8–2.5 mmol/l (7.2–10 mg/100 ml) and parathormone concentrations, indicating that one important factor involved in the control of PTH release is the blood calcium level. Indeed, the direct negative feedback by calcium ions on the parathyroid glands is the principal regulatory mechanism on PTH release. Other stimuli for PTH production include various amines such as the catecholamines (β-receptor-mediated action) and dopamine. These stimuli appear to induce the release of pre-formed PTH from membrane-bound granules through a cAMP–protein kinase mechanism, an effect that can be abolished by β-blockers such as propranolol (Fig. 10.4).

When the parathyroids are stimulated the secretion of PTH follows a biphasic pattern. The early, rapid phase occurs within five minutes, is puromycin-insensitive, and is due to the release of hormone from a pre-formed, and therefore immediately available, pool. The second phase is slower and delayed, is puromycin-sensitive, and represents newly synthesized PTH. Calcium influences

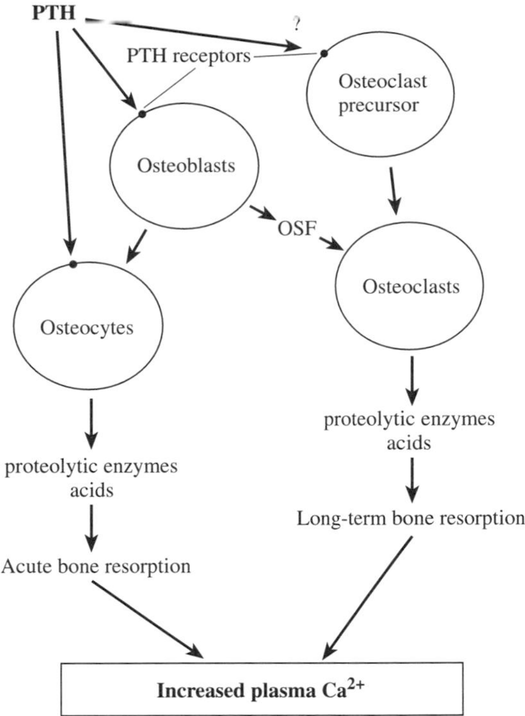

Fig. 10.3. The actions of parathormone (PTH) on bone cells. OSF = osteoclast stimulating factor.

both of these phases of PTH production, but the mechanism(s) of action through which these effects are induced are still unclear. It is likely that calcium ions decrease cAMP formation thus inhibiting PTH release; thus the stimulatory effect of a decreased plasma calcium ion concentration on PTH release is associated with a decrease in this cAMP inhibition. Also, various ion channels are activated by an increased intracellular calcium ion concentration. For example, activation of a calcium-sensitive potassium channel may explain the depolarization of the chief cell membrane in the presence of a raised extracellular calcium concentration.

Hypomagnesaemia has also been linked to increased PTH production and the effect of this ion would appear to be directed at the releasing mechanism rather than on the synthesis pathway. However, the changes in plasma magnesium concentration which are associated with increase PTH release are outside the normal physiological range. Also, the blood PTH concentration is apparently not increased when hypocalcaemia occurs with a severe hypomagnesaemia, which would suggest that a certain magnesium level is necessary for the normal feedback mechanism by calcium to operate.

The active vitamin D_3 metabolite $1,25(OH)_2D_3$ inhibits the release of PTH, partly by inhibiting PTH synthesis and perhaps partly because its own actions are mediated by an increase in intracellular calcium ion concentration which inhibits

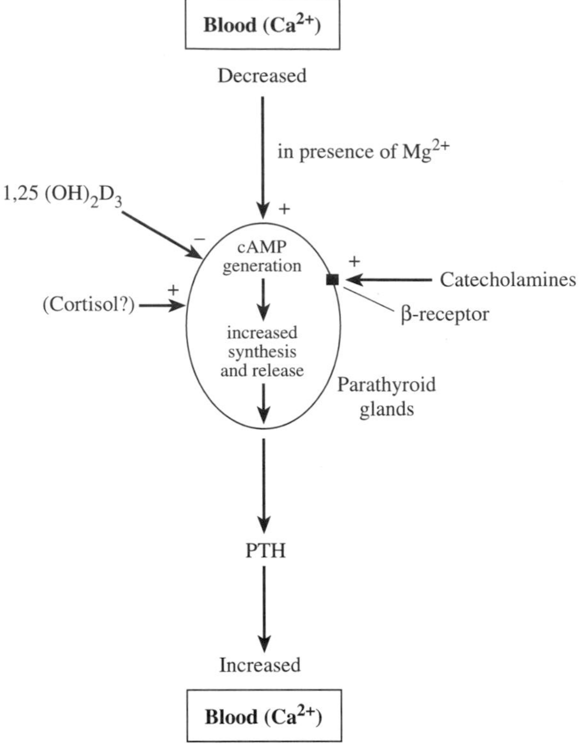

Fig. 10.4. The control of parathormone (PTH) production.

cAMP activation. Another steroid, cortisol, has a stimulatory effect on PTH secretion but the physiological role of this effect is unclear.

Vitamin D_3 and its metabolites

In humans, the natural form of vitamin D is cholecalciferol (vitamin D_3) which is absorbed in the small intestine with other fat-soluble components, or is synthesized in the skin from the cholesterol derivative 7-dehydrocholesterol by a reaction initiated by ultraviolet radiation. Skin pigmentation decreases the efficiency of this synthesis pathway. The extent of exposure of the skin to sunlight may not be sufficient to meet the body's requirement for vitamin D_3, particularly in urban areas in northern climates, and supplementary quantities can be ingested in the diet. The effects of vitamin D_3 on calcium metabolism are not direct, however, and the vitamin must first be converted to certain metabolites. The first conversion is a 25-hydroxylation which occurs mainly in the liver. The product, 25-hydroxycholecalciferol [or 25-hydroxy-vitamin D_3 — $25(OH)D_3$], is stored in the liver and to a lesser extent in other tissues. The parent molecule, cholecalciferol, is stored in adipose tissue to a large extent. The 25 $(OH)D_3$ is not biologically active *in vitro*, or in patients with severe renal damage, unless given in very large quantities.

However, the kidneys contain a 1α-hydroxylase enzyme which converts $25(OH)D_3$ to 1,25 dihydroxycholecalciferol ($1,25(OH)_2D_3$) and it is this metabolite which is the principal known active form of the vitamin. The plasma concentrations of $25(OH)D_3$ and $1,25(OH)_2O_3$ have been measured as 6–40 ng/ml and 30–40 pg/ml, respectively.

When 1α-hydroxylase activity is suppressed another enzyme, 24-hydroxylase, is stimulated and $25(OH)D_3$ is converted to $24,25(OH)_2D_3$ instead of $1,25(OH)_2D_3$. The 24,25-dihydroxy metabolite may have some biological activity but there is no substantial support for this possibility at present. In addition, $25(OH)D_3$ can be converted to $25,26(OH)_2D_3$ mainly in the kidneys. The dihydroxy metabolites of vitamin D_3 can be further hydroxylated to trihydroxy metabolites [e.g. $1,24,25(OH)_3$ D_3 and $1,25,26(OH)_3D_3$] but the physiological significance of these compounds is unknown; certainly, they appear to be biologically inactive with respect to calcium metabolism (Fig. 10.5).

Of the various vitamin D_3 metabolites formed in the body, the biologically potent $1,25(OH)_2D_3$ is the one which is considered as a hormone since it is

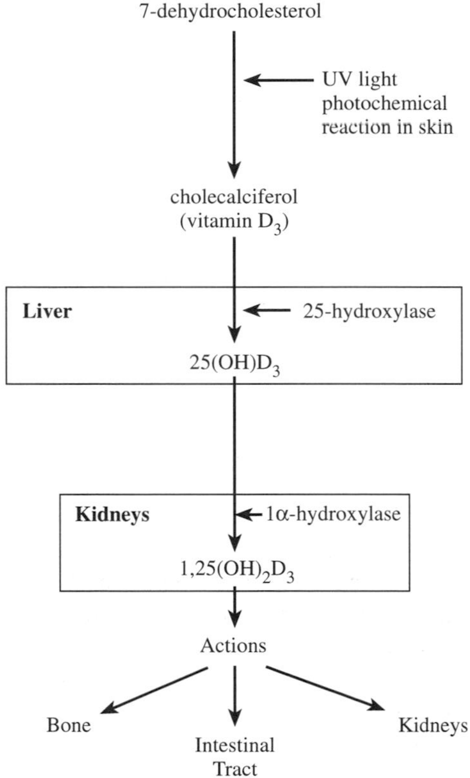

Fig. 10.5. The synthesis of vitamin D3 (cholecalciferol) and its metabolites (for further details, see text).

synthesized in the kidneys and exerts its effects on the small intestine and bone, in addition to the kidneys themselves. In the blood it is transported in the chylomicrons, or mostly bound to a globulin synthesized in the liver. This protein, called 25(OH)D_3-binding globulin, acts as a general transporting protein for cholecalciferol and its various metabolites, but seems to have a particularly high affinity for the 25-hydroxy forms.

Actions of 1,25 dihydroxycholecalciferol

The actions of the hormone 1,25$(OH)_2D_3$ are mainly directed towards raising the plasma calcium concentration in conjunction with PTH. In this respect, it acts directly on bone, renal tubules, and the small intestine (Fig. 10.6).

Bone

In bone, 1,25$(OH)_2D_3$ increases calcification of the matrix. At least part of this effect is indirect, and is probably due to the intestinal absorption of calcium and phosphate ions which is stimulated by the metabolite (see later section). In addition, there is evidence that it can directly stimulate an increase in bone mass by increasing osteoblast proliferation and osteoblast protein synthesis. One protein which is present in the bone matrix and is secreted by the osteoblasts is called osteocalcin. This protein is detected in plasma and changes in plasma levels have been considered to be markers of altered osteoblastic activity. While its physiological role is unclear, it certainly increases with vitamin D treatment.

Kidneys

The reabsorption of calcium from the distal tubules of the renal nephrons may be stimulated by 1,25$(OH)_2D_3$. There is also evidence to suggest that proximal tubular

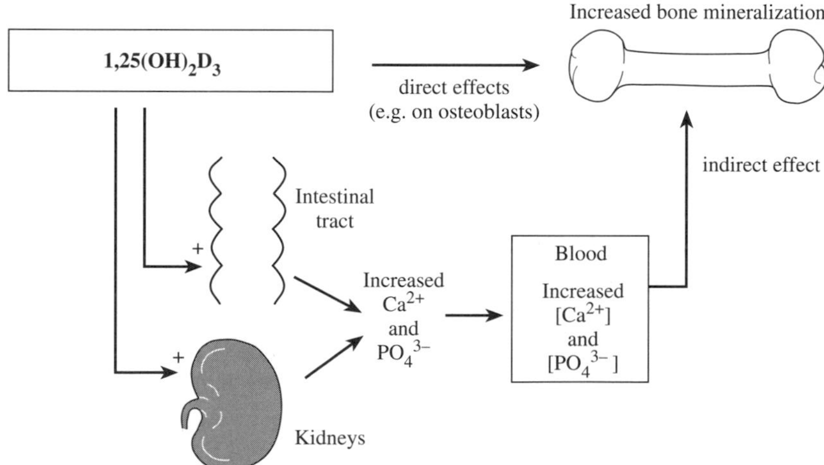

Fig. 10.6. The actions of 1,25-dihydroxycholecalciferol (1,25(OH)2D3).

calcium and phosphate reabsorption are increased within one hour of infusion with either $25(OH)D_3$ or $1,25(OH)_2D_3$. It can also inhibit the action of 1α-hydroxylase activity in the proximal tubule, and thus it has a negative feedback influence on its own production.

Gastrointestinal tract

The active absorption of calcium and phosphate from the small intestine, by separate mechanisms, is stimulated by $1,25(OH)_2D_3$. As mentioned earlier, this hormone is the principal regulator of calcium absorption along the small intestine, and this is certainly the most important physiological role of the steroid on calcium metabolism.

Other actions

In addition to bone, the kidneys and the gastrointestinal tract $1,25(OH)_2D_3$ receptors are present in many other tissues (including brain, skin, and pancreas), and other physiological roles have been indicated. Certainly, it inhibits PTH secretion (see earlier), but it also appears to influence prolactin release. It increases 7-dehydrocholesterol accumulation in the skin, and it can induce differentiation in certain leucocyte cell lines. Indeed, a role in immunoregulation is currently one particularly exciting area of vitamin D research.

Mechanism of action

The vitamin D_3 metabolites, being steroids, enter their target cells and bind to cytoplasmic receptors. The hormone-receptor complex then enters the nucleus where mRNA synthesis can be induced. It is possible to demonstrate the presence of $1,25(OH)_2D_3$ within the nuclei of various cells including intestinal cells osteoblasts, osteocytes, and renal tubular cells. As a consequence of its nuclear action, protein synthesis is stimulated by $1,25(OH)_2D_3$ and these new proteins are probably involved in calcium transport mechanisms across cells and across cell and/or mitochondrial membranes. Actinomycin D blocks the effect of this vitamin D metabolite on bone calcium mobilization indicating that the hormone acts at the transcription stage of protein synthesis. Various proteins are synthesized as a result of the steroid action in the nucleus, and these include osteocalcin and calcium-binding protein, a specific protein identified in intestinal cells which is associated with calcium transport across the intestinal mucosa.

Control of release

The regulation of $1,25(OH)_2D_3$ production occurs principally at the second hydroxylation stage in the kidneys. Parathormone stimulates 1α-hydroxylase enzyme activity while calcitonin inhibits it. Changes in the calcium concentration influence the nature of the dihydroxymetabolite formed. For instance, hypocalcaemia is associated with increased 1α-hydroxylase activity resulting in raised $1,25(OH)_2D_3$ production, while 24-hydroxylase activity is reduced. Hypercalcaemia has the opposite effect, namely increased $24,25(OH)_2D_3$ (biologically inactive) production instead of the active metabolite. The effect of a change in calcium concentration is probably mediated by the hormones PTH and calcitonin and is therefore not direct. However, plasma phosphate levels have an effect on 1,25$(OH)_2D_3$ production such that hypophosphataemia results in an accumulation of this metabolite in the plasma. This may be a direct effect on the synthesis of 1,25$(OH)_2D_3$ in the kidneys, and indicates a direct link between the need for phosphate and the stimulation of the intestinal absorption of this anion by the dihydroxy D_3 metabolite. As mentioned above, the 1,25$(OH)_2D_3$ metabolite has a direct inhibitory influence on renal 1α-hydroxylase activity.

Calcitonin (CT)

Calcitonin is a polypeptide of 32 amino acids synthesized in the parafollicular cells (or C cells) situated between the follicles of the thyroid. These cells originate in the neural crests; they then migrate to the pharyngeal pouches which are incorporated into the developing thyroid. As with other peptide hormones, calcitonin is initially synthesized as a larger precursor prohormone sequence. A related molecule which is also derived from the calcitonin gene has been isolated and is called calcitonin gene-related peptide (CGRP). It is found in the nervous system and the gastrointestinal tract; its physiological role is currently unknown.

Actions

The net effect of calcitonin is to lower the blood calcium concentration should it rise above 2.5 mmol/l. It acts on bone and kidney cells directly, and its receptors have been identified on osteoclasts and in the cells of the lower thick segment of the ascending limb of the loop of Henle and the early part of the distal convoluted tubule (Fig. 10.7).

Bone

Bone is the primary target organ for calcitonin, which inhibits osteoclast activity and hence prevents bone resorption. Virtually all bone resorptive effects, such as release of lysosomal enzymes, degradation of collagen, and release of calcium, are inhibited. Indeed, the greater the initial osteoclastic activity the greater the effect of calcitonin in inhibiting bone resorption. The result of this inhibitory action on bone resorption is a decrease in the supply of calcium to the extracellular compartment which is reflected by a hypocalcaemia. This is accompanied by a hypophosphataemia and a decrease in alkaline phosphatase activity. The inhibitory effect of calcitonin is generally self-limiting and is followed by what is known as an 'escape phenomenon', a likely explanation of which is a receptor down-regulation.

Kidneys

Calcitonin increases the urinary excretion of sodium, chloride, calcium, and phosphate. A mild hyperphosphaturia can augment the hypophosphataemic effect of calcitonin on bone resorption. The effect on sodium chloride can be sufficient to cause a saline diuresis although this is unlikely to occur with physiological concentrations of circulating hormone.

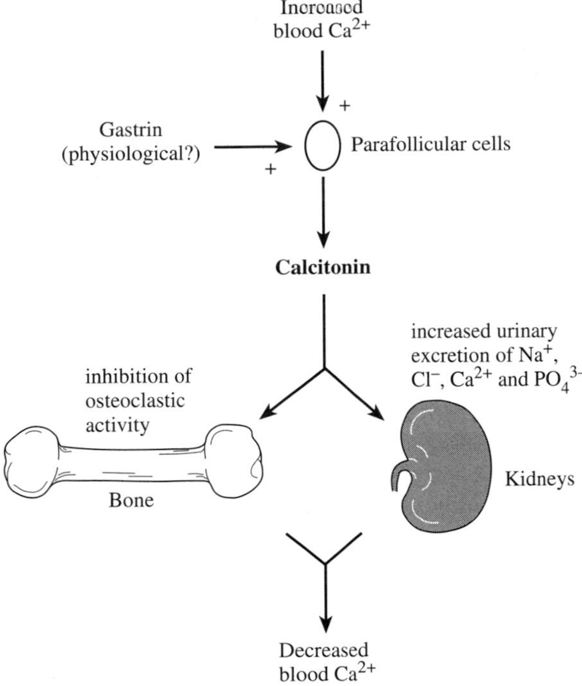

Fig. 10.7. The actions and control of calcitonin.

Mechanism of action

Cyclic AMP is generally believed to act as the intracellular second messenger in the renal target cells and osteoclasts. However, observations concerning the mechanism of action of CT indicate an initial release of calcium ions (e.g. from bone cells) into the surrounding extracellular fluid. This effect follows the binding of the hormone to its specific plasma-membrane receptors and may indicate a direct action on the cell membrane resulting in a decreased cytoplasmic Ca^{2+} concentration.

Control of release

The only established physiological control mechanism involved in the regulation of calcitonin secretion is the plasma calcium level. If the plasma level rises above 2.4 mmol/l (9.5 mg/100 ml) the rate of secretion of CT rises proportionally. High concentrations of magnesium ions have also been shown to stimulate calcitonin release but this effect is probably not physiological. Another biologically active molecule, the gastrointestinal hormone, gastrin, has a somewhat surprising stimulatory effect on calcitonin release. This effect only occurs in response to large amounts of gastrin and thus is probably not of physiological significance.

Other hormonal influences on calcium regulation

Various other hormones influence calcium ion regulation and bone metabolism to some extent. Gonadal steroids and corticosteroids are two pertinent groups of hormones. For example, the protective effect of oestrogens is well established, even though the precise nature of their involvement remains unclear. This protective effect is lost at menopause, and increased likelihood of bone fractures is a consequence. The possible physiological role of parathormone-related peptide (PTHRP) in the fetus has been mentioned in an earlier section.

CLINICAL DISORDERS

Many patients with abnormalities of parathyroid function or of vitamin D action are first identified following the discovery of either hypercalcaemia or hypocalcaemia. Sometimes these biochemical changes are discovered quite by chance in patients with a variety of non-specific presenting symptoms. This clinical section will therefore be introduced by a brief consideration of the differential diagnosis of these two extremes of disordered serum calcium homeostasis.

It will be immediately re-emphasized that less that 50 per cent of serum calcium is present in the biologically significant ionized form. Conversely, the 50 per cent or more protein-bound fraction may be altered by any disorder affecting protein metabolism generally, and this will be reflected by reduction or increase in the customarily measured total serum calcium, without any influence on its biological effects. Furthermore, blood pH is relevant, acidosis increasing and alkalosis decreasing the ionized fraction. It would be more relevant to measure ionized calcium direct. However, this is not as readily measured, as it does not lend itself to the automated processes which are now standard in all service (as distinct from research) laboratories.

In practice, it is necessary to 'compensate' for the apparent hypocalcaemia produced by reduced serum proteins, especially albumin. Hypo-albuminaemia is very common in renal, hepatic disease, and in a wide variety of acute and chronic illnesses. Although a number of normalizing algorithms have been proposed, albumin levels are usually 'corrected' to 40 g/l. Thus in a patient with a (low) measured serum calcium of 2.05 mmol/l and serum albumin of 30 g/l, corrected calcium is: $(40–30) \times 0.02 = 0.2$ higher. Thus, corrected calcium is $2.05 + 0.2 = 2.25$ mmol/l (normal). It is worth noting that for similar reasons, hypercalcaemia may be masked: an apparently normal measured serum calcium of 2.48 mmol/l with a serum albumin of 28 g/l provides a corrected serum calcium of $2.48 + (12 \times 0.02) = 2.72$ mmol/l (raised).

Table 10.1 shows some of the clinical situations which must be considered before proceeding with more detailed evaluation. Specifically to be excluded in the case of measured hypercalcaemia is poor venesection technique. Samples should always be taken without stasis. In clinical practice, investigation of the cause of hypercalcaemia must sometimes await initial intervention therapy, especially if serum calcium exceeds 3.5 mmol/l, above which patients are usually

Table 10.1. Principal causes of hypercalcaemia

1. *Endocrine*
   - Primary and tertiary hyperparathyroidism
   - Ectopic (paraneoplastic) hypercalcaemia
   - Hyperthyroidism
   - Adrenocortical insufficiency
   - Familial hypocalciuric hypercalcaemia
2. *Other metabolic factors*
   - Vitamin D excess
   - Milk-alkali syndrome
   - Sarcoidosis
3. *Primary bone disease*
   - Metastatic carcinoma, myeloma, reticulosis
   - Paget's disease — immobilized
   - Immobilization hypercalcaemia
4. *Other causes*
   - Drugs: thiazide diuretics and ion-exchange resins
   - Venous stasis/venesection induced haemoconcentration (ionized calcium level normal)

symptomatic. Rehydration (by increasing renal calcium clearance) may be all that is required to lower serum calcium to a safer level, but other approaches are sometimes called for. Similarly, hypocalcaemia when symptomatic usually requires prompt therapy and investigations need to be delayed until initial symptomatology has been corrected.

Primary hyperparathyroidism and hypercalcaemia

Although previously considered a rare disease, it is now assessed from population studies that between 1 in 500 and 1 in 1000 of Western populations have hyperparathyroidism. Similarly high rates of apparently asymptomatic disease can be identified on routine multichannel screening which is now so widely performed. Indeed, such serendipitous diagnosis is now more common than a symptomatic presentation of hyperparathyroidism.

In 5–10 per cent of cases there is an association with other endocrine tumours, including phaeochromocytoma, pituitary tumours either non-functioning or functioning (e.g. acromegaly) and medullary thyroid carcinoma (see Chapter 16): thus hyperparathyroidism can be part either of multiple endocrine neoplasia (MEN) type 1 or 2 syndromes, and identifies a significant genetic factor in some cases. In addition, there is an association with Von Recklinghausen's disease (neurofibromatosis).

In approximately 80 per cent of patients with this disorder, the cause is an adenoma of a single gland. In almost 20 per cent of cases, either multiple adenomas or hyperplasia are responsible, while in less than 2 per cent of cases carcinoma of the parathyroid is found. Histologically, the distinction between these pathological variants may be difficult.

Hypocalcaemia due to vitamin D deficiency (of various aetiologies) is associated with a compensatory hypersecretion of parathormone (the secondary hyperparathyroidism referred to later in this chapter). After a period of time, the parathyroids in some of these cases undergo a transition to autonomous hyperfunction (adenoma or hyperplasia), which initially corrects but subsequently over-corrects serum calcium, resulting in hypercalcaemia. This is usually termed 'tertiary hyperparathyroidism'. However, the underlying and initiating hypocalcaemia may have not been apparent (e.g. minor degrees of small bowel malabsorption) and the condition may therefore masquerade as (apparent) primary hyperparathyroidism.

Clinical features

As indicated above, the current most common single presentation is the incidental discovery of hypercalcaemia with multichannel screening. Such patients usually have modest hypercalcaemia (less than 2.8 mmol/l). This entity is customarily referred to as 'asymptomatic hyperparathyroidism'. Although there are often one or more associated vague symptoms which are theoretically attributable to hypercalcaemia, at this level of serum calcium they cannot be confidently ascribed to hyperparathyroidism. More significant clinical features can be subdivided into those due to the effects of parathormone excess and those directly attributable directly to hypercalcaemia.

Effects of parathormone excess

Renal calculi occur as a consequence of increased intestinal calcium absorption and enhanced bone reabsorption with a consequent hypercalciuria. Phosphate excretion by the renal tubules is also stimulated by parathormone, and this may increase the crystallization potential of urinary calcium salts.

Nephrocalcinosis reflects a deposition of multifocal calcium salts within the kidney parenchyma which is also based on the events described above. It is usually found with more severe hypercalcaemia of longer duration and is normally associated with a significant reduction of tubular, and more importantly renal glomerular function.

Gastrointestinal effects Parathormone and hypercalcaemia together have a stimulating effect on gastric acid secretion; accordingly, dyspepsia and duodenal ulceration are both more common in hypercalcaemic states.

Bone lesions are due to a generalized rarefaction of bone due to enhanced resorption, and in more severe cases to bone cyst formation, often in long bones and the jaw. The generalized bone lesions probably account for the bone pains of which some patients complain. The more localized so-called 'osteitis fibrosa cystica' is in fact quite rare, but is often responsible for the pathological fractures which occur in this condition.

Direct effects of hypercalcaemia Varying degrees of tiredness and lethargy may result from serum calcium elevations between 2.8 and 3.0 mmol/l. This degree of hypercalcaemia is also often associated with usually reversible impairment of tubular water reabsorption, sometimes resulting in polyuria: essentially a form of nephrogenic (ADH-resistant) diabetes insipidus. After a period of time which is highly variable, persisting hypercalcaemia of this order results in additional and largely irreversible impaired glomerular function, leading to progressive renal glomerular failure.

At higher levels of serum calcium (greater than 3.0 mmol/l), the clinical features are mainly those of vague ill health and lethargy. Tiredness together with muscle weakness, due to proximal myopathy are prominent. An organic psychosis may develop and clinical depression may also be seen. At levels greater than 4.0 mmol/l mental confusion becomes common, leading if untreated to coma and even death. This progression is enhanced by the dehydration which results not only from the renal water loss, but also from vomiting, which is common in severe hypercalcaemia and is due to a direct effect on subcortical brain centres. Cardiac arrhythmias, especially heart block, may supervene in terminal states and contribute to the fatal outcome of unrecognized and untreated cases.

Clinical examination may often be entirely negative at all levels of hypercalcaemia, so that a high index of suspicion is necessary. Ectopic calcification of the conjunctivae, corneal margins (band keratopathy: Plate 10.3), and tympanic membranes are a clue to the chronicity of hypercalcaemia. These features are more commonly seen in association with renal failure; phosphate retention coupled to hypercalcaemia exceeds the solubility product so that crystallization and soft tissue deposition occurs.

Differential diagnosis of hypercalcaemia All the features mentioned above may be encountered with other causes of hypercalcaemia mentioned earlier in this chapter, the precise diagnosis being reached on clinical and laboratory grounds. Thus, in the milk-alkali syndrome, a history of excess intake of absorbable alkali (commonly sodium bicarbonate) is obtained and there is coexistent hyperphosphataemia and alkalosis; patients with sarcoidosis are known to synthesize vitamin D analogues within their sarcoid granulomata, and usually have other manifestations of this multisystem disease. They may also have hyperphosphataemia, and show a striking responsiveness to the effects of synthetic corticosteroids, which inhibit vitamin-D-mediated absorption of calcium from the small bowel. Tumour-associated hypercalcaemia is not usually directly due to lytic effects of bone metastases, except in multiple myeloma and in the presence of very numerous secondary bone deposits as are sometimes encountered in breast and prostatic carcinoma. More frequently it is due to the production, by both the tumour and its metastases of a parathyroid hormone related peptide (PTH-RP), which has a different amino acid sequence to human parathormone, but almost identical biological effects. Standard investigation usually identify one of the more common (e.g. bronchus, breast) malignancies. Hyperthyroidism increases bone turnover, and as in the case of Paget's disease, immobilization will exacerbate the hypercalcaemia.

Investigation

Detailed investigation is normally initiated if three or more sequential serum calcium levels, ideally taken fasting and without stasis are significantly elevated

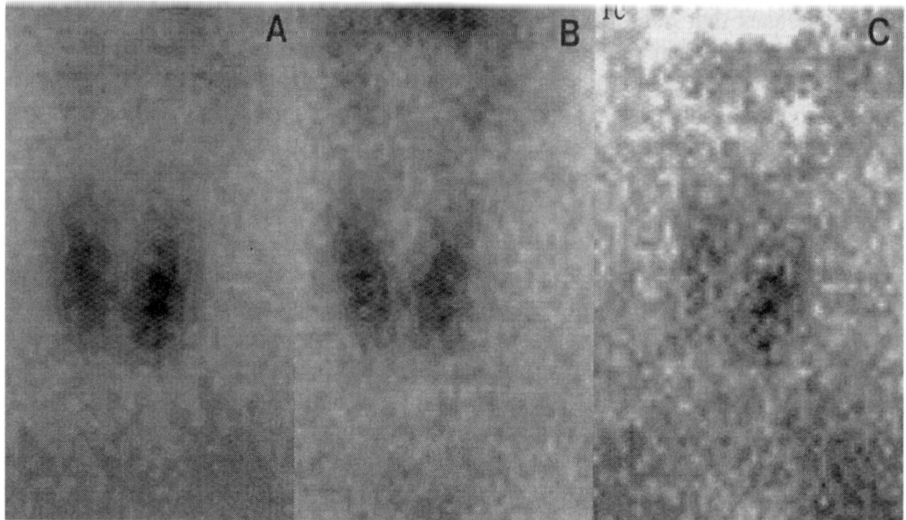

Fig. 10.9. Thallium–technetium subtraction scan. Thallium (A) localizes to both thyroid and parathyroid (adenoma) tissue; technetium (B) only to thyroid. In this instance, a left lower parathyroid adenoma is disclosed in left lower pole in subtraction scan (C).

hypocalcaemia, since hypomagnesaemia inhibits both parathormone secretion and receptor affinity. After the immediate post operative period, permanent hypoparathyroidism still remains the major complication of parathyroid surgery. Replacement therapy with vitamin D analogues, either 1α-hydroxycholecalciferol (alfacalcidol) or 1:25 dihydroxycalciferol (calcitriol), with or without calcium supplements, is then necessary (see below).

Non-operative treatment of hypercalcaemia

Other forms of therapy have been introduced which are occasionally useful in patients with primary hyperparathyroidism in whom surgery is contraindicated, for pre-operative stabilization or in cases with malignancy-associated hypercalcaemia. Thus, the administration of oestrogens (which decreases parathormone receptor affinity), frusemide (a diuretic which enhances calcium excretion), and phosphate preparations (which interfere with calcium absorption, complex calcium, and directly inhibit bone resorption) can all be used in appropriate cases.

Intravenous phosphate can be used in patients in whom the serum calcium level needs to be lowered rapidly: 50 mmol of phosphate in 500 ml of saline infused over a period of 8 hours usually produces a fall of 1–1.5 mmol/l which lasts 24 hours or more, and can be repeated as necessary. Glucocorticoids are only rarely effective except for the acute hypercalcaemia of sarcoidosis, vitamin D intoxication and occasionally myeloma, exerting their effect by inhibiting both intestinal calcium absorption and bone resorption.

Pamidronate (one of the family of biphosphonates) directly inhibits bone resorption, whatever its aetiology. An infusion of 30 mg is highly effective in severely hypercalcaemic patients, reduces serum calcium significantly with 24 hours and needs to be repeated every 2–4 days. The effect can be prolonged, in some cases by giving oral biphosphonates which are usually very well tolerated. Calcitonin can be used but is expensive and must be given by daily injection. The antibiotic, mithramycin, which inhibits osteoclastic activity, has been used in a wide variety of clinical situations with good results although it carries some of the obvious adverse effects of a cytotoxic agent. Infusions of 10–20 μg/kg are given every two to three days.

Secondary hyperparathyroidism

As mentioned above, any clinical situation (other than parathyroid deficiency itself) which results in hypocalcaemia with or without hyperphosphataemia, will result in secondary stimulation of parathormone secretion. This is most frequently encountered in chronic renal failure, and is due to multiple causes. These include an defective intestinal calcium absorption due to reduced synthesis of calcitriol by the abnormal kidney, and the effect of phosphate retention. It also occurs in primary vitamin D deficiency, whatever the cause (see below).

The classical findings are those of a low but occasionally normal serum calcium (maintained by compensatory parathormone secretion), an elevated or normal serum phosphate, and often an elevated serum alkaline phosphatase. Serum parathormone concentration is elevated, often to very high levels. Bone lesions are frequent. Usually, these consist of generalized demineralization, but osteosclerosis is occasionally seen in vertebral bodies (particularly in renal osteodystrophy), giving rise to the so-called 'rugger-jersey' spine. Soft tissue and arterial calcification is also sometimes noted due to calcium salt deposition. The changes of osteomalacia are also found, including pseudo-fractures in long bones and scapulae. The administration of calcitriol to these patients is capable of treating the bone lesions, and is also being increasingly used prophylactically when renal function deteriorates in patients with chronic renal failure (usually above a serum creatinine level of 180 μmol/l.

Tertiary hyperparathyroidism

This term is usually applied to the autonomous development of parathyroid hyperplasia or multiple adenomatosis after prolonged periods of secondary stimulation. It is most frequently seen during long-term dialysis for renal failure, and occasionally as a consequence of the secondary hyperparathyroidism consequent on vitamin D deficiency. More effective treatment in the early stages of secondary hyperparathyroidism probably helps to prevent it, but for established cases, parathyroidectomy provides the only treatment. Total parathyroidectomy is usually necessary, and the difficulty in locating the occasionally aberrant glands provides a major surgical challenge. Re-implantation of part of the excised parathyroid tissue into forearm muscle (from which it may be readily retrieved if necessary) is sometimes used to prevent postoperative hypoparathyroidism.

Parathormone deficiency and hypocalcaemia

The effectiveness of the normal control system for serum calcium implies that for hypocalcaemia to occur, absolute or relative parathormone deficiency must be present. As in the previous section,. the clinical features of hypocalcaemia will be dealt with under this heading. (The principal causes of hypocalcaemia are shown in Table 10.2.)

Parathyroid deficiency may occur as a primary disorder, immunologically linked to the thyrogastric immune group of disorders (see Chapter 16). In this form, it may occur even in childhood. The most common cause however is iatrogenic, resulting inadvertently from thyroid surgery (especially total thyroidectomy for thyroid carcinoma), or as a consequence of surgery for hyperparathyroidism.

Clinical features

Mild hypocalcaemia (serum calcium 1.9–2.1 mmo/l) is often asymptomatic, at worst leading over a period of years to cataract formation, ectopic calcification in basal ganglia, or a mild organic brain syndrome. More severe hypocalcaemia (usually less than 1.8 mmo/l) is almost always associated with symptoms related mainly to increased neuromuscular excitability. These symptoms include paraesthesiae, cramps, and with more severe degrees of hypocalcaemia (less than 1.6 mmol/l), spontaneous tetany, as manifest by carpopedal spasm and by epileptiform convulsions.

Examination may reveal this increased excitability, even in the absence of spontaneous symptoms either by the development of a twitch when the facial nerve is

Table 10.2. *Principal causes of hypocalcaemia*

1. *With normal ionized calcium* (i.e. hypocalcaemia due to decreased calcium-binding proteins)
   (a) Nephrotic syndrome
   (b) Hepatic cirrhosis
   (c) Malnutrition and chronic debility
   (d) Protein malabsorption

2. *With reduced ionized calcium*
   (a) Endocrine/metabolic
   - Hypoparathyroidism: surgical, auto-immune.
   - Magnesium deficiency
   - Hungry-bone syndrome (postparathyroidectomy)
   - Pseudo-hypoparathyroidism
   - Drugs: biphosphonates, phosphate, antineoplastic drugs

   (b) Vitamin D: deficiency or altered metabolism
   - Deficient intake or solar exposure
   - Malabsorption of fat soluble vitamins
   - Anticonvulsant therapy
   - Chronic hepatic disease.
   - Renal failure

   (c) Acute pancreatitis

percussed (Chvostek's sign), or by induction of carpal spasm within 3–5 minutes of inducing arm ischaemia with a sphygmomanometer cuff (Trousseau's sign).

Investigations

1. In hypoparathyroidism, serum calcium is low and serum phosphate elevated and the primary cause is often obvious. Parathormone assay is usually helpful: all cases other than hypoparathyroidism have raised levels. The presence of hypophosphataemia as well as hypocalcaemia suggests a primary defect of vitamin D action, with phosphaturia induced by the renal action of parathormone compounding defective phosphate absorption. Serum alkaline phosphatase is then usually raised. These findings should lead to consideration of those factors listed in the section on osteomalacia and rickets (p. 264).

2. Hypomagnesaemia may be present, particularly following parathyroidectomy for adenoma or hyperplasia, since such patients may be already magnesium-depleted. The additional fall is due to magnesium flux into bone. Since hypomagnesaemia inhibits both parathormone secretion as well as target-organ effects, it may become clinically significant. Other causes of hypomagnesaemia, such as alcoholism, diabetic ketoacidosis, and severe small intestinal malasorption, may also be important metabolically.

3. Radiology may demonstrate subcutaneous and basal ganglion calcification in rare cases.

Treatment

Symptomatic hypocalcaemia calls for the administration of intravenous calcium gluconate or chloride in doses of 10–20 ml of a 10 per cent solution. This may need repeating hourly or less frequently. Transient hypocalcaemia is common following parathyroid adenomectomy but only requires correction if symptomatic. The persistence of hypocalcaemia beyond 48 hours usually indicates the need for life-long therapy. Since the administration of parenteral parathormone is expensive and uncomfortable, long-term hypoparathyroidism is usually treated by one of the vitamin D analogues, such as alfacalcidol or calcitriol 1–3 μg daily, usually without any need for calcium supplementation. These compounds are safer than 'native' calciferol, since they have shorter biological half-lives and show less variation in biological activity. The effect of a particular dose change is usually fully reflected by serum calcium level repeated after 7–10 days. There are substantial dangers in over-treatment, including hypercalcaemia, hypercalciuria (leading to nephrocalcinosis and nephrolithiasis), and ultimately renal failure.

Pseudo-hypoparathyroidism

This is a familial syndrome characterized by parathormone unresponsiveness in bone, renal tubules, and possibly small intestine. Some cases appear to be secondary to a defect resulting in reduced intracellular synthesis of cyclic AMP, a mediator of parathormone action. There are typical phenotypic changes, not all of which may be present in the one patient. These include a round face, short stature, short fourth or fifth metacarpal and metatarsal bones, and subnormal intelligence.

Investigation shows low serum calcium and an elevated serum phosphate, with elevated serum parathormone concentrations. Some patients appear to have a selective renal tubular unresponsivess, so that they may have paradoxical hyperparathyroid bone lesions. Almost certainly, the syndrome represents a heterogeneous group of genetic abnormalities affecting parathormone receptors.

Treatment consists of calcitriol to which the syndrome appears to be mostly responsive even when physiological doses (0.5 μg) are used. This suggests that a defect of renal dihydroxylation is an essential element of some examples of the syndrome.

Osteomalacia and rickets

Any interference with the metabolic cascade of vitamin D metabolites is theoretically capable of inducing defective mineralization of bones resulting in rickets (in children) and osteomalacia (in adults).

This syndrome is histologically definable by characteristic bone morphology, readily demonstrated by examination of stained undecalcified sections of bone obtained by iliac crest biopsy. Total bone matrix is normal in quantity, but osteoid seams are actually widened and defectively calcified, resulting in bone structure which is biomechanically unsound, and subject to both bowing (in childhood) and pathological fracture (in adulthood). The syndromes may result from a variety of causes as outlined in Table 10.3.

Table 10.3. Principal causes of osteomalacia or rickets

1. *Defective substrate*
   - Lack of solar exposure (especially in Asians)
   - Dietary vitamin D deficiency (especially vegetarians)
2. *Defective absorption*
   - Small bowel malabsorption
   - Gastrectomy or bypass surgery
   - Other causes of steatorrhoea
   - Phytate excess (found especially in chupattis)
3. *Defective 25-hydroxylation*
   - liver disease
   - alcoholism
   - other causes of P-450 microsomal enzyme induction (e.g. phenytoin, barbiturates)
4. *Defective 1,25-hydroxylation*
   - Chronic liver disease
   - Hypoparathyroidism
   - Hyperparathyroidism
   - Vitamin D-resistant rickets (autosomal recessive, X-linked dominant variety)

In addition, phosphate depletion due to laxative abuse (which decreases phosphate absorption) or excess aluminium hydroxide-containing antacids (which bind phosphate) may induce osteomalacia. In primary hyperparathyroidism, significant osteomalacia is also present, the uncalcified osteoid tissue reflecting increased calcium resorption rather than the decreased deposition which is so characteristic of vitamin D-deficient states. Finally, a variety of malignant tumours (commonly bronchial) have been associated with hypophosphataemic osteomalacia, the nature of the responsible humoral agent being as yet unidentified.

Clinical features

Some signs and symptoms are secondary to the underlying disease process responsible for the osteomalacia. In addition, in children, there is defective longitudinal growth, outward bowing of weight–bearing long bones, and general debility: the condition of rickets.

In adults, generalized bone pain is the predominant clinical feature, with muscle weakness and pathological fractures occurring in long bones even with minimal trauma. However, many cases of early or mild osteomalacia are entirely asymptomatic or have vague ill-health which may be overlooked. Particularly in the very elderly, the combination of reduced solar exposure and poor diet has been shown to result in a high prevalence of undiagnosed vitamin D deficiency. It is also realized that among (particularly vegetarian) Asians, both in Asia and more so in immigrant UK populations, the prevalence of osteomalacia may be as high as 15 per cent. Particularly in this ethnic group, the increased demand for vitamin D during pregnancy may precipitate symptoms, and neonates may suffer from tetany.

Investigations

1. The biochemical hallmarks of rickets and osteomalacia are hypocalcaemia, hypophosphataemia, and reduced serum 25-hydroxy-vitamin D concentrations, coupled to invariable elevations of parathormone to values which are usually much higher than are found in primary hyperparathyroidism. Because of the parathormone response to the hypocalcaemia, serum calcium may be maintained within the normal range, accompanied by hypophosphataemia which is aggravated by the phosphaturic effect of parathormone excess.

2. Radiological findings are variable and may be absent even in symptomatic osteomalacia. However, there may be some general reduction in bone density, best appreciated in lateral radiology of the dorsilumbar spine. In children, characteristic cupping of the metaphyses, together with abnormal epiphysial lines are seen. In adults, hairline micro-or pseudo-fractures are sometimes seen in the upper femoral shafts and medial aspects of the scapulae, running at right angles to the periosteal surface. These are usually referred to as Looser's zones or Milkman's fractures.

3. Bone biopsy is sometimes necessary to confirm mild degrees of osteomalacia which may be present even in the absence of biochemical change. Particularly in the elderly patient with femoral neck fractures, histology frequently shows a mixed

picture of osteomalacia and osteoporosis, due to multiple dietary and hormonal deficiencies.

Treatment

In patients with nutritional deficiency, defective solar exposure, steatorrhea, and drug-induced osteomalacia, comparatively small doses of vitamin D or one of its synthetic analogues are almost universally successful in effecting a total cure. Ergocalciferol can be used in doses of 400 to 1200 units per day. Alternatively, alfacalcidol or calcitriol has been used in doses of 0.25 to 0.5 μg daily, supplemented by calcium, usually in effervescent form in order to provide an extra 500–1000 mg of elemental calcium daily.

Consideration has been given to prohylactic administration of vitamin D analogues in susceptible populations; Asians and in the elderly (particularly institutionalized). The cost-effectiveness of this approach has not been adequately examined.

The autosomal recessive variant of vitamin D-resistant rickets (see Plate 10.1) responds either to alfacalcidol or calcitriol but not to ergocalciferol. The X-linked dominant variety is difficult to treat, even with very large doses, due to a presumed reduced receptor affinity. In both disorders, supplemental phosphate is necessary for adequate bone mineralization.

The osteomalacia of chronic renal failure may also be treated with alfacalcidol, which has direct bone mineralization effects. More rationally calcitriol is used, since renal di-hydroxylation is defective in this situation, Indeed, early therapy of this condition probably minimizes the risk of developing the secondary and tertiary hyperparathyroidism referred to earlier.

Osteoporosis

In contrast to osteomalacia, this disorder represents an overall loss of bone mass (including osteoid matrix), resulting in biomechanical failure with the consequences of bone pain and pathological fracture. Central to the understanding of this disorder is the realization of the normal age-related changes in bone mass.

Bone mass, as revealed either by bone biopsy or quantitative radiological or radioisotopic studies, is consistently lower in females, and shows a rise to a maximum at 25–30 years of age in both sexes. This peak bone mass may be genetically determined: some studies show a relationship to vitamin D receptor status. There is a subsequent decline in bone mass, which is accelerated in females at the time of menopause.

Any conditions listed in Table 10.4 occurring at any point of the age curve will result in a steeper 'decay', enhancing the risk of symptoms or pathological fractures later in life as bone mass reduces below the theoretical fracture threshold. However, in all cases, the process of fracture is due equally or in greater part to trauma (falls, tripping, etc.) which, by their very nature, are more common in the elderly. Restoration of lost bone mass, even after correction of the underlying disease process is only occasionally achieved.

Table 10.4. Major causes of osteoporosis

1. *Endocrine*
   - Postmenopausal (especially premature menopause)
   - Cushing's syndrome
   - Hyperthyroidism
   - Male hypogonadism
2. *Drugs*
   - Corticosteroid osteoporosis
   - Heparin osteopenia
3. *Miscellaneous*
   - Simple osteoporosis of ageing (senile)
   - Immobilization
   - Dietary deficiency of calcium, protein, or vitamin C
   - Malabsorption syndrome
   - Idiopathic juvenile osteoporosis
   - Idiopathic adult osteoporosis

Postmenopausal osteoporosis is a common problem, and responsible for a significant proportion of recurrent back pain in the elderly. Premature menopause, either spontaneous or induced by oophorectomy is associated with a substantially higher risk of osteoporosis, which can be totally prevented by oestrogen replacement.

Loss of bone mass with immobilization is quite rapid, especially in weight-bearing bones: in young patients (with their more rapid bone turnover), this may also result in hypercalcaemia despite normal renal function. Studies of the biological effects of space flight indicates that bone loss is substantial and not invariably reversible when weightlessness is corrected.

Chronic corticosteroid therapy is a common cause of severe osteoporosis. In some susceptible individuals, spinal symptoms may occur within 6–12 months of commencing treatment. Heparin-induced osteopenia (so called because bone histology reveals disordered bone structure in addition to simple osteoporosis) appears to be an idiosyncratic response to long-term heparin therapy, as occasionally used in the prophylaxis of thromboembolism.

When all known causes are excluded, there still remains a subgroup, unsatisfactorily called 'idiopathic'. The juvenile form is, however, interesting in that it often appears to be familial and non-progressive. Fractures occur around the age of puberty, but subsequently heal, leaving disability and deformity, but without pain.

Clinical features

Substantial bone loss can occur before symptoms appear. Pain is customarily in the lower dorsal and lumbar regions, and vertebral collapse is associated with a loss of height and a progressively stooped posture. There is an increased incidence both of Colles' (lower radius) and femoral neck fracture. Some patients with the idiopathic adult variety have an associated poor musculature. This has led to the suggestion that reduced muscular tone, weightlessness, and immobilization act through a common mechanism altering the biophysical state of bone below a level which is critical to the maintenance of normal bone mass. Currently, research is active in this very important area.

Investigations

1. Serum calcium, phosphate, and alkaline phosphatase are typically normal. However, biochemical studies can shed light on the activity of the osteoporosis, and may be useful in monitoring response to treatment. Specifically, serum osteocalcin rises in response to increased bone formation, while urinary hydroxyproline concentration as well as urine or serum pyridoline cross-links reflect the rate of bone resorption.

2. Radiological changes are not usually apparent in the spine and long bones until around 30 per cent of the bone mass has been lost. Hence the absence of radiological abnormality does not exclude the diagnosis in a patient with symptoms. Even before there is obvious bone 'thinning' radiologically, it can be shown that the anterior vertebral height is reduced. In gross osteoporosis there is diffuse demineralization and 'cod fish' deformity of vertebrae due to increased concavity of the vertebral plates due to pressure of the intervertebral discs. There is often nterior 'wedging' of vertebra, and finally compression fractures affecting the whole vertebra. (See Fig. 10.10.)

The most common method for documenting bone density is dual energy X-ray absorption (DEXA), a comparatively inexpensive and reproducible method of measuring bone density, with low radiation risk. Density can also be measured non-invasively by quantitative CT scanning and by ultrasound techniques.

3. Bone biopsy is not often required, but can be performed for quantitative histomorphometry. This is less appropriate for diagnosis than as a research method for assessing responses to new drugs and other therapeutic approaches.

Treatment

Prevention is probably the most promising approach in the management of osteoporosis. Oestrogen replacement in early onset menopause is considered mandatory, although there are divided views about the merits of routine oestrogen replacement after a normal menopause. Although there is no doubt that bone density is maintained compared with untreated patients, the benefits of reduced fracture risk are partially offset by an increased risk of endometrial malignancy (if unwisely used without progestogen) and of breast cancer. However, it is likely that longer-term studies will provide support for universal oestrogen–progestogen replacement (with very few contraindications): such therapy is also associated with a reduced incidence of myocardial infarction and cerebrovascular accidents (strokes).

Physical exercise and a high dietary calcium intake has also been shown to both reduce osteoporosis risk, although with less evidence that these measures are thera-

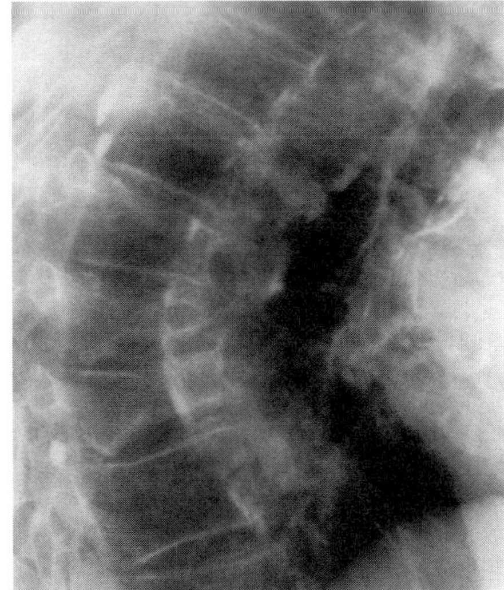

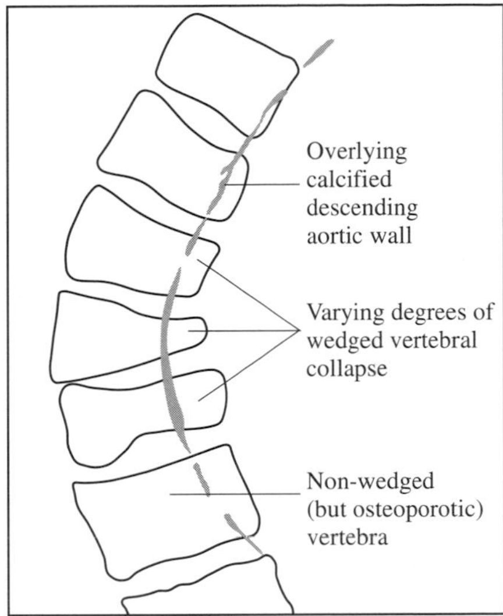

Fig. 10.10. Typical multiple vertebral wedge fractures in a woman aged 65, with premature (age 38) menopause.

peutically useful in established cases. It has been suggested that both weight-bearing and muscular 'tension' on bones enhances mineralization.

Corticosteroid-induced osteoporosis is a potentially serious problem. The concurrent use of biphosphonates, such as editronate or pamidronate, has been shown to reduce the risk of bone loss, and the same approach can be used in treatment, once the problem has arisen. Earlier expectations that alternate-day steroid therapy might reduce bone loss have not been realized.

The use of combined calcium and low-dose alfacalcidol or calcitriol as a prophylactic and therapeutic approach to menopausal and 'senile' osteoporosis has recently shown beneficial effects.It is relevant that large scale epidemiological studies reveal lower calcium intakes in eventual osteoporosis sufferers.

Treatment directed towards increasing bone mass has been mostly unsuccessful. Calcitonin, fluoride, and anabolic steroids have all been tried. Although minor densitometric stabilization and even improvement can be documented, the clinical benefits are unimpressive: increased bone mass does not necessarily equate to reduced proneness to fracture. Intensive physical exercise and retraining have been shown to be one of the few modalities capable of helping to restore bone mass. This may be particularly helpful with the osteoporosis of space flight. Continuous or cyclical biphosphonates (2 weeks in every 3 months) have been shown both to prevent and also partially restore bone density. It is not yet clear whether the benefits are maintained either with ongoing treatment beyond 4 years, or once therapy is discontinued.

Paget's disease of bone: osteitis deformans

Although not strictly an endocrine-related disorder, the classification of Paget's disease of bone (osteitis deformans) is difficult, and most cases requiring metabolic therapy are managed in departments of endocrinology or metabolic medicine. The cause of Paget's disease is unknown. A significant genetic component seems likely from family studies: even the pattern of skeletal involvement shows familial patterns.

Either single-bone (monostotic) or multiple-bone (polyostotic) involvement is seen, and radiological and isotopic screening has shown that more than 10 per cent of the population over the age of 60 is affected, with only a minor proportion of affected individuals having sufficient abnormality to induce symptoms. The pathological characteristics include increased vascularity and coexistent osteolysis and osteogenesis, reflecting both increased osteoclastic and osteoblastic cell proliferation. Structurally, the osteolytic component often predominates early in the disease, so that the bones undergo softening deformity and may fracture. Later, the increased osteoblastic activity and density results in the thickened deformed bone which is responsible for the dominant symptom of pain.

Clinical features (see Plate 10.2)

As indicated, the disorder is mostly asymptomatic, being diagnosed coincidentally from radiology carried out for another purpose, or by the elevated alkaline phosphatase (reflecting osteoblast activity) measured as part of a multichannel screening procedure.

In symptomatic cases, pain is produced by one of three mechanisms: (1) expansion of the periosteum: (2) by entrapment of nerves and spinal cord; or (3) by the presence of abnormal bone in proximity to a joint space. No skeletal region is immune to involvement: the skull, spine, tibia, and pelvis are probably the major involved areas. The skin overlying affected bones may be warm to touch, and in polyostotic disease, the extent of hypervascularity is occasionally enough to provide substantial arteriovenous shunting, a consequent hyperdynamic circulation, and in the most severe cases congestive cardiac failure may occur.

Paget's disease appears to be a premalignant condition, but the incidence of osteogenic sarcoma, or more rarely fibrosarcoma is probably nor higher than 1 per cent of cases.

Investigations

1. Serum calcium is usually normal, although more immobile patients with polyostotic disease may have increased osteolysis resulting in hypercalcaemia and

hypercalciuria and consequent nephrolithiasis. Serum alkaline phosphatase is usually increased with polyostotic disease in proportion to the mass of abnormal tissue, but may quite often be normal with single-bone involvement. It forms a useful marker of disease activity and for monitoring the response to therapy.

2. Radiology demonstrates variable features, including loss of trabecular structure, areas of bone lucency, but a dominant picture of increased density and deformity. The only significant diagnostic confusion arises with diagnosis of multiple bone metastases of the sclerotic type as seen particularly in prostate and breast carcinoma.

3. Radioisotope scanning is a more sensitive indicator of bone involvement than radiology; quantitative isotope uptake has been used to provide a guide as to response to therapy, but is not strictly essential for management. (See Fig. 10.11.)

Treatment

Most cases require some form of pain relief: standard analgesia is often insufficient. Where pain or pressure symptoms occur, a number of methods can

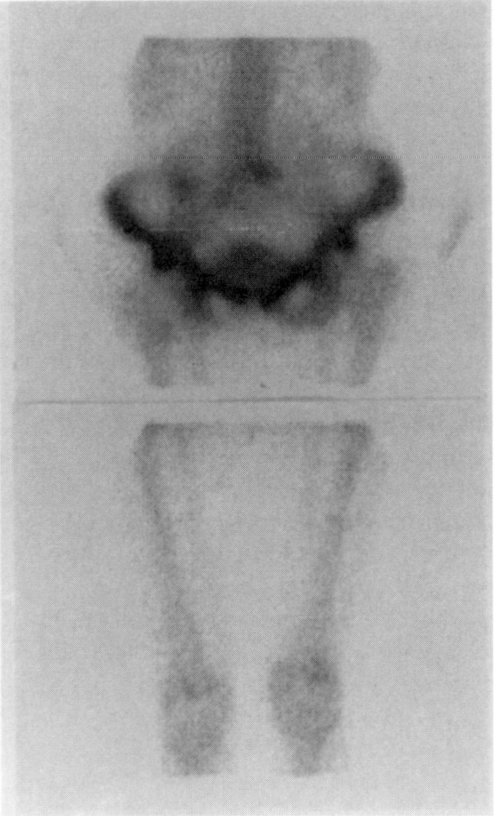

Fig. 10.11. Technetium bone scan showing high concentrations of isotope in areas of Pagetic involvement (pelvic bones only).

now be used to reduce bone turnover, and specifically osteoclastic and osteoblastic activity. Nevertheless, many of these approaches fail to provide pain relief, largely because Paget's disease often affects juxta-articular regions of bone. With even moderately advanced disease, the involvement of joints results in associated non-reversible degenerative changes.

Calcitonin (salmon, porcine, or synthetic human) specifically suppresses osteoclastic activity. It must be given parenterally, initially daily, and the duration of benefit even after several months therapy is not long. The discomfort and cost must be carefully weighed against unspectacular treatment benefits.

The group of biphosphonates act by inhibiting osteoclastic activity, and are currently the most useful drugs in the treatment of Paget's disease. However, these compounds significantly inhibit calcification of osteoid, partly by inhibiting renal 1-hydroxylation, resulting in an osteomalacia-type picture if given in excessive doses. The usual approach is to give infusions of biphosphonates daily or weekly for a finite period, observing the clinical and biochemical course before initiating further therapy.

Cytotoxic agents, such as actinomycin-D and mithramycin, inhibit RNA synthesis in the hyperactive osteoclasts, and produce effective pain relief. However, they suffer from nephrotoxicity and hepatotoxicity and are accordingly infrequently used. Similarly, radiotherapy, possibly by inhibiting RNA synthesis, also has a small place in the treatment of this disorder.

Finally, it has not been proven that any form of treatment inhibits the occasional progression to malignant disease.

FURTHER READING

PHYSIOLOGY

Orloff, J.J., Reddy, D., De Papp, A., Yang, K.H., Soifer, N.E., and Stewart, A.F. (1994). Parathyroid hormone-related protein as a prohormone: posttranslational processing and receptor interactions. *Endocrine Reviews*, **15**, 40–60.

Walters, M.R. (1992). Newly identified action of Vitamin D endocrine system. *Endocrine Reviews*, **13**, 719–64.

CLINICAL

Bilezikian, J.P. (1993). Management of hypercalcaemia. *Journal of Endocrinology and Metabolism*, **77**, 1445–9.

Finch, P.J., Ang, L., Eastwood, J.B., and Maxwell, J.D. (1992). Clinical and histological spectrum of osteomalacia among Asians in south London. *Quarterly Journal of Medicine*, **83**, 439–48.

Fraser, D.R. (1995). Vitamin D. *Lancet*, **345**, 104–7.

Gutierrez, G.E. Poser, J.W., Katz, M.S., *et al.* (1990). Mechanism of hypercalcaemia of malignancy. *Clinical Endocrinology and Metabolism*, **4**, 119–38.

Heath, D.A. (1995). Localization of parathyroid tumours. *Clinical Endocrinology*, **43**, 523–4.

Mundy, G.R. (1988). Hypercalcaemia of malignancy revisited. *Journal of Clinical Investigation*, **82**, 1–6.

Nuovo, M.A., Dorfman, H.D., Sun, C.C. *et al.* (1989). Tumor-associated osteomalacia and rickets. *American Journal of Surgery and Pathology*, **13**, 588–94.

Pols, H.A.P., Birkenhaeger, J.C., and Van Leeuwen, J.P (1994). Vitamin D analogues: from molecule to clinical application. *Clinical Endocrinology*, **40**, 285–92.

Rebel, A. (1987). Paget's disease. *Clinical Orthop.* **217**, 2–170.

Recker, R.R. (1993). Current therapy for osteoporosis. *Journal of Clinical Endocrinology Metabolism*, **76**, 14–16.

Riggs, B.L. and Melton, L.J. (1993). The prevention and treatment of osteoporosis. *New England Journal Medicine*, **327**, 620–7.

11

The pancreas (1): control of metabolism, diabetes, and hypoglycaemia

PHYSIOLOGY

The pancreas has both exocrine and endocrine functions. The latter is limited to the islets of Langerhans, small clumps of glandular tissue dispersed throughout the pancreas first described by Langerhans in 1869. The islets form less than 2 per cent of the pancreatic tissue but their endocrine secretions nevertheless play an important role, particularly concerning blood glucose regulation. The two principal hormones produced from the islet cells are insulin and glucagon. Other physiologically relevant polypeptide hormones have also been identified within the islets and these include somatostatin and pancreatic polypeptide (PP).

Anatomy, histology, and development

The pancreas develops from the endoderm of the foregut close to the junction with the midgut; a dorsal and ventral outgrowth form a typical exocrine gland connected by a duct to the gut. Cells bud off to form isolated clumps, which are the islets of Langerhans, within the exocrine tissue of the pancreas. While the islets are present throughout the pancreas, they are more common in the tail end. The arterial blood supply is provided by the splenic, hepatic, and superior mesenteric arteries while the venous blood drains directly into the portal vein thus reaching the liver directly. Nerve fibres to the pancreas terminate on the islet cells as well as on the exocrine cells.

In humans, three main types of cell have been identified in the endocrine pancreas and these are called α-, β-, and δ-cells (A-, B-, and D-cells). The α- and β-cells synthesize, store, and secrete the hormones glucagon and insulin, respectively, while the δ-cells are associated with somatostatin (somatotrophin release-inhibiting hormone, see Chapter 4). In humans, the α- and δ-cells are located peripheral to the more central β-cells which account for approximately 60 per cent of the total (Fig. 11.1). All three types of cell contain secretory granules in their cytoplasm, as well as the usual intracellular components such as rough endoplasmic reticulum, Golgi complex, and microtubules. The α-cells contain greater concentrations of granules than the β-cells but they are generally smaller. The α-cell granules are also denser than those of the β-cells. The δ-cells contain numerous, more uniform, granules which are less dense than those of either the α- or the β-cells. A fourth cell type, the F-cell, is scattered apparently randomly

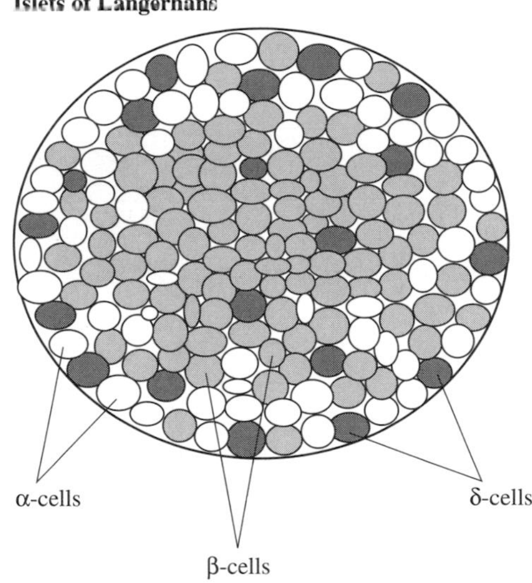

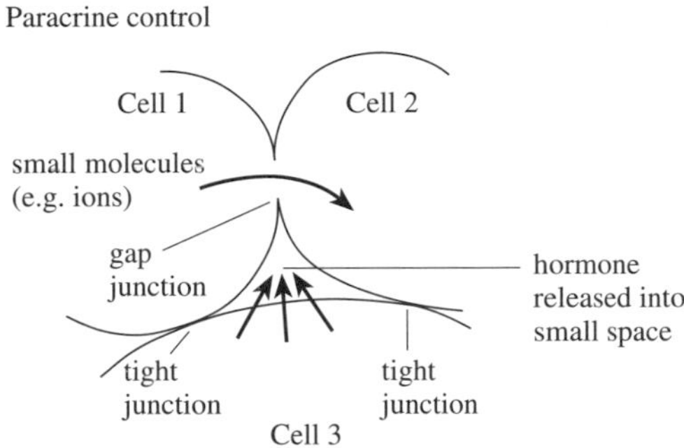

Fig. 11.1. Diagram illustrating the type of cell distribution in a cross sectional view of a pancreatic islet of Langerhans, and below it a diagram illustrating the possible paracrine control which may exist between adjacent cells in a pancreatic islet.

throughout the islets; they are associated with the production of pancreatic polypeptide (see Chapter 12).

Gap junctions have been observed between the various cells of the islets, these being points of cellular contact which could represent areas of direct intercellular communication. Ions and small molecules can cross from cell to cell through these gap junctions so that when one cell is stimulated it can influence adjacent cells through these pathways. In addition, tight junctions, which consist of constantly changing contact points involving fusions of the outer cell membranes, have also been observed. These tight junctions may close off some of the intercellular space from the remaining interstitial fluid; hormones secreted by particular islet cells could then be concentrated in these temporarily isolated fluid compartments, and

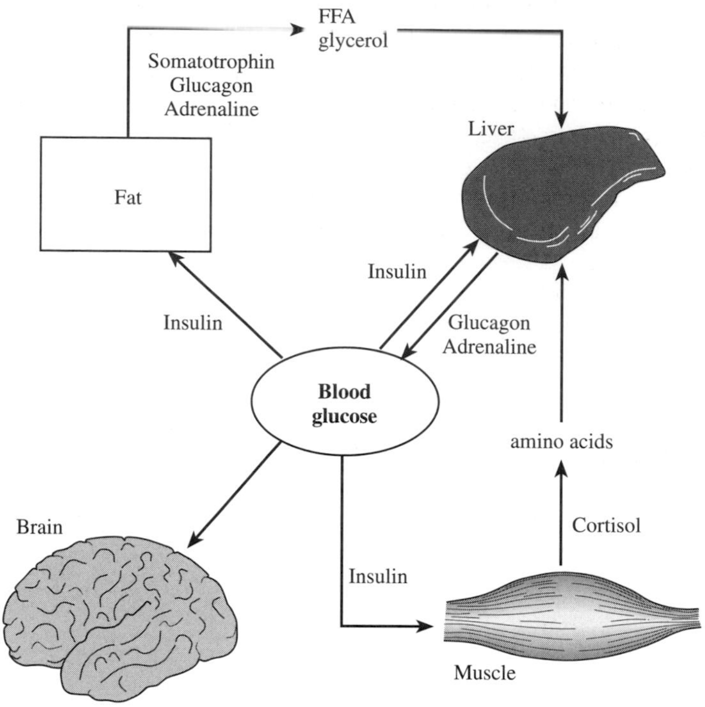

Fig. 11.2. An overview of the hormonal control of glucose and its distribution to the principal organs of the body.

thus exert powerful controlling influences over the secretions of other islet cells. This possible mechanism for intercellular communication is called paracrine control. The physiological relevence of paracrine control over islet cell function is still uncertain, particularly since minute circulating concentrations of pancreatic hormones are quite capable of exerting profound effects directly. The local circulation within each islet may be at least as important, with some evidence for blood flow from central (β-cell) regions to outer (α-cell) areas.

Unmyelinated sympathetic and parasympathetic nerve fibres terminate close to all three types of islet cell and synaptic connections have been suggested. The islets are surrounded by basement membranes separate from the capillary membranes and when hormones are released from any particular group of cells, they have to cross these two membranes before entering the general circulation.

Before describing the pancreatic hormones in more detail the role of glucose and the importance of its regulation in the blood will be considered briefly.

Blood glucose regulation

Glucose is a vital energy substrate primarily because the central nervous system depends almost entirely on this molecule as its source of energy. Neurones have very small reserves of the glucose storage form, the polymer glycogen, and the brain does not concentrate glucose from the general circulation. Thus, the concentration gradient from blood to the brain extracellular fluid and the neurones has to be maintained, and special carrier-mediated transport systems involving glucose transporting (GLUT) proteins are present. The blood glucose concentration is normally maintained within a reasonably narrow range (approximately 4–8 mmol/l). In cells glucose is metabolized by enzymes involved in the glycolytic pathway. A key product is pyruvate which enters the tricarboxylic acid (TCA) cycle and is metabolized to produce various adenosine triphosphate (ATP) molecules. Most cells can store glucose as glycogen (glycogenesis) to varying degrees and can break down glycogen to glucose (glycogenolysis) for their own utilization. However, the enzyme necessary for glucose to be released back into the circulation (glucose-6-phosphatase) is only present in the liver and kidneys. In addition, the liver and the kidneys are the only organs which can synthesize glucose from non-carbohydrate precursors, such as glycerol, lactate, and certain glucogenic amino acids (particularly alanine), by a process generally called gluconeogenesis. The kidneys only become relevant as a source of glucose for the general circulating pool in conditions of starvation, and it is the liver which plays this crucial role under normal circumstances. Muscle can either store or utilize glucose, metabolism of which provides lactate; this metabolic product enters the general circulation and reaches the liver where it acts as a gluconeogenic precursor. During fasting, muscle glucose utilization almost ceases; fatty acids are oxidized for energy requirements and proteolysis provides amino acids (e.g. alanine) which also enter the hepatic gluconeogenic pathway. Adipose tissue can also switch from glucose metabolism to fatty acid oxidation for its energy requirement under fasting conditions (see Fig. 11.2). Thus, the liver plays a crucial role in supplying the brain with the glucose on which it depends. In the brain, glucose is metabolized to carbon dioxide and water. Ketone bodies in the circulation (acetoacetic acid, dihydroxybutyric acid and acetone) formed in peripheral cells from acetyl coenzyme A can also be utilized by the brain. These substrates become increasingly important during prolonged fasting.

From the above brief description it is clear that the blood glucose concentration is vital for the normal functioning of the body with particular reference to the central nervous system. A decrease in the blood glucose concentration (hypoglycaemia) is usually quite rare, however. This is because there are many endocrine systems which can influence metabolic pathways such that the concentration of glucose in the blood is maintained. Of the numerous hormones known to influence the blood glucose concentration, nearly all of them act on metabolic pathways so that the end result is to *increase* it. These glucogenic hormones include the rapidly acting catecholamines (adrenaline and noradrenaline) and glucagon, and the longer-term glucocorticoids (cortisol), and certain pituitary hormones (particularly somatotrophin). In contrast, only one hormone acts in opposition to these glucogenic hormones and *decreases* the blood glucose concentration: insulin. This hormone nevertheless plays a crucial role in blood glucose regulation in addition to its other important metabolic effects. It will be appreciated that it, too, can increase the blood glucose concentration whenever its actions are inhibited or otherwise reduced.

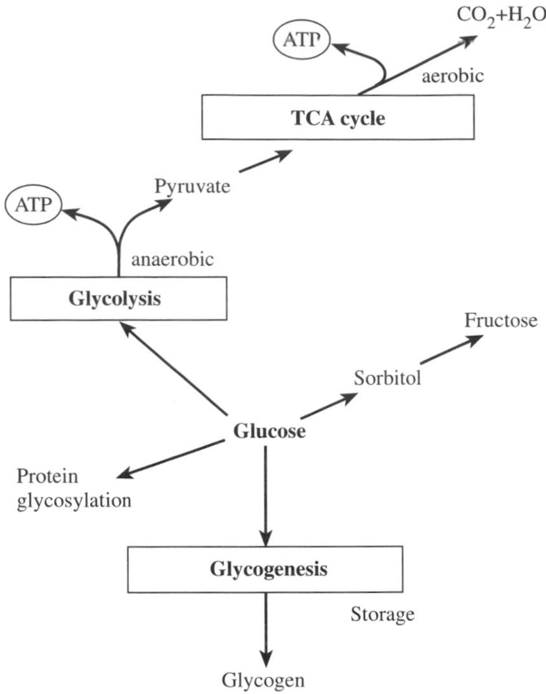

Fig. 11.3. The principal pathways involved in glucose metabolism (ATP, adenosine triphosphate; TCA cycle, tricarboxytic acid cycle)

Hence, insulin is the one key hormone most commonly associated with the disease diabetes mellitus which has, as its chief characteristic, an increased blood glucose concentration. This disease is usually associated with an impaired insulin system, either involving decreased insulin production or a tissue defect making it unresponsive to the hormone. The effects of a lack of insulin are compounded by the relatively raised levels of glucagon which may exist in this condition.

Not surprisingly, the nervous system has an important influence over the release of the various hormones involved in the regulation of the blood glucose concentration, and this will be considered later.

The principal metabolic pathways involving glucose either as the source of energy (in the form of ATP) by glycolysis, or as a source of energy storage by glycogenesis, are shown in Fig. 11.3. Two other pathways of glucose metabolism which become relevant in diabetes mellitus are worth considering briefly here: protein glycosylation and the polyol pathway.

Protein glycosylation

Some proteins are glycosylated, and this process is normally regulated by specific enzymes (e.g. for the glycoprotein hormones of the adenohypophysis). However, non-enzymatic protein glycosylation (called glycation) can also occur, and this is in proportion to the blood glucose concentration. Thus, when the blood glucose level is raised chronically, the amount of glycosylated haemoglobin becomes a good indicator of the degree of regulation of glucose metabolism.

Polyol pathway

Glucose can also be converted to the polyol sorbitol (the polyol pathway) in the presence of an enzyme called aldose reductase which is found in the retina, the lens, the kidneys, Schwann cells, and the aorta — all tissues frequently affected in diabetes mellitus. The sorbitol can then be oxidized slowly to fructose. In those tissues such as the retina and the lens which contain aldose reductase, sorbitol accumulates and exerts an osmotic force which results initially in swelling and later in Na^+ K^+-ATPase inhibition. This process, in addition to general protein glycosylation in the lens, may account for the retinopathy and cataracts which are complications of chronic diabetes.

The pancreatic hormones

In this chapter only the main pancreatic hormones, insulin and glucagon (also somatostatin), are considered but from the above description of blood glucose regulation it will be apparent that other endocrine systems are part of the physiological and clinical story and should be referred to when necessary.

Insulin

Synthesis, storage, and release

Insulin is synthesized in the β-cells, initially as a large precursor molecule called pre-proinsulin (approximately 12 kDa) this being the initial product of translation from messenger RNA. The 23-amino acid signal (leader) sequence is lost as it enters the rough endoplasmic reticulum. The remaining precursor molecule, called proinsulin, is a single-chain polypeptide containing 86 amino acids (approximately 9 kDa) which folds spontaneously upon itself so that two disulphide bonds can be formed. The proinsulin molecules are incorporated into granules at the Golgi complex. Once within the granules proteolysis occurs with the formation of insulin (approximately 5.8 kDa) and a cleavage peptide (the C peptide). The insulin molecule consists of an α-chain of 21 amino acids and a β-chain of 30 amino acids, with the two chains linked together by the disulphide bridges (Fig. 11.4). The insulin gene is on chromosome 11 in humans.

Insulin is stored within the granules, partly as polymers and partly complexed with zinc. The pancreatic cells normally contain a reasonably large store of insulin (about 10 times the normal daily requirement). The synthesis and storage of the hormone are not directly coupled to its release, so that the processes are independently regulated.

The release of the granule contents (insulin and C peptide in equimolar amounts) by exocytosis into the portal blood is calcium-dependent and probably involves microtubules. These are two types of insulin release, basal and stimulated. Basal

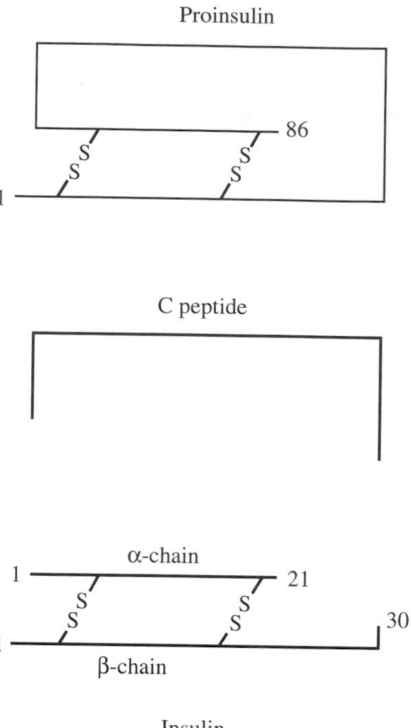

Fig. 11.4. A diagram of the precursor proinsulin and the products (insulin and C-peptide) which are derived from it.

release occurs even during fasting, when the blood glucose concentration may be below 4–5 mmol/l. Various stimuli act on the β-cells to increase insulin secretion, but it appears (from *in vitro* studies) that they are only effective provided that some glucose is available. Indeed, glucose itself is the main stimulus for the release of insulin and will be considered in greater detail in the section on control of release. Insulin secretion is associated with changes in the plasma membrane potential. Variations in extracellular glucose concentration within the physiological range alter the frequency of action potentials recorded from the cells; a rise or a fall in the glucose concentration of the perfusion fluid in an *in vitro* system increases or decreases respectively the number of action potentials recorded.

The current view on the mechanism of release of insulin is that a stimulus such as a raised blood glucose concentration increases the influx of calcium ions into the β-cell, presumably associated with the membrane depolarization. The increased intracellular calcium concentration then triggers a contractile process, probably involving the microtubular network which could participate in the movement of granules from the cell interior to the plasma membrane. The intracellular second messenger cAMP has also been implicated in the release process and could modulate the islet cell response to the primary stimulus. The ultimate release of insulin into the general circulation is brought about by exocytosis, involving the fusion of granular and cellular membranes with the subsequent expulsion of the granule contents into the surrounding fluid. Some insulin may be released by a variety of other mechanisms including the intracellular rupture of granules or the release of hormone from a soluble cytoplasmic pool. The half-life of insulin is approximately 5 minutes, with most of the insulin degraded by the liver and kidneys, mainly by cleavage of the two chains.

Some proinsulin is also secreted with the insulin and approximately 15 per cent of the total immunoreactive insulin-like activity in plasma is attributed to this molecular component. Its biological activity, estimated to be approximately 7 per cent of that of insulin, is negligible. Other molecules which have insulin-like activity are the somatomedins, also known as insulin-like growth factors I and II (IGF-I, IGF-II). They are synthesized in the liver, mainly, following stimulation by somatotrophin (growth hormone) from the adenohypophysis (see Chapters 4 and 13).

Actions

Insulin is a hormone which is primarily involved in the regulation of metabolic processes, the principal manifestation being the control of the blood glucose concentration. Insulin has membrane and intracellular effects on its target cells, and some of its actions are listed in Table 11.1.

Carbohydrate

Glucose is rapidly metabolized to glucose 6-phosphate once it has entered a cell and therefore its intracellular concentration is kept very low. The arterial blood glucose concentration is normally maintained within a range of 4–8 mmol/l (72–144 mg/100 ml), so that a concentration gradient across the cell membrane is always present. However, relatively little glucose actually enters many peripheral cells by simple diffusion, despite the presence of this large concentration gradient. The small quantities of glucose entering these cells by diffusion are insufficient to

Table 11.1. Some of the actions of insulin

Membrane effects

1. Increased glucose transport (and some other monosaccharides)
2. Increased amino acid transport (especially arginine)
3. Increased fatty acid transport
4. Increased cellular uptake of K^+ and Mg^{2+}*

Intracellular effects

1. Increased RNA and DNA synthesis
2. Increased protein synthesis
3. Increased stimulation of glycogen synthase (glycogenesis)
4. Stimulation of glucokinase
5. Inhibition of glucose 6-phosphatase
6. Stimulation of lipogenesis
7. Decreased lipolysis (inhibition of cyclic AMP synthesis)
8. Increased nucleic acid synthesis*
9. Increased Mg^{2+}-activated Na^+/K^+ ATPase activity*

*Little is known of the importance of these actions of insulin.

meet the metabolic requirements of the cells, even when the concentration gradient is raised by a marked elevation of the blood glucose level. In the presence of insulin, on the other hand, the net movement of glucose into these peripheral cells is greatly increased. This action of insulin only occurs when a concentration gradient favouring the inward movement of glucose is present, is subject to competitive inhibition by other monosaccharides such as galactose, and follows saturation kinetics. Insulin therefore stimulates a facilitated diffusion process for the transport of glucose which involves a hormone-sensitive glucose transporter (GLUT) protein molecule located in the cell membrane. Glucose is transferred across the cell membrane by this process in both directions, the net movement of glucose being dependent on the concentration gradient which normally is from extracellular to intracellular compartments. Various different GLUT proteins have been identified in different cells, but only one of them — GLUT4 — is insulin-sensitive, and this is found in the membranes of skeletal and cardiac muscle and adipose tissue.

Some tissues obtain their glucose requirements entirely by insulin-independent mechanisms. For example, the cells of the liver and the central nervous system receive their glucose requirements by a mechanism, involving insulin-independent GLUT proteins, and are therefore purely dependent on the maintenance of an adequate blood glucose concentration. In addition, erythrocytes, renal, and intestinal cells transfer glucose across the cell membranes in association with sodium ions by cotransport carrier mechanisms driven by the passive diffusion of sodium ions into the cells down their concentration gradient.

Insulin also has effects on intracellular metabolic pathways. Glycogen synthesis is stimulated in hepatic and other cells by an action involving enhanced glycogen synthase activity, resulting in an increased incorporation of glycosyl units into glycogen. Insulin also stimulates hepatic glucokinase activity, this enzyme catalysing the phosphorylation of glucose to glucose 6-phosphate. The hormone also inhibits hepatic phosphatase, which dephosphorylates glycose 6-phosphate to glucose. These actions on hepatic cellular enzymes result in a decreased production of glucose which, together with the stimulated peripheral cell uptake of this substrate produces the blood glucose-lowering effect of insulin. In addition, the increased utilization of glucose by the cells spares other energy substrates such as fats and proteins.

Protein metabolism

Insulin stimulates the active transport of amino acids into peripheral cells, and also stimulates protein synthesis directly. Since these two effects can be dissociated from each other insulin has separate membrane and intracellular actions. The enhanced protein synthesis induced by the hormone occurs subsequent to an observed increase in mRNA activity and this provides evidence for a second messenger-mediated nuclear effect. Protein synthesis is also stimulated indirectly by the increased amounts of amino acid entering the cells in the presence of insulin. In addition, the increased glucose utilization induced by insulin results in decreased protein catabolism, hence the protein-sparing effect of the hormone.

As a result of these various effects of insulin on protein metabolism, the hormone plays an important role in the processes of growth and development.

Fat metabolism

The cellular uptake and oxidation of glucose by adipose tissue are stimulated by insulin. Also, insulin stimulates the synthesis of lipoprotein lipase of endothelial cells; this enzyme catalyses the hydrolysis of triglycerides bound to circulating lipoproteins and stimulates the movement of fatty acids into adipocytes. These effects, together with a direct stimulation of lipogenesis in hepatic and adipose tissues, result in the increased storage of fats in these tissues. In addition, insulin inhibits cAMP-mediated lipolysis by inhibiting the hormone-sensitive intracellular lipoprotein lipase enzyme.

Potassium

The presence of insulin is necessary for the maintenance of the intracellular potassium ion concentration, presumably by a membrane effect.

Mechanism of action

Insulin binds to specific dimeric receptors which span the target cell membranes, and these have inherent tyrosine kinase activity (Fig. 11.5). The receptors belong to a family of related proteins including the receptors for IGF-I and IGF-II with which they have some homology. Each receptor has extracellular, transmembrane,

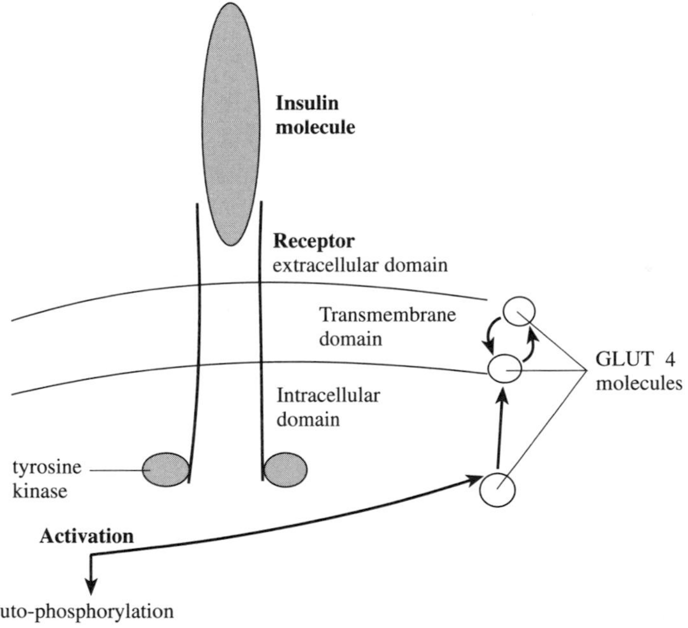

Fig. 11.5. The dimeric insulin receptor and the actions of insulin which are produced following tyrosine kinase activation (GLUT, glucose transporter;)

and intracellular domains, the last having intrinsic tyrosine kinase activity. The extracellular domains confer specificity for the various binding molecules (ligands) so that while insulin is the main ligand, IGF-I and IGF-II also bind to the insulin receptors to some extent. This accounts at least partly for some of the shared effects of insulin, IGF-I and IGF-II.

Tyrosine kinase activity is stimulated immediately following binding of the hormone to its receptor, and subsequent phosphorylation of intracellular proteins mediates the various actions of insulin. Auto-phosphorylation of the receptor tyrosine kinases and cross-phosphorylation of neighbouring receptors (e.g. for IGF-I) provides scope for amplification of the initial signal. Some of the membrane effects of the hormone may be due to direct actions on the membrane. However, the translocation of glucose transporters from intracellular sites to the plasma membrane suggests the involvement of intracellular mechanisms being activated, for example.

Certainly, other mechanisms almost certainly mediate the intracellular effects of insulin. In adipose tissue, lipolysis is associated with an increased cytoplasmic cAMP concentration. Insulin may block lipolysis by inhibiting cAMP formation. Insulin also decreases the cAMP concentration in hepatic cells, thus reducing glycogenolysis and gluconeogenesis. In addition, other second messenger systems such as cGMP and calcium ions have been the subject of much investigation, but little is known about the role of these substances in mediating any of the effects of insulin.

Finally, there is evidence to suggest that the insulin-receptor complex may be internalized by endocytosis. The insulin can be inactivated by proteolysis or disulphide bond cleavage, and the receptors can be recirculated back to the membrane or be degraded. This process may be particularly relevant for the regulation of receptor numbers. There is a negative correlation between the number of insulin receptors and the insulin concentration. Thus, in type II (non-insulin-dependent) diabetes mellitus, the receptor number in adipose tissue for instance may be decreased despite a raised plasma insulin concentration (down-regulation) resulting in tissue insensitivity to the hormone (see later sections on diabetes).

Control of secretion

The release of insulin from the β-cells is regulated by the integration of the numerous stimulatory and inhibitory factors which participate in the process (see Fig. 11.6). As mentioned earlier, insulin is secreted even in the absence of a specific stimulus. This basal release may partly determine the response of the β-cells to a particular stimulus. Following such a stimulus the release of insulin is biphasic: there is an immediate response detectable within seconds; this secretion then decreases, and a second more gradual increase in insulin secretion develops to reach a peak level which can be sustained indefinitely. The initial increase is due to the release of immediately available insulin, stored within the granules closest to the cell membrane. The second phase is related to another intracellular pool of insulin which is less readily available. Newly synthesized hormone probably adds to this pool continually when the stimulus is prolonged.

The principal stimulus for insulin release is an increased blood glucose concentration. As the blood glucose level rises above 4 mmol/l it stimulates not

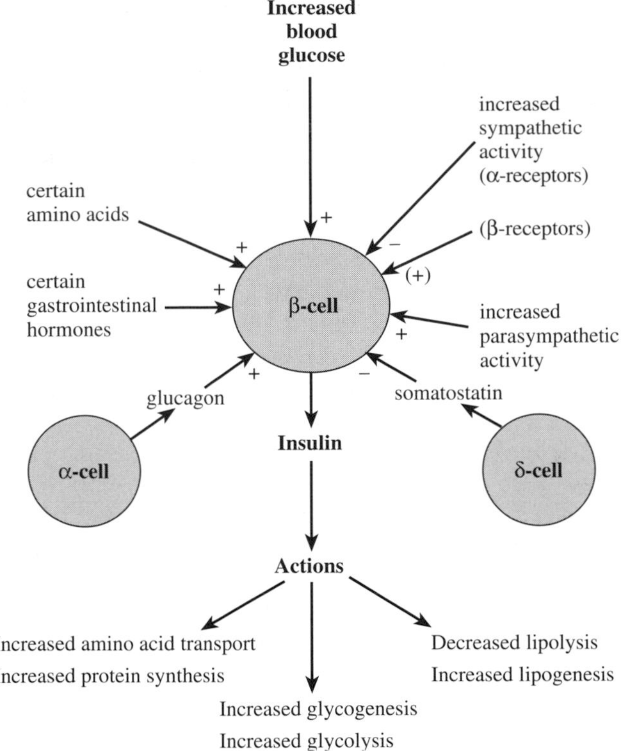

Fig. 11.6. The control of insulin production.

only the release process but also the synthesis of new hormone. Precisely how changes in the extracellular glucose level produce their effects on insulin synthesis and release is not yet known although glucose metabolism within the islet cell appears to be an important step. A glucose receptor located in the β-cell membrane has also been suggested but failure to detect it casts doubt on its existence. Certain amino acids are also potent stimulators of insulin release (e.g. arginine) but fatty acids only appear to stimulate the process slightly in humans and therefore probably play a minor role in the control system.

The autonomic nervous system is clearly implicated in the regulation of insulin release. Sympathetic nerve stimulation produces a net inhibition of its release and this effect is mediated by α-receptors on the β-cell membrane. On the other hand, there is evidence to suggest that β-receptor stimulation produces an enhanced release of insulin, but only when the β-cell is subsequently stimulated by some other stimulus. This implies that the β-receptor effect is associated with an increased pool of readily available hormone. It should, nevertheless, be emphasized that the dominant effect of sympathetic stimulation is inhibitory. Stimulation of the parasympathetic fibres produces the opposite effect, namely an increased release of insulin.

Stress has been shown to be associated with an inhibition of insulin release, probably mediated by increased sympathetic activity. Since stressors cause the release of various glucogenic hormones (e.g. the catecholamines, cortisol, somatotrophin) which consequently increase the blood glucose concentration, it is perhaps not surprising that the glucose-decreasing hormone insulin is inhibited. These efferent pathways illustrate how the central nervous system can clearly influence pancreatic hormone release and hence the blood glucose concentration.

Various hormones influence the release of insulin and for some of them the effect is probably at least in part indirect, and is consequent upon the increase in blood glucose concentration that they produce. Somatotrophin is one such hormone which can indirectly stimulate the release of insulin. Catecholamines such as adrenaline and noradrenaline could have complex effects on insulin release (see above), but the dominant effect is undoubtedly inhibitory via the α-receptors, thus participating in the raising of the blood glucose level. Glucocorticoids, oestrogens, and progesterone can all stimulate the release of insulin partly by decreasing peripheral tissue responsiveness to insulin which results in an increase in the main stimulus for its release, the blood glucose level.

The gastrointestinal hormones gastrin, secretin, and pancreozymin-cholecystokinin stimulate the release of insulin. Indeed, an oral glucose load will stimulate a greater release of the hormone than the load given intravenously. This effect by the gastrointestinal hormones probably prepares the insulin system for the forthcoming sudden increase in portal blood glucose following a meal. They will also amplify the dietary glucose signal by greatly increasing the amount of insulin released for a given oral stimulus.

The other islet hormones glucagon and somatostatin also influence the release process. While these effects can be brought about by the hormones released into the general circulation, it is more likely that both glucagon and somatostatin exert their effects on the β-cells directly. For instance hormones released into the interstitial spaces between the islet cells could exert their effects directly, at local concentrations far higher than those present in the bloodstream, a point particularly relevant for somatostatin. Paracrine effects could therefore be of great importance in the control of insulin release.

Glucagon

Synthesis, storage, and release

Glucagon is a polypeptide of 29 amino acids (approximately 3.5 kDa) synthesized in the α-cells of the islets of Langerhans. The synthesis of the molecule occurs on the rough endoplasmic reticulum and involves an initial large precursor molecule called pre-proglucagon which is modified in the granules formed at the Golgi complex first to a proglucagon molecule and then finally to glucagon. The hormone is then stored in the granules in the cell cytoplasm until released by exocytosis.

Various immunoreactive glucagons (IRG) have been identified in the plasma and other glucagon-containing areas of the body in addition to the pancreas (such as the fundus of the stomach, at least in dogs). These IRG molecules partly represent proglucagon precursors and degradation products, in addition to glucagon itself.

Actions

Glucagon exerts its actions on carbohydrate, protein, and fat metabolism, and the principal consequent effect of the hormone is to raise the blood glucose concentration. It plays an important frontline role in maintaining available energy substrates in the circulation during times of fasting.

Carbohydrate

Glucagon stimulates glycogenolysis in the liver which results in an increased production of glucose which can then be released into the general circulation. The hormone also stimulates hepatic gluconeogenesis.

Protein

Glucagon has been reported to stimulate the transport of various glucogenic amino acids into the liver, at least in *in vitro* experiments. This effect would contribute to the activity of the gluconeogenic pathway in hepatic tissue.

Fats

Lipolysis in adipose tissue is stimulated by glucagon-sensitive lipase and consequently the plasma level of fatty acids and glycerol increases. Glycerol can be used as a glucose precursor in the hepatic gluconeogenic pathway, and fatty acids can be metabolized, for instance, to ketone bodies, thus sparing glucose as an energy substrate.

Mechanism of action

Glucagon binds to specific receptors located in the plasma membranes of its target cells. The actions of glucagon in hepatic and adipose tissues are associated with increases in adenyl cyclase activity and consequently increased cytoplasmic cAMP concentration. The generation of this second messenger is believed to mediate all the effects of the hormone.

Control of release

Even under basal conditions the secretion of glucagon is relatively high, in contrast to insulin. Hyperglycaemia inhibits, while hypoglycaemia stimulates the release of glucagon, although the mechanism by which changes in the blood glucose concentration alter the level of glucagon secretion remains unclear. In addition to the important stimulus of a decreased blood glucose concentration, other energy substrates also have a profound influence on glucagon release.

Various amino acids (e.g. arginine, alanine) stimulate glucagon secretion. It is interesting to note that these amino acids also stimulate insulin release. A teleological explanation for this apparently paradoxical effect is that glucagon will tend to counteract the effect of insulin on the blood glucose concentration while enabling the latter hormone to stimulate the entry of amino acids into cells and to promote protein synthesis. There is some evidence to suggest that decreased circulating levels of fatty acids are also associated with an increased glucagon release and that hyperlipidaemia causes a slight decrease in the plasma glucagon con-

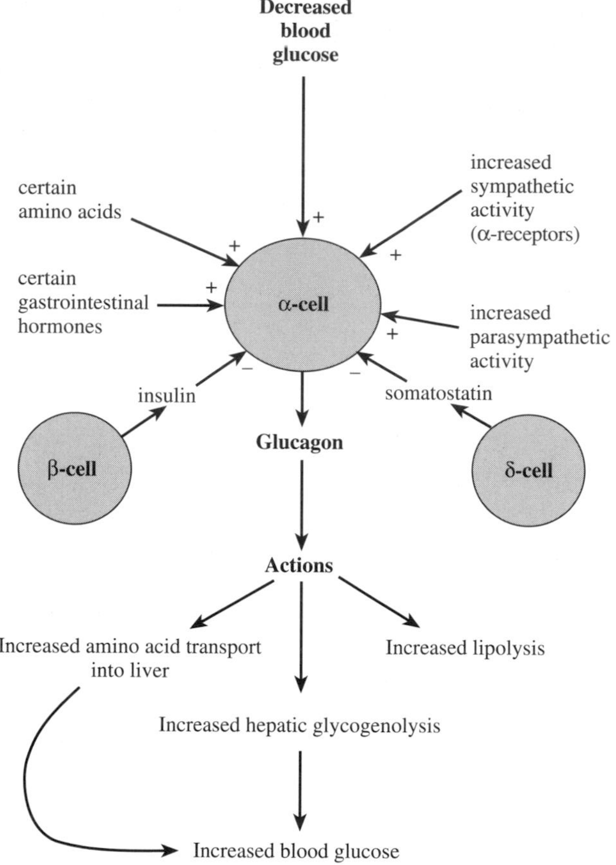

Fig. 11.7. The principal actions of glucagon and the control of its production.

centration. However, the physiological importance of these effects remains speculative (see Fig. 11.7).

The sympathetic nervous system influences glucagon secretion in a manner which is diametrically opposed to its effects on insulin release; thus sympathetic stimulation (which inhibits insulin release) increases the secretion of glucagon. However, acetylcholine appears to stimulate glucagon release and increase the secretion of insulin. The 'push-pull' control of α- and β-cell secretions by the sympathetic nervous system is undoubtedly of considerable importance in the regulation of blood glucose levels under specific conditions such as those associated with various stressors.

Various gastrointestinal hormones, in particular pancreozymin-cholecystokinin (PZ-CCK), stimulate the release of glucagon. Thus, a protein meal elicits a greater glucagon response than can be accounted for by the increased plasma amino acid level, and this 'amplification' is presumably mediated by the release of PZ-CCK.

Glucagon release is also inhibited by insulin and somatostatin, and a possible 'paracrine' system relating the different types of islet cells has already been mentioned in an earlier section. One important consequence of this effect of insulin is seen in diabetes mellitus when insulin levels are low so that the inhibitory effect on glucagon release is reduced. The glucagon concentration is then inappropriately high in relation to the blood glucose level and certainly contributes to the excessive blood glucose concentration in this metabolic disorder.

Hyperglycaemia of diabetes mellitus

In the relative or total absence of insulin (diabetes mellitus) blood glucose concentrations rise, sometimes reaching levels in excess of 35 mmol/l (about 600 mg/100 ml plasma). The renal proximal tubules normally reabsorb all the glucose filtered by the glomeruli unless the blood level exceeds 10 mmol/l (180 mg/100 ml plasma). The hyperglycaemia of diabetes exceeds this threshold allowing glucose to be excreted in the urine (glycosuria) inducing an osmotic diuresis (polyuria), although the osmotic change induced by the glucose is small. The diuresis may also be partly due to an inhibition of vasopressin release from the neurohypophysis. The excessive water loss causes dehydration and thirst resulting in a large fluid intake (polydipsia).

A net increase in protein catabolism raises blood amino acid levels, resulting in an enhanced load of these substances to the liver. Here they are deaminated, and the carbon residues of the glucogenic amino acids contribute to the formation of glucose (increased gluconeogenesis) which further exacerbates the hyperglycaemia. The protein depletion contributes to the weakness and loss of weight found in this condition.

Lipolysis is stimulated with a resulting increase in free fatty acid and glycerol concentrations in the blood (the latter raising the blood glucose level through gluconeogenesis). An excess of acetyl coenzyme A accumulates in the liver as it cannot be fully utilized in the tricarboxylic acid cycle. It is then converted in enhanced quantities to acetoacetic acid. This substance is reduced to β-hydroxybutyric acid, or is decarboxylated to form acetone; these three substances are called 'ketone bodies'. Thus, the production of ketone bodies increases and peripheral utilization is unable to cope with this excess; the blood concentration of ketone bodies rises (ketonaemia). Hence the enhanced fat catabolism is responsible for the acidosis (ketoacidosis) and also contributes to the loss of body weight in diabetes mellitus.

CLINICAL DISORDERS

Insulin excess: insulinoma

Insulinoma is one of the more common causes of spontaneous hypoglycaemia. Usually benign, but in 10 per cent a malignant tumour, it may present at any age with a wide variety of symptoms. A family history of diabetes is common, while following removal of an insulinoma, diabetes subsequently develops in over 10 per cent of cases. This suggests a common set of genes for both conditions, modified by other as yet undetermined factors. There is also a 10 per cent incidence of multiple pancreatic tumours and an association with adenomas in adrenal, pituitary, and parathyroid glands in some patients, or in members of their family (see MEN-I: Chapter 16). The tumour is usually located in the body or tail of the pancreas and is usually 1 cm or smaller at the time of diagnosis. Little is known of the aetiology of these tumours.

Clinical features

Symptoms of hypoglycaemia usually occur when blood glucose concentrations fall below 2.2 mmol/l (40 mg/100 ml). This is obviously more likely to occur in the fasting state or as a result of exercise, which has a direct, and partially insulin-independent effect on muscle glucose uptake. Symptoms of hypoglycaemia may be due to cerebral glycopenia with hunger, dizziness, confusion (including bizarre behaviour), and even convulsions and coma. Symptoms may also be caused by sympathetic activation in response to hypoglycaemia, and manifest by tremor, sweating, and palpitations (tachycardia). Occasionally, patients identify for themselves that sweet foods are capable of aborting an attack. Because of the vague nature of the symptoms, they may be present for many months or years before the true diagnosis is even suspected.

Differential diagnosis of hypoglycaemia

Two levels of differential diagnoses are necessary. First, that of the 'fits, faints, or funny turns' which initially provoked consideration of hypoglycaemia as a possible cause, and secondly that of the hypoglycaemia, once it has been confirmed that this biochemical abnormality is the actual cause of the symptoms. (See Tables 11.2 and 11.3.)

Severe liver failure is usually clinically apparent. Cortisol or growth hormone deficiencies may not be so obvious, and specific pituitary and adrenal function testing (see appropriate section) may need to be carried out if any supportive clinical features are present. Patients with galactosaemia or glycogen storage disease usually present in childhood, and frequently have hepatomegaly, while, in addition, galactosaemic subjects have premature cataract. Both conditions, as well as fructose intolerance tend to occur in younger age groups than other causes of hypoglycaemia.

Alcohol blocks glycogenolysis, and this can induce hypoglycaemia in susceptible individuals especially in the extended fasting state, during which glycogen

Table 11.2. Principal differential diagnoses of a presumed hypoglycaemic episode

- Vaso-vagal syncope
- Postural hypotension
- Hyperventilation syndrome
- Anxiety/panic attack
- Temporal lobe epilepsy
- Carotid/vertebrobasilar ischaemia
- Phaeochromocytoma

Table 11.3. Major causes of hypoglycaemia

Spontaneous (fasting) hypoglycaemia	Reactive hypoglycaemia
Insulinoma	Gastroenterostomy
Severe liver cell failure	'Reactive' hypoglycaemia
Glycogen storage disorders	Early diabetes
Cortisol or growth hormone deficiency	
Galactosaemia	
Alcohol hypoglycaemia	
Fructose intolerance	
Tumour-associated hypoglycaemia	
Auto-immune hypoglycaemia	

stores are additionally depleted. Indeed, the symptoms of hypoglycaemia may readily mimic the features of alcoholic intoxication.

Large tumours, commonly mesotheliomas of pleura and peritoneum are sometimes associated with hypoglycaemia. The mechanisms for induction of hypoglycaemia in these cases are not clear (see Chapter 15). In some patients, excess somatomedins (IGF-II) have been identified and are assumed to be released from the tumour. Other tumours appear to induce their effects by increased glucose consumption, via mechanisms which are still obscure. In all cases serum insulin levels are very low.

Factitious hypoglycaemia reflects surreptitious administration of insulin or oral hypoglycaemic agents. This usually occurs in people with a significant, but not necessarily readily identifiable psychiatric disorder.

'Reactive hypoglycaemia' is a term used to describe a fall of blood glucose which follows one to two hours after ingestion of refined carbohydrate. Symptoms have in the past often been attributed to this phenomenon. However, it is now recognized that such swings to a blood glucose as low as 2.5 mmol/l occur quite asymptomatically in about 20 per cent of normal subjects given an oral dextrose load. Only after gastrectomy, when rapid monosaccharide transit to, and absorption from the small bowel occurs, is it likely that reactive hypoglycaemia is sufficient to induce symptoms. True reactive hypoglycaemia also occurs in early diabetes, when the characteristic delay in insulin release may very occasionally induce a 'reactive' and symptomatic lowering of blood glucose.

Auto-immune hypoglycaemia is a recently identified syndrome encompassing a series of aetiological processes. The auto-immune insulin syndrome represents the abnormal formation of insulin–antibody complexes which dissociate in the post-prandial state, releasing insulin. Other auto-immune syndromes may also be present in these patients. The second type of anomaly is the development of antibodies to the insulin receptor which are themselves stimulatory (analogous to the abnormal thyroid stimulator in Graves' disease). Finally, islet cell-stimulating antibodies have been proposed as a cause of hypoglycaemia in some cases, but not uneqivocally identified. Confirmation of all these causes requires highly specialized analyses.

Investigations

1. During a spontaneous episode of suspected hypoglycaemia blood should be taken both for glucose and insulin assay. If blood glucose concentration is less than 2.2 mmol/l (40 mg/100 ml) and insulin is simultaneously detectable at a level greater than 10 mU/l, the only diagnoses to be considered are insulinoma or the self-administration of insulin or a sulphonylurea drug. In addition, insulinoma patients have plasma C-peptide concentrations (reflecting endogenous insulin release) which cannot be suppressed by the induction of hypoglycaemia using an insulin infusion.

2. In patients with insulinoma, prolonged fasting for a period of 48–72 hours should normally induce the typical symptoms associated with verified biochemical hypoglycaemia. The test must be performed under the closest supervision. The development of the relevant symptoms coincident with documented hypoglycaemia, their immediate correction by intravenous glucose, and the identification of hyperinsulinaemia coincident with the hypoglycaemia are essential elements of diagnosis.

3. Specific procedures may be indicated to define the other causes of hypoglycaemia.

4. Plasma proinsulin is very frequently elevated (greater than 20 pmol/l) in insulinoma, its absence suggesting other pathologies, such as factitious hypoglycaemia.

Treatment.

Treatment is by surgical removal of the tumour. However, this is not always easy, as the tumours may be small and/or multiple. Localization may be achieved by coeliac axis angiography (Fig. 11.8) or a complex transhepatic venous sampling technique, but isotope scanning has been generally unrewarding. Occasionally, the tumour may be ectopically situated in the hilum of the spleen or in the wall of the duodenum. A careful inspection and, if need be, a dissection is required. If no tumour can be identified, 'blind' pancreatectomy is not considered advisable. Recently, the technique of intraoperative ultrasound has enabled the tumour to be localized when it has been inapparent to manual exploration.

Patients can also be treated medically with the hyperglycaemic agent diazoxide (5–15 mg/kg body weight/24 hours). With this dose, side-effects such as severe hypotension, nausea, fluid retention or vomiting are usually avoided. The hyperglycaemia induced by this drug is enhanced, and adverse effects are reduced by the addition of an thiazide diuretic. This treatment can also be used in the rare syndromes of nesidioblastosis and islet cell hyperplasia, both conditions not being otherwise amenable to surgery other than total pancreatectomy. Metastases occur relatively early in cases of malignant insulinoma: the drug streptozotocin (a β-cytotoxic antibiotic which is used experimentally to induce diabetes in experimental animals) has been used successfully in many patients with inoperable disease. As indicated earlier, the removal of tumour in some patients results in later development of overt diabetes mellitus; accordingly, long-term follow-up is essential.

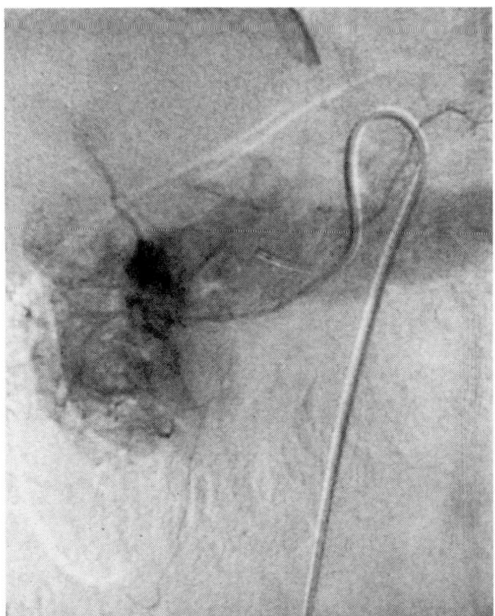

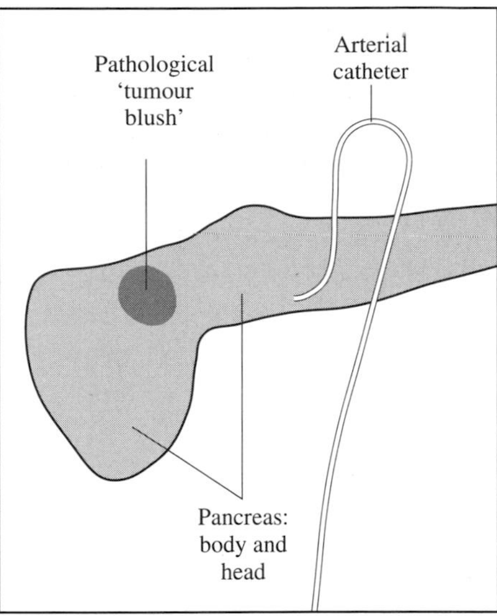

Fig. 11.8. Digital subtraction angiography of coeliac axis in a patient with insulinoma: tumour circulation shown as dense area in comparison with normal remaining pancreas.

Deficiency

Diabetes mellitus

Contrary to many disorders described in this book, diabetes was already well described over 2000 years ago. The word 'diabetes' is derived from a Greek word signifying a siphon, reflecting the increased urine output (polyuria) and thirst (polydipsia) which represent two of its major symptoms.

The syndrome is now recognized as representing a heterogeneous group of disorders, based on different genetic and environmental factors; even further subdivisions are likely to become apparent as identification of genetic markers becomes more precise. Approximately 1.5–2 per cent of populations of industrialized nations are diabetic, but some ethnic groups (Australian Aboriginals, North American Indian groups, and South Pacific Islanders) have a prevalence exceeding 15 per cent. Incidence is age-related, so that over the age of 60, prevalence rises to between 5 and 10 per cent in the majority of developed countries for which adequate epidemiological data is available.

Although earlier descriptions drew attention to the common denominator of hyperglycaemia, it is now clear that although the primary defect is either an absolute or relative deficiency of insulin, other biochemical abnormalities are mostly present which modulate the effect on blood glucose. Furthermore, the metabolic consequences of insulin deficiency and hyperglycaemia are complex and widespread, producing secondary functional and structural changes in almost every system of the body.

Aetiology

Secondary diabetes

Review of the various physiological factors which control blood glucose within the normal range allows prediction of the effects of primary excesses of these hormones. Thus, hyperglycaemia may be a consequence of cortisol (Cushings' syndrome), catecholamine (phaeochromocytoma), or growth hormone (acromegaly) excess, or to the rare disorder of glucagon-producing pancreatic tumours, (glucagonoma). Furthermore, destructive lesions of the pancreas such as chronic relapsing pancreatitis, haemochromatosis (due to abnormal tissue iron deposition), and pancreatic carcinoma may cause 'secondary' diabetes. Although difficult to prove, it is likely that these disorders probably require a additional genetic predisposition of β-cell incompetence, before the clinical syndrome of diabetes can become manifest.

Primary diabetes

This has been subclassified, based on different genetic factors and clinical behaviour.

Type I (insulin-dependent) diabetes: IDDM This accounts for approximately 25–30 per cent of all diabetic cases. Epidemiological studies reveal the higher prevalence of class I histocompatibility antigens HLA-B8, -BW15, DR-3, and -4. Certain class II (DQ) haplotypes confer even stronger susceptibility. All alleles are also found commonly in the related group of thyrogastric immune disorders mentioned earlier in this book (see also Chapter 16). Accordingly, an increased incidence of these disorders is seen both in type I diabetics as well as in their first degree relatives. The highly significant genetic component is highlighted by the 30 per cent concordance rate in identical twins and the 5–8 per cent prevalence in first degree relatives (compared with 0.3 per cent in the general population).

The nature of the putative environmental precipitant(s) is still unclear. The association of onset with epidemics of cocksackievirus B4 virus infection, and the isolation of viruses (including cocksackievirus and mumps) from the pancreatic islets in the occasional fatal case, point to a viral trigger in some cases. Congenital rubella is also associated with a high incidence of type I diabetes. These triggers are thought to act by causing presentation of surface antigen on β-cells, subsequently initiating both a cell and antibody-mediated immune response from an abnormally primed immune system. Islet cell (ICA) and insulin (IAA) antibodies are frequently found in newly diagnosed cases: they are also present in a significant proportion of (unaffected) first degree relatives. Together with other markers such as antibodies to a 64kDa β-cell antigen (probably glutamic acid dehydrogenase, GAD), presence of these antibodies are a strong predictor of later development of IDDM. This may prove to be important in terms of identifying candidates for preventive immunotherapy when appropriate agents become available.

Symptoms may be of quite sudden onset, at any age from one year onwards, although 90 per cent of cases present before the age of 35, thereby giving rise to, the now outdated and imprecise term of 'juvenile-onset diabetes'.

Type II (non-insulin-dependent) diabetes: NIDDM This represents the majority of all diabetics seen in most populations. No clear-cut genetic marker has been identified, although gene mapping has identified some familial clusters of cases where defective glucokinase genes are likely to be responsible for the disorder. There are likely to be multiple gene defects involved, affecting such diverse steps as glucose receptors on islet cells, glucose transporters, insulin receptors, and intracellular glucose signalling. Genetic factors are accordingly of greater importance in type II than in type I diabetes, as evidenced by the higher concordance rate (more than 90 per cent) for type II diabetes when identical twin pairs are examined. Approximately 40 per cent of first degree relatives of NIDDM patients will show either impaired glucose tolerance (IGT) or an overtly diabetic pattern on glucose tolerance testing.

Whether this currently unidentifiable genetic anomaly is rendered clinically significant depends on additional and largely non-genetic hyperglycaemic factors. Of greatest importance among these is obesity; it has been shown that muscle glucose uptake is inversely proportional to skin-fold thickness. The mechanism of this insulin 'resistance' is unclear, although obesity is associated with a reduction of both number and affinity of insulin receptors in a variety of target tissues.

In addition, relative inactivity (which directly reduces muscle cell glucose uptake) and over-eating (which provides excessive substrate) often play a part in precipitating hyperglycaemia as do the stress hormones (somatotrophin, cortisol, glucagon, and catecholamines).

A number of drugs may induce diabetes, particularly in the genetically predisposed. These include corticosteroids (which enhance gluconeogenesis), phenytoin (which suppresses insulin secretion), thiazide and other diuretics (which have both direct suppressive effects on insulin secretion as well as on peripheral glucose uptake), and the contraceptive pill (whose oestrogenic component is thought to be the major factor), inducing mild peripheral insulin resistance by a mechanism which is currently unclear.

Age of onset may be from 15 years upwards: hence the often-used term 'maturity onset diabetes' is misleading. A small and strongly familial form of type II diabetes, so-called maturity-onset diabetes of youth (MODY) has been identified, but not yet genetically characterized. Most cases are under the age of 30 at diagnosis.

The onset of type II diabetes is usually less dramatic than in type I diabetes: at the time of diagnosis, many cases have undoubtedly had asymptomatic hyperglycaemia for many years. This concept is central to the understanding of the relationship of hyperglycaemia to mode of presentation and natural history of the non-metabolic complications of diabetes.

Pathophysiology

It is clear that for hyperglycaemia to occur, there must be relative or absolute insulin deficiency at key cell sites.

Type I diabetes reflects a state of almost complete insulin deficiency, and this can be verified by insulin or C-peptide assay at any stage from 3 months following diagnosis onwards. A very small proportion of apparent type I diabetics continue to release some insulin for up to 3 years following diagnosis. If death occurs in the first few weeks of type I diabetes (fortunately a rare event), pancreatic islets may be found enlarged and degranulated. Later in the course of the disease, islets are individually smaller and are reduced in number and show evidence of a lymphocytic infiltrate, representing the hallmark of the thyrogastric immune group of disorders. The question of concomitant glucagon deficiency has arisen. It is now clear that glucagon (and incidentally growth hormone) secretion is actually elevated in uncontrolled diabetes, potentiating the hyperglycaemia. However, normalizing blood glucose invariably lowers plasma glucagon concentrations into the normal range. Rare cases of primary glucagon producing tumours of the pancreatic α-cells have been described, and are dealt with in the next chapter.

The consequence of insulin deficiency is shown in Fig. 11.9, which illustrates the basis of the major symptoms of diabetes. Attention is drawn to the additional insulin-independent metabolic pathways which are activated as a result of untreated or inadequately controlled hyperglycaemia. These important pathways are partly responsible for the long-term vascular and neurological complications of diabetes, which in turn form the major morbidity and mortality determinants of this disease.

In type II diabetes, a similar biochemical and physiological sequence of events occurs to that outlined above. However, in contrast to type I diabetes, circulating insulin is always present and often increased: lipolysis and ketogenesis remain inhibited, explaining the low prevalence of ketonaemia and ketonuria in this type of diabetes. Nevertheless, acute superimposed illness, possibly acting via increased circulating catecholamines can further reduce insulin secretion and induce acute metabolic decompensation identical to an acute type I diabetic. Histology of the pancreas may show essentially normal islets, occasionally enlarged and more numerous. An eosinophilic-staining amyloid-like substance has been often noted. Recent work shows that a peptide named amylin, which can be extracted from this material has opposing effects to insulin in terms of blood glucose regulation. Accordingly, there are some data to support a pathogenetic role for amylin.

There is little doubt that insulin resistance in a variety of tissues plays a major role in the genesis of type II diabetes. The term 'Syndrome-X' or 'Reaven's syndrome' is applied to the insulin resistance, hyperlipidaemia, and hypertension which frequently coexist with non-insulin-dependent diabetes, and are collectively responsible for the high prevalence of atherosclerotic macrovascular disease and its consequences. The nature of this association is currently unclear.

Symptom profile

Non-diabetic subjects rarely exceed a blood glucose of 8 mmol/l (145 mg/100 ml), which is also the approximate renal threshold for glucose. If blood glucose continuously exceeds the renal threshold for glucose by more than 5 mmol/l (90 mg/100 ml), polyuria and polydipsia will logically ensue in both types of diabetes. However, particularly in type II diabetes, blood glucose may initially oscillate between 8 and 14 mmol/l (or intermittently even higher) for months or even years and therefore without significant symptoms. During this 'subclinical' phase, the biochemical consequences of combined hyperglycaemia and relative insulin

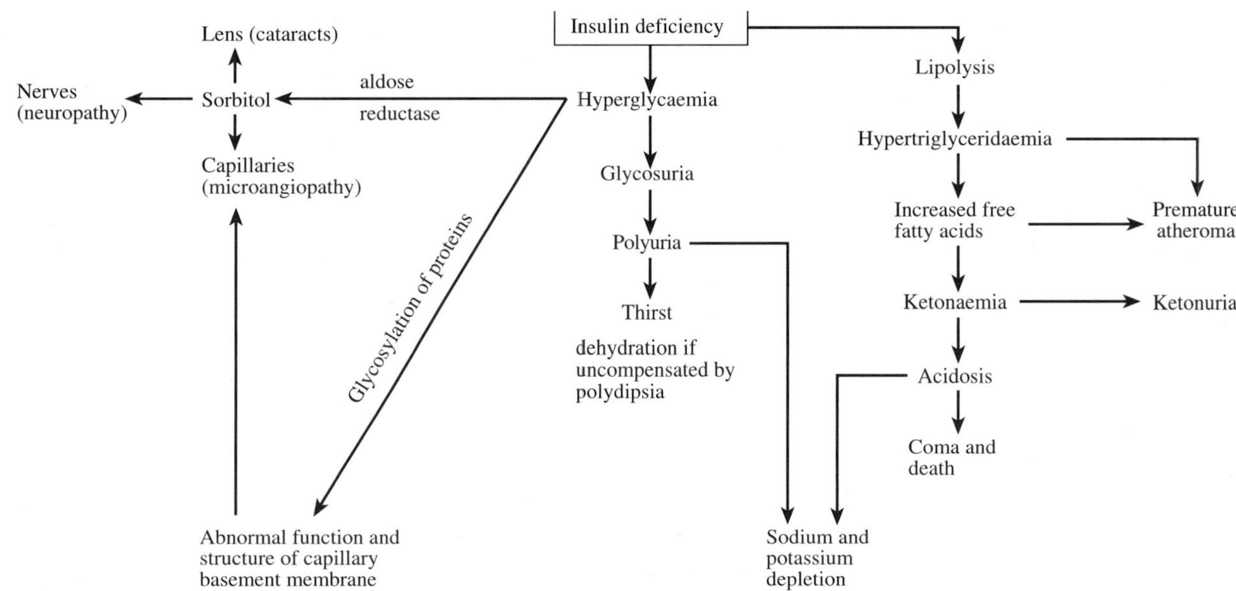

Fig. 11.9. Consequences of insulin deficiency in the diabetic syndrome.

deficiency result in irreversible structural changes. Microvascular, macrovascular, and neurological lesions may then actually be the presenting features of diabetes.

Significant dehydration is common only in type I diabetes. At the cellular level, this results in further insulin resistance leading ultimately to the ketonaemia (which may cause nausea and vomiting) and abnormal acid–base balance characteristic of diabetic ketoacidosis. Before this event however, patients may complain of visual blurring (due to osmotic lens changes), muscle cramps (due to electrolyte imbalance), and general tiredness and weakness (due to loss of muscle glycogen).

Proneness to skin, urine, and chest infections (particularly tuberculosis in countries where this is endemic) is due to the inhibition of normal leucocyte function which may be a consequence of activated leucocyte aldose reductase pathways.

Diagnosis of diabetes

In practice, a random or postprandial blood glucose above 12 mmol/l (215 mg/100 ml) is diagnostic of diabetes, and is sufficient to justify initiation of treatment. Fasting blood glucose is a less reliable criterion, although values above 7 mmol/l (125 mg/100 ml) are probably abnormal.

The diagnostic classification of diabetes has been standardized by the World Health Organization (WHO), based on a 75 g oral dextrose load (oral glucose tolerance test) given after an overnight fast. The critical measurement is the 2-hour postload serum glucose level:

Less than 7 mmol/l	(125 mg/100 ml):	non diabetic	see also p. 384
7.1–11.1 mmol/l	(200 mg/100 ml):	impaired glucose tolerance (IGT)	
Above 11.1 mmol/l	(200 mg/100 ml):	diabetic	

The entity of impaired glucose tolerance (IGT) is important. Approximately 50 per cent of such individuals become overtly diabetic in later life; macrovascular complications (see later) are as common as in overt diabetics, and as mentioned earlier, IGT is present in about 40 per cent of first degree relatives of type II diabetics.

With the development of assays for a variety of glycosylated proteins, it was hoped that these might prove as useful for diagnosis as for monitoring glycaemic control. To date, neither glycosylated haemoglobin (Hb A_{1c}) nor fructosamine have been shown to be reliable for this purpose.

Treatment of diabetes mellitus

Education of the patient is all-important. This has justified the establishment of hospital and community-based diabetes centres incorporating educational facilities which allow diabetics to learn from specialist nurses, doctors and dietitians, and even from each other. Bearing in mind that diabetes is a life-long disorder, there are also emotional consequences of following the necessary disciplines, and ongoing support at this level is also important.

Glycaemic control requires self-monitoring by the patient. Urinary glucose can be measured by strips incorporating a glucose-oxidase-dependent colour reaction (e.g. Diastix). However, glycosuria is obviously dependent on factors other than plasma glucose; specifically, glomerular filtration rate and tubular glucose reabsorption. Although this renal 'threshold' has a mean value of around 8 mmol/l

(145 mg/100 ml), it is highly variable (from 5 to 15 mmol/l) between individuals, and to a lesser extent within a single individual. Accordingly, the more relevant blood glucose monitoring is used, particularly in IDDM. This involves comparatively inexpensive and portable colorimeters or biosensors requiring a drop of capillary blood obtained by the patient. There is evidence that such monitoring (although more expensive) provides superior long-term control, providing that patients record the values and act on them.

Ketone-sensitive strips are used for monitoring the urine when heavy glycosuria develops. This represents the best method of identifying the earliest phase of ketoacidosis so that appropriate treatment can be undertaken.

Circulating levels of red cell glycosylated haemoglobin (Hb A_1c) or fructosamine, circulating by-products of non-enzymic glycosylation of proteins (one of the insulin-independent metabolic pathways) are regularly used as tests which reflect quality of control. Glycosylated haemoglobin accumulates irreversibly over the lifespan of the red cell, and therefore reflects a retrospective 8–10 week period, while fructosamine has a shorter circulating half-life, and reflects an approximate 2-week control period. The higher the levels, the worse the control.

Diet is all-important in both types of diabetes. Education on diet principles by a trained dietitian, both to the patient and his immediate family is mandatory at the time of diagnosis, and at repeated intervals thereafter. The important principles can be summarized as follows:

1. Achievement and maintenance of body weight within the 'ideal' range by calorie control.
2. Reduction of total dietary fat to supply no more than 30 per cent of total calories (and tighter restriction if an abnormal lipid pattern is present).
3. Increase of dietary fibre to at least 15 g daily.
4. Reduction of 'neat' refined carbohydrate, although limited admixture with other macronutrients is acceptable.

Increasing attention is being paid to the serum lipid profile in diabetes. The role of hyperlipidaemia in the genesis of atherosclerosis is clear (see Chapter 14) and the relevance may be greater in diabetics. Prevalence of dyslipidaemia is higher in diabetics (especially type II) than in non-diabetics, involving a high prevalence of raised LDL-cholesterol, triglyceride and lipoprotein (a), and reduced HDL-cholesterol. Poor glycaemic control in both diabetic subtypes induces a further component of reversible combined hyperlipidaemia. Diet has been an important tool for modifying dyslipidaemia in diabetics, and it is likely that more meticulous control of serum lipids will prove to be necessary in order to limit the gross excess of macrovascular occlusive events which are so life-threatening to diabetics. Further research is likely to confirm the need for more widespread use of the lipid-lowering drugs referred to in Chapter 14.

Type I diabetes

Since insulin deficiency is usually absolute, only insulin itself can be used in therapy. The species employed was originally bovine. Porcine insulin has greater homology with human insulin with only one (compared to three) amino acid difference, and hence less antigenicity. More recently introduced insulins are synthesized by recombinant DNA technology and have a precise human amino acid sequence. Since they are not biological extracts, they are free of α- and β-chains and C-peptide which were unnecessary and immunologically undesirable constituents of the earlier animal insulin preparations. Although human insulins will probably displace porcine, there is no evidence to suggest that they provide superior diabetic control or carry additional advantages.

The action of insulin can be prolonged by complexing with zinc and various proteins in crystalline form, so that a variety of insulins with different time/dose response curves are available to individualize therapy. The objective of insulin therapy is to provide the lowest (most normal) blood glucose levels consistent with the avoidance of hypoglycaemia; as will be discussed below, this philosophy is based on experimental and human evidence linking such good control to a reduction in the frequency of microvascular and neurological complications. It has been shown that twice daily or more frequent dosage is needed to achieve this aim. Continuous infusion of insulin by a portable or remotely controlled and programmable implantable infusion pump is now possible, using either subcutaneous or intraperitoneal catheters. The quality of control achieved is usually good, but a significant hypoglycaemia risk has been reported by some groups. An appropriate helpline is mandatory to provide operating support for patients using this approach.

Meanwhile, pen-type injectors, either prefilled or reloadable with insulin refill ampoules have simplified insulin administration. Using these pens to give short-acting (soluble) insulin three times daily preprandially, with a longer acting (usually isophane) insulin at bedtime, produces a flexible regime. This system is capable of allowing the patient to adapt to the moment-to-moment reduced insulin needs of exercise and increased demands of extra food, while still maintaining satisfactory glycaemic control. In most studies, the quality of control achievable by this multiple injection therapy approaches and sometime equals the level of control seen with infusion pumps.

Future approaches to type I diabetes

Immunosuppression can be carried out both on newly diagnosed diabetics (where the immunodestructive process is usually still incomplete), as well as 'prediabetic' individuals with high-probability antibody markers (derived from family studies or population screening). In the former group, the insulin-requiring state can be deferred by several years. In the latter group, development of diabetes can be delayed. For either of these concepts to be successful, immunosuppression regimens will need to improve beyond the current non-specific approaches with their attendant dangers of compromising responses to infection: the development of anti-idiotype antibodies may allow specific components of the immune system to be targeted.

The peptide amylin, originally purified from amyloid-type material found in the pancreas of patients with type II diabetes is cosecreted with insulin in response to glucose (and arginine). However, its hypoglycaemia-opposing effect suggested that it may have a buffering effect on blood glucose, and might be used therapeutically as an adjunct to insulin to reduce hypoglycaemia risk. This substance is still under review.

Segmental pancreas transplants (with immunosuppression) are being increasingly performed with simultaneous renal transplantation, when this is required for end-stage nephropathy. Allogeneic and even xenogeneic islet cell transplants may also prove to be more consistently successful, when appropriate methods of islet isolation and recipient immunosuppression have been further improved. Gene therapy also offers a theoretical solution, once the appropriate genes have been identified. As indicated above, totally implantable insulin pumps, remotely controlled by telemetry, are under investigation in a number of centres. The algorithms for insulin pump secretion in response to ambient glucose dynamics have been well-researched. If a reliably stable, implantable glucose sensor also becomes available, the concept of an implantable artificial pancreas will at last be realized.

Type II diabetes

Since these patients have some circulating insulin, the primary objective is to reduce substrate load and peripheral insulin 'resistance' by dieting and weight reduction, respectively. This can usually be achieved by a combination of caloric restriction (often as low as 1000 calories daily) and an increased activity pattern, the latter also increasing glucose utilization. Approximately 50 per cent of all type II diabetics can be controlled in this way, even with presenting hyperglycaemia exceeding 20 mmol/l (360 mg/100 ml). If diet alone is unsuccessful after a several week trial period, or if dictated by severity of presenting osmotic symptoms, oral drugs are introduced:

1. Sulphonylurea drugs (e.g. tolbutamide 0.5–3.0 g, glibenclamide 2.5–15 mg, gliclazide 40–320 mg daily). These all have the effect of enhancing β-cell responsiveness to glucose, also inhibiting insulin uptake into the liver and partly enhancing muscle glucose uptake directly.
2. Biguanides (e.g. metformin 0.5–2.0 g daily) act by stimulating muscle glucose uptake and by inhibiting both gluconeogenesis and glucose absorption from the gut.
3. α-glucosidase inhibitors (e.g. acarbose 150–600 mg daily or miglitol) inhibit starch digestion and therefore retard monosaccharide absorption.

Most patients unresponsive to diet can be controlled on a sulphonylurea regime. Apart from a tendency to hypoglycaemia with the more potent agents, these drugs are remarkably safe with only rare occurrences of skin rash, nausea, and liver dysfunction. Acarbose and related compounds often cause unpleasant flatulence. In contrast, unless introduced in gradually increasing dosage, biguanides may induce quite unpleasant upper and lower gastrointestinal symptoms, which may be transient or persistent. In the presence of renal dysfunction or with any potential for excess lactate production (ischaemic heart disease, cardiac failure, hypoxia) metformin may rarely induce potentially fatal lactic acidosis, and this drug must be avoided in these high-risk situations. In practice, there is little difference in clinical effectiveness between any of the different sulphonylureas, non-responsiveness being more closely related to dietary non-compliance. Failure to completely respond to either biguanide or sulphonyurea can be dealt with by combining all three groups of drugs if necessary, or supplementing either group with once-daily insulin.

With the increasing emphasis on achieving near normal blood glucose levels, insulin alone is being increasingly used in type II diabetics with oral drug failure. Especially using the prefilled pens referred to earlier, even the most elderly patient can adapt to the regime, perhaps with the support of close family or community nurse. The transition to insulin is often made reluctantly, but the resulting improved well-being is often striking.

Future approaches to type II diabetes

The major focus of research is the possibility of identifying patients at risk. Multiple genes are likely to be responsible for clinical expression of the disease. As these become identified, subsequent individually directed preventive strategies (i.e. weight reduction, exercise, drugs) may prove feasible, in 'genetically positive' individuals. Similarly, 'gene therapy' is a theoretically feasible approach. Even the earlier identification of the disorder would be an advantage, bearing in mind that at present, 20 per cent of type II diabetics already have complications at the time of diagnosis. Even within the present state of knowledge, awareness that 40 per cent of first degree relatives either have diabetes or impaired glucose tolerance should facilitate earlier case finding.

The knowledge that insulin resistance plays an important part in the genesis of type II diabetes (and its complications to be described later) has prompted the development of drugs which are specifically capable of reversing this phenomenon. One such group, the thiazolidine-diones are promising at least in the experimental setting: the drug, troglitazone, has been shown to simultaneously reduce insulin levels and improve glucose tolerance both in non-insulin-dependent diabetes and simple obesity. Particularly in Reaven's syndrome X, where insulin resistance appears to be present to a greater degree than in other type II diabetics, such drugs may prove to have substantial benefits on morbidity and mortality.

Finally, a glucagon-like peptide (GLP-1) is released into the circulation from the small bowel in response to meals. This substance, also called incretin, is the most potent secretagogue for insulin and may theoretically supplant sulphonylurea-type drugs in the future.

The complications of diabetes

These can be divided into acute problems, and those which most commonly develop over a period of years following diagnosis.

Acute metabolic complications

Hypoglycaemia Blood glucose levels of less than 2 mmol/l are usually associated with symptoms of sweating and tremor (due to the acute autonomic response to hypoglycaemia). These normally precede the hunger, confusion (and ultimately coma) which are due to cerebral glycopenia. In insulin-treated patients, hypoglycaemia may arise because of an accidentally excessive dose, a missed meal, acute exercise or the use of beta-adrenergic blocking drugs. By blocking glycogenolysis, alcohol excess, especially associated with a temporary low food intake may also induce hypoglycaemia; as indicated earlier, this phenomenon may also be seen in non-diabetics.

A loss of the early warning (autonomic) symptoms of hypoglycaemia is seen after many years of diabetes, probably due to autonomic neuropathy. Although it was originally suggested that the use of human insulins was also associated with reduced warning symptoms, there is little objective support for this view. However, it has been shown that the maintenance of lower blood glucose (resulting from a natural enthusiasm for avoiding complications) itself reduces warning symptoms, and this can be reversed by allowing blood glucose to run a little higher. Over-enthusiastic blood glucose control or a casual approach to diabetes can also lead to repeated (and if occurring at night, unrecognized) hypoglycaemia, with the consequence of brain damage. This may take the form of a cerebrovascular attack (stroke) brought about by further jeopardizing brain tissue which has already been subjected to chronic ischaemia. It may also cause dementia.

Good patient education minimizes the risks of hypoglycaemia, since a diabetic patient must be prepared to have a dextrose sweet or cube at all times to cope with unexpected eventualities. In most instances, patients may learn to decrease their insulin dose when a high exercise level is anticipated. Hypoglycaemia may also occur in patients on oral drugs. Thus, the elderly may often casually omit a meal; this may result in severe and intractable hypoglycaemia, because of the age-related loss of homeostatic release of catecholamines and somatotrophin. Such patients sometimes present as cerebrovascular accidents, incorrectly diagnosed as a primary thrombotic or haemorrhagic episode. Once again the situation is preventable by effective education and the use of short-acting drugs, such as tolbutamide, although no sulphonylurea is totally immune from such risk.

Significant hypoglycaemia should be preventable by improving the understanding of patients, appropriate anticipation of those circumstances known to acutely lower blood glucose, and the immediate taking of dextrose at the earliest warning symptom. An established hypoglycaemic episode can be treated by force-feeding of a sweet drink, intravenous dextrose (20 ml of 50 per cent concentration): occasionally even a dextrose infusion is necessary. Patients who live remote from medical care can be given glucagon (1 mg in 1 ml) subcutaneously by a family member or a friend in the event of severe hypoglycaemia. Carrying of diabetes identification is an important method of ensuring early diagnosis in the setting of unexplained coma.

Diabetic ketoacidosis Ketoacidosis represents the end point of insulin deficiency, as indicated in Fig. 11.9. A number of factors may be responsible:

1. Accidental omission or reduction of insulin dosage.
2. Infection, stress, or other intercurrent illness (which promote the release of the hyperglycaemic stress hormones cortisol, glucagon, catecholamines, and somatotrophin).

3. Use of hyperglycaemic drugs: corticosteroids, thiazide-type diuretics, diazoxide, and phenytoin.
4. A lack of patient recognition of polyuria and polydipsia as signs of poor control.
5. A failure to increase insulin dose in response to (2) or (4).
6. Overlooking the importance of urine ketone measurement when heavy glycosuria develops.
7. Incorrect diagnosis of the cause of vomiting (often an early sign of ketoacidosis).
8. Delayed referral of unstable diabetes patients into hospital for initiation of therapy.

It is often possible to identify multiple factors being responsible for the occurrence of ketoacidosis in a single case. It is also clear that ketoacidosis is essentially a preventable disorder. The clinical features consist of dehydration, lethargy, and vomiting, followed by drowsiness, coma, and occasionally death. In the earlier stages, hyperventilation of the Kussmaul type (deep sighing respirations) is quite common and has been mistaken for the (psychologically based) hyperventilation syndrome, with disastrous consequences.

Investigations show hyperglycaemia, a low serum bicarbonate, and an arterial blood pH usually below 7.3 (unless compensated by the alkalotic effects of hyperventilation). The diagnosis can be easily and more precisely confirmed by testing the patient's plasma with ketostix strips, and if a positive reaction is obtained, confirming that the reaction persists with a plasma dilution of 1 in 4. Neutrophil leucocytosis is common even in the absence of infection. Further tests are sometimes required to determine the underlying cause. These depend to some extent on the history, if available, together with other clinical features. However, most hospitals follow a specified protocol which aims to automatically screen for the likely triggering conditions.

Management of ketoacidosis Therapy consists of correcting the major abnormalities of acidosis, dehydration, and hyperglycaemia. Intravenous bicarbonate (400–800 ml of 1.35 or 2.7 per cent sodium bicarbonate, repeated if necessary) is generally used only in comatose patients, or when the blood pH is less than 6.8: the administration of insulin is usually associated with sufficiently prompt suppression of ketogenesis as to make bicarbonate therapy unnecessary in less severe cases. Furthermore, administration of bicarbonate can produce a disequilibrium between blood and cerebrospinal fluid pH, in turn causing persisting disturbed consciousness. Insulin is given as an intravenous infusion at 4–6 units per hour, using an infusion pump and with one or two hourly monitoring of blood glucose concentrations.

Fluids are given initially to reverse hypovolaemia. In addition, cellular dehydration is known to induce insulin resistance, and rehydration alone is often associated with a 'spontaneous' fall in blood glucose. Treatment customarily involves normal saline 4–6 litres over the first 24 hours, since the prolonged diuresis preceding ketoacidosis is associated with substantial whole-body sodium and potassium depletion (although serum potassium may be misleadingly normal due to acidosis-induced extracellular movement of potassium).

Colloid in the form of Haemaccel or similar is sometimes required when hypovolaemia is severe enough to reduce renal perfusion. Hydration level must be closely monitored, especially in the elderly so as to avoid circulatory overload. Serum potassium levels are also monitored at 1- to 4-hourly intervals since administration of insulin and the correction of the acidosis are associated with a major intracellular potassium shift; indeed the routine replacement of 20–30 millimoles of potassium per litre of infused fluid is usual, even in anticipation of a subsequent lowering of serum potassium.

With careful therapy, the mortality of ketoacidosis should now be restricted to that of the underlying cause. Regrettably, the occasional management by medical teams with inadequate experience of this condition may result in needless morbidity and mortality.

It is important to stress again that it is possible to prevent almost every case of ketoacidosis by appropriate steps. Education of the patient (and the medical profession) is the key factor.

Hyperosmolar non-ketotic coma In some elderly patients, ketogenesis appears to be suppressed, probably by a residual circulating insulin. Accordingly, the clinical features are dominated by progressive dehydration, coma, and ultimately death.Predictably, investigation shows hyperglycaemia, which is usually of greater degree than in ketoacidosis, a normal serum bicarbonate and blood pH, gross hypernatraemia (due to disproportionate loss of water compared to sodium), and estimated or measured serum osmolality as high as 400 millimoles per kilogram. Occasionally, this metabolic state represents the presenting feature of diabetes, precipitated by the use of thiazide-type diuretics which are, as indicated earlier, hyperglycaemic.

Treatment consists of rehydration, initially with normal saline, transferring to half normal saline as osmolality falls from the simultaneous correction of the hyperglycaemia. Excessively rapid rehydration can be dangerous, inducing circulatory overload or cerebral oedema. In the absence of ketoacidosis, these patients are often exquisitely insulin-sensitive. Accordingly, insulin is usually infused at the rate of no more that 2 units per hour and intravenous dextrose-saline solution is substituted as a rehydration fluid when glucose levels approach normal.

Despite apparently effective therapy, the mortality remains approximately 30 per cent, due to the development of myocardial infarction and stroke as consequences of the severe and often prolonged hypovolaemia and haemoconcentration.

Lactic acidosis This is an unusual consequence, mostly of the use of the biguanide drug, metformin, which enhances anaerobic glycolysis and inhibits lactate recycling in the liver. Both these pharmacological actions are normally of little adverse consequence. However, when renal or hepatic disease are present (inhibiting lactate handling) particularly with an additional cause of hypoxia which induces excess lactate production (such as myocardial or mesenteric infarction, severe infection or septicaemia), a major risk of lactic acidosis exists.

Patients show the features of acidosis without significant hyperglycaemia or dehydration. Investigations reveal the expected low serum bicarbonate concentrations and low blood pH, but the semiquantitative ketone test is usually negative, and if measured, serum lactate levels are extremely high. Additional tests usually show evidence of significant renal or hepatic impairment. Treatment consists primarily of avoidance of metformin in the elderly (who are clearly more prone to ischaemic episodes), and in those patients with renal, cardiac, or hepatic disease. The related drug, phenformin, produced a disproportionately large number of reported cases of fatal lactic acidosis, and is no longer used.

Once established, correction of acidosis is the basic therapy, together with attempted correction of any underlying disorder. Dialysis of the excess lactic acid, or conversion of lactic to pyruvic acid both by methylene blue and other methods have been tried, all with comparatively little benefit. The mortality remains approximately 80 per cent.

Diabetes and infection It is common for the stress of infection either to precipitate clinical diabetes, or to unstabilize previously well-controlled diabetes. Accordingly, a site of infection should always be sought in unstable or newly presenting diabetics. Although less common today, pulmonary tuberculosis is still occasionally diagnosed in this way, and is a frequent concomitant of newly diagnosed diabetes in Asian countries.

The reciprocal relationship is of even greater importance: hyperglycaemia predisposes both to the development and the progression of bacterial, mycotic, and monilial (but not viral) infections. This phenomenon is closely related to the quality of control; indeed a chronic vulvitis due to *Candida albicans* infection is often a presenting feature of diabetes in women. Leucocyte migration, phagocytic and bactericidal activity are only some of the infection defence factors which are impaired in hyperglycaemic patients. It has been shown that the aldose reductase pathway is active in leucocytes, and enhanced activity of the pathway induced by hyperglycaemia may be one of the causative mechanisms. These observations underline the serious nature of infections when they occur in diabetics, and the importance of maintaining normoglycaemia when infection is present.

Long-term complications

Diabetic microvascular disease A major element of diabetic morbidity depends on the development of diabetic microangiopathy. Structurally, this is represented by thickening of the basement membrane of capillaries, affecting both their permeability and structural integrity. By light and electron microscopy, changes can be identified in almost all body tissues, but most relevantly in the poorly supported capillaries in the retina and in the kidney.

The nature of the substance responsible for this basement membrane abnormality is still unclear. Most studies support an increased synthesis and decreased catabolism of normally present glycoproteins, rather than a distinctly abnormal compound. Evidence has accrued for a role of both the sorbitol pathway and non-enzymic glycosylation in the genesis of this basement membrane abnormality.

Work in animals rendered diabetic demonstrates a major dependence of renal basement membrane thickening on glycaemic control. In such models, islet transplantation is capable of halting or even reversing thickening. Some studies actually show reversibility of microangiopathy when glycaemic control is improved or the kidney is transplanted from a diabetic to a non-diabetic animal.

Some diabetic patients show comparatively little evidence of microangiopathy despite two or three decades of poor control, suggesting that other factors, possibly genetic, play a part in the expression of microvascular disease: families of unique proneness or resistance have been described, and both high- and low-risk class I and II histocompatibility antigens have been associated with these patterns.

Recent Swedish and North American (DCCT, see Heidden 1994) studies have documented a 60–75 per cent reduction in the incidence of microvascular complications in groups of patients intentionally treated aggressively with multiple dosage insulin regimes, to achieve lower levels of Hb A_1. Such findings endorse the view that achievement of near-normoglycaemia is of the highest importance, although this requires a major commitment both from the patient as well as health professionals. Similar conclusions are likely to be drawn from prospective studies in type II diabetics, when these are finally completed.

Around 20 per cent of type II diabetics have microangiopathic changes already present at the time of diagnosis. In these cases diabetes has clearly been of longer duration, evading earlier diagnosis because modest blood glucose elevations were still asymptomatic.

Diabetic retinopathy (see Plate 11.1 to 11.6)

Approximately 10 per cent of all diabetics will have symptoms from, or require treatment for diabetic retinopathy. However, over 80 per cent of all insulin requiring diabetics can be shown to have some degree of retinopathy during their lifespan. Fluorescein angiography, which demonstrates areas of abnormal leakage and vascular disorganization often provides a dramatic picture of the extent of circulatory disruption. The retinal microcirculation therefore provides a very valuable site for assessing both structural and functional microangiopathy. (See Fig. 11.10.) Retinopathy is customarily graded into two types: background and proliferative retinopathy.

Background retinopathy This is represented by dot and blot haemorrhages, and areas of exudate (some of which are, in fact, areas of retinal ischaemia). Unless these lesions encroach on the macula, visual defect is unusual. Approximately 20 per cent of these cases will progress to proliferative retinopathy.

Proliferative retinopathy This describes the essential component of neovascular proliferation, which represents a response to retinal ischaemia. Some ophthalmologists describe a preproliferative phase, highlighted by intraretinal microvascular abnormalities (IRMA). The new vessels are fragile, poorly supported, and bleed readily into the vitreous, producing sudden visual loss. Organization of the thrombus is followed by fibrosis, which may in turn cause traction detachment of the retina and blindness. About 50 per cent of cases with this

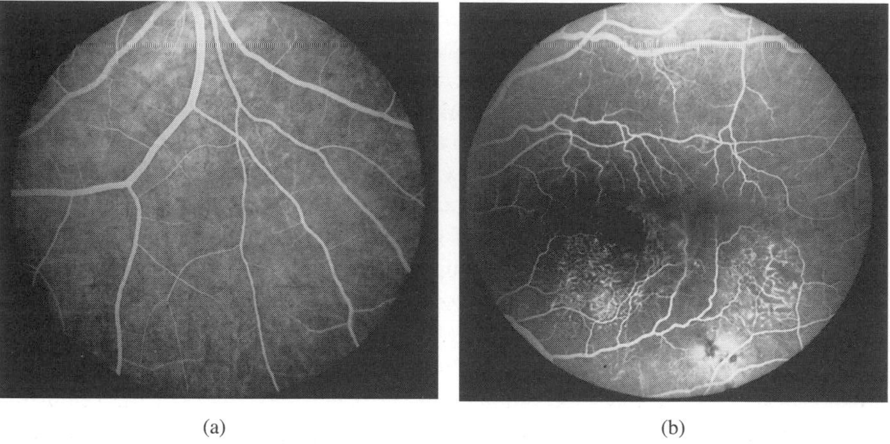

(a) (b)

Fig. 11.10. Fluorescein retinal angiogram in an (a) non-diabetic and (b) diabetic of 15 years duration. In lower sectors, note near vessel formation: also focal areas of minor and major fluorescein dye diffusion due to increased capillary permeability.

type of retinopathy, if untreated will progress to blindness within a period of five years.

Additional forms of retinopathy are sometimes seen. Maculopathy is the name given to the macular aggregation of both haemorrhage and exudate: because of its location, there is often impairment of central vision. Macular oedema also occurs in association with active retinopathy and occasionally as an apparent consequence of acute or prolonged hyperglycaemia.

Treatment of retinopathy consists of multiple-area photocoagulation usually with a laser source applied to the peripheral retina and to areas of major vessel proliferation and leakage. Carefully controlled studies demonstrate the benefits of this treatment in both forms of retinal disease. Vitrectomy is sometimes performed for the visual defect resulting from substantial vitreous haemorrhage.

Other non-microangiopathic eye problems

Cataract is more common and appears to progress more rapidly than in non-diabetics. This is almost certainly due to the aldose–reductase pathway: cataract can be delayed experimentally by the use of aldose reductase inhibitors, which reduce formation of sorbitol which is toxic to lens protein. Optic neuritis and a neovascular lesion of the iris (rubeosis iridis) may also occasionally be seen.

Diabetic nephropathy

Electron microscopic abnormality of the basement membrane of the renal glomerulus can be seen within 12 months of diagnosis of diabetes. Nevertheless, clinically apparent renal disease rarely occurs before diabetes has been present for 10 years.

Microalbuminuria (20–200 mg excretion/24 hours) is often the first sign of developing renal disease (representing initially functional and later structural disruption of the glomerular sieve), progressing to classical nephrotic syndrome as manifest by 'dipstick-positive' proteinuria, hypoalbuminaemia, and oedema.

Microalbuminuria is present in approximately 10 per cent of all patients with diabetes, and has been used as a warning sign of the predisposition to microvascular complications (which may also have a genetic component). Accordingly, a more aggressive approach to both glycaemic and blood pressure control in this subgroup is often adopted. In fact macrovascular events, mainly myocardial infarction are also 20–40 times more likely to occur in patients with microalbuminuria: the reason for this latter relationship remains unclear.

Ultimately, glomerular 'fall out' occurs with progressive renal glomerular failure, with rising serum urea and creatinine levels, and giving rise to symptoms of lethargy, weakness, polyuria, and if untreated, fatal uraemia. At the stage of proteinuria, renal biopsy commonly shows quite gross changes including the classical Kimmelstiel–Wilson lesion (nodular intercapillary glomerulosclerosis).

The advent of chronic ambulatory peritoneal dialysis (CAPD), haemodialysis programmes and renal transplantation have materially altered the outlook for this group of patients, since renal failure was at one time the major cause of death in type I diabetics. With longer survival times however, nephropathy is itself complicated by a strikingly accelerated form of atherosclerosis, affecting coronary, cerebral, and peripheral vascular territories. Hypercholesterolaemia and hypertriglyceridaemia are often present: treatment may delay the progression of the vascular lesions.

Rigorous control both of blood glucose and the frequently associated hypertension, as well as protein restriction, have all been shown to delay progression of the renal lesion. There is also evidence to suggest that the angiotensin-converting enzyme (ACE) inhibitors have significant advantages over other hypotensive agents when hypertension is present, and also carry benefit in normotensive patients, particularly with microalbuminuria.

Other non-microangiopathic renal disorders

Proneness to infection increases the rate both of asymptomatic bacteriuria and overt pyelonephritis. Together with arteriosclerotic renovascular disease (see below) and analgesic abuse, there is an increased risk of renal papillary necrosis, inducing renal colic and urinary tract obstruction.

Diabetic large vessel disease

It is now well recognized that atherosclerosis is more common, occurs at an earlier age, and appears to progress more rapidly in diabetics than in non-diabetics. However, there is no evidence that this depends on glycaemic control. Indeed, the very dietary factors which themselves determine the clinical appearance of type II diabetes (high calorie and fat intake) may themselves by responsible for the high prevalence of arterial disease which so frequently accompanies this type of diabetes. Furthermore, the high prevalence of dyslipidaemia contributes in a major way to macroangiopathy, and and highlights a means by which the prevalence and severity of these complications may be diminished in due course.

The clinical manifestations of atherosclerosis are similar to the non-diabetic: cerebrovascular accidents, myocardial ischaemia and infarction, mesenteric

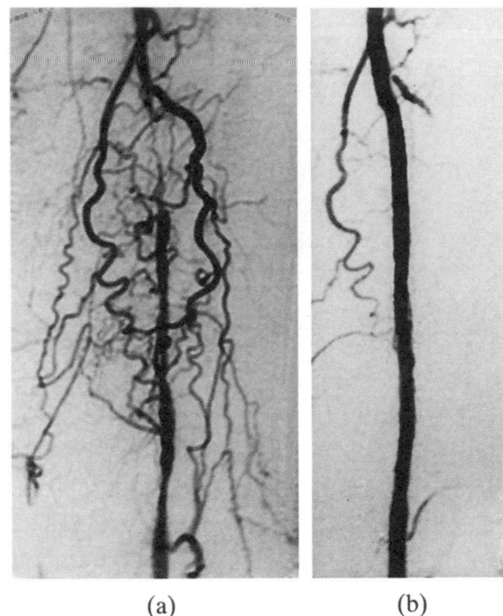

Fig. 11.11. Segmental femoral vascular occlusion (a) causing intermittent claudication (for anatomical description see (c)). Dilatation of occluded segment confirmed by repeat angiography (b) following transfemoral angioplasty. Claudication cured.

insufficiency, and, most characteristically, lower limb arteriopathy that particularly affects the more peripheral arteries which can become heavily calcified. Renal vessels can also become involved, causing hypertension and renal failure. As in the non-diabetic, cigarette smoking increases even further the likelihood of development of these complications. Progression of peripheral vascular disease leads ultimately to the classical symptoms of calf pain on exercise (intermittent claudication) and gangrene.

It has been shown that diabetics with microalbuminuria (see above) have a 20–40 times greater risk of having myocardial infarction than those without. The precise link between these phenomena is not presently known.

The diabetic foot (see Plates 11.9, 11.10)

The foot constitutes a major risk area for both types of diabetic. Peripheral sensory neuropathy (see below) predisposes the foot to unnoticed injury, arterial ischaemia induces tissue vulnerability, and microangiopathy and uncontrolled hyperglycaemia affect resistance to infection and subsequent tissue healing. Plantar ulceration (occasionally unnoticed until very far advanced) proceeds rapidly to deep tissue infection and osteomyelitis. Antibiotics and immobilization may fail to achieve healing in the more chronic lesions: amputation of toes or more extensive resection then become necessary.

Much of this problem is preventable through patient education on basic foot care and personal hygiene, and the routine employment of a chiropodist/podiatrist where visual difficulty is present, and where vascular/neurological deficit has been identified so as to render feet ‘at risk’.

Neuropathic complications

Every part of the peripheral nervous system is vulnerable to diabetic involvement. The common denominator is thought to be the insulin-independent aldose–reductase pathway which is operative in all neural tissue: neurotoxic sorbitol is accordingly formed. Studies with aldose-reductase inhibitors (which prevent neuropathy in experimental diabetes) show that this is likely to be a significant mechanism, although other factors, such as microangiopathy of the vasa nervorum, have been implicated in certain cases. Again, tight glycaemic control has been shown to reduce the prevalence and severity of these changes.

Motor neuropathy

Delay in motor nerve conduction velocity, often reversible by achieving glycaemic control, can be demonstrated in almost every newly diagnosed diabetic. Indeed a motor neuropathy affecting cranial (especially 3rd, 4th, 6th, or 7th nerves) or peripheral (often the peroneal and anterial tibial) nerves may be a presenting feature of the diabetes, or may occur at any later stage of life. The onset is frequently rapid. Together with the histological changes in the responsible nerves accompanying these clinical changes, microvascular occlusion rather than a metabolic process is likely to be the underlying pathology. The clinical lesions are frequently totally reversible, irrespective of therapy.

Sensory neuropathy

Minor reversible deficits in sensory nerve conduction velocity can also be identified particularly at the time of initial diagnosis. However, clinical sensory neuropathy is a comparatively late complication, and manifest by loss of sensation (anaesthesia) and/or abnormal sensation (paraesthesia). The neurological damage is likely to be mediated by metabolic factors consequent upon activation of non-insulin dependent pathways (aldose–reductase and non-enzymic glycosylation). In all studies, the incidence and severity of neuropathy can be linked to the degree and duration of poor glycaemic control. Sensory neuropathy is one of the major factors leading, as indicated earlier, to foot ulceration. At this level of involvement, reversibility is not seen.

Neurogenic arthropathy

Denervation of joints leads to a Charcot-type arthropathy, characteristically affecting the ankle and tarsal joints, with gross disruption of foot, swelling, and loss of stability and normal gait. Immobilization in a plaster cast sometimes produces partial correction.

Autonomic neuropathy

Many manifestations may be present, particularly in longstanding diabetics. The relationship to the severity or duration of hyperglycaemia is unclear. The more common features are listed below:

1. Postural hypotension (due to involvement of autonomic arteriolar control). Fludrocortisone and ephedrine have been successfully used in treatment.

2. Delayed gastric emptying (due to vagal inhibition). Metoclopramide and cisapride have both been used to enhance gastric emptying.

3. Diabetic diarrhoea (due to defective gut innervation); reduced or increased motility results in subsequent bacterial overgrowth and often steatorrhoea. Metronidazole and broad-spectrum antibiotics are often capable of controlling symptoms.

4 Pupillary abnormalities (due to involvement of the ciliary ganglion).

5. Neurogenic bladder (due to poor sensation and autonomic motor dysfunction): this also predisposes to infection. Bladder-neck surgery can be used to correct this problem.

6. Impotence (due to involvement of nervi erigentes). This can be dealt with by intracavernosal papaverine or prostaglandin injections, vacuum methods, or implantation of rigid or semi-rigid prostheses.

The diagnosis of autonomic neuropathy can be made by a series of ECG-monitored cardiovascular function studies: pulse rate fails to rise despite postural blood pressure drop, there is a loss of beat-to-beat variation in response to deep breathing, and a loss of the bradycardia-tachycardia response to the Valsalva manoeuvre.

Diabetes and pregnancy

Effect of diabetes on pregnancy

A history of large babies, and the consequent complications of cephalopelvic disproportion are some of the major problems encountered. This phenomenon is probably due entirely to maternal hyperglycaemia, which by transplacental glucose passage induces fetal hyperinsulinaemia. Since insulin is a significant growth factor, fetal overgrowth (macrosomia) is induced.

Apart from this effect, there is an increased prevalence of miscarriage, pre-eclamptic toxaemia, and intrauterine death with neonatal respiratory distress syndrome and hypoglycaemia (the latter being again due to maternal hyperglycaemia and subsequent hyperinsulinaemia in the fetus). Tight control of blood glucose during pregnancy has been shown to almost eliminate many of these problems. In the requisite 9-month period, appropriate motivation and patient compliance can be remarkably good. However, the high prevalence of congenital malformations (10 per cent) is unlikely to be reduced unless normoglycaemia can be achieved actually at the time of conception.

Effect of pregnancy on diabetes

Acting through enhanced secretion of corticosteroids, oestrogen, somatotrophin, and probably chorionic somatotrophin, pregnancy reflects a major diabetogenic event. Pre-existing diabetes requires higher doses of insulin, and cases previously controllable on oral hypoglycaemic agents are transferred to insulin.

As indicated previously, the term 'gestational diabetes' defines the spontaneously reversible subtype (although some cases remain permanently hyperglycaemic in the postnatal period). Follow-up studies suggest that even if postnatal normoglycaemia returns, diabetes may develop in later life in as many as 50 per cent of cases of gestational diabetes. Routine screening for diabetes in the second and third trimester is increasingly performed, both as an aid to early diagnosis as well as for the benefit of the pregnancy itself.

It should be noted that glycosuria is common even in normoglycaemic pregnancy, and was originally used as a test for pregnancy. This phenomenon is due to the increased glomerular filtration rate of pregnancy which in turn induces glucose filtration in excess of tubular reabsorptive capacity.

Other complications

A wide variety of less common conditions may complicate diabetes. Skin problems include the atrophic and occasionally ulcerative lesions of necrobiosis lipoidica diabeticorum, as well as fat hypertrophy (or rarely atrophy) at the site of injections: these latter problems can be prevented or reversed by more effective rotation of injection sites. A specific cardiopathy has been suggested as a cause of heart failure in the absence of apparent ischaemia. Unusual 'myopathies' (sometimes called amyotrophy) can occur due to anterior nerve root neuropathy: they mostly revert spontaneously.

Coping with diabetes

One of the biggest challenges to both patients with diabetes and their carers is the problem of emotional adjustment to diabetes as a life-long commitment. The threat to vision, limb, and life represented by the diabetic syndrome, the ever-present hazard of hypoglycaemia, the potential problems with pregnancy all add up to a threatening profile which psychologically unstabilizes a significant proportion of people with diabetes. The families of diabetics also participate in this uncertain future.

Dealing with such patients requires experience, understanding, and considerable patience: more extreme emotional decompensation often calls for the participation of a clinical psychologist. Not surprisingly, depression is also quite common, affecting about two to three times as many diabetics as the general population.

FURTHER READING

PHYSIOLOGY

Baron, A.D. (1994). Hemodynamic actions of insulin. *American Journal of Physiology*, **267**, E187–E202.

Bergman, R.N., Steil, G.M., Bradley, D.C. and Watanabe, R.M. (1992). Modelling of insulin action in vivo. *Annual Review of Physiology*, **54**, 861–84.

Kimball, S.R., Vary, T.C. and Jefferson, L.S. (1994). Regulation of protien synthesis by insulin. *Annual Review of Physiology*, **56**, 321–48.

Schwartz, M.W., Figlewicz, D.P., Baskin, D.G., Woods, S.C. and Porte, D. Jr. (1992). Insulin in the brain: a hormonal regulator of energy balance. *Endocrine Reviews*, **13**, 387–414.

CLINICAL

Abecassis, M. and Corry, R.J. (1993). An update on pancreas transplantation. *Advances in Surgery*, 163–88.

Atkinson, M.A. and Maclaren, N.K. (1994). The pathogenesis of insulin-dependent diabetes mellitus. *New England Journal of Medicine*, **331**, 1428–36.

Dineen, S., Gerich, J., and Rizza, R. (1992). Carbohydrate metabolism in non-insulin dependent diabetes mellitus. *New England Journal of Medicine*, **327**, 707–13.

Drury, P.L. and Watkins, P.J. (1993). Diabetic renal disease and its prevention. *Clinical Endocrinology*, **38**, 455–50.

Field, J.B. (1989). Hypoglycaemia. *Endocrinology Metabolism Clinics North America*, **18**, 27–43.

Hadden, D.R. (1994). The diabetes control and complication trial (DCCT): what every endocrinologist needs to know. *Clinical Endocrinology*, **40**, 293–4.

Hammond, P.J., Jackson, J.A., and Bloom, S.R. (1994). Localization of pancreatic endocrine tumours. *Clinical Endocrinology*, **40**, 3–14.

Kohner, E.M. (1993). Diabetic retinopathy. *British Medical Journal*, **307**, 1195–9.

Laws, A, and Reaven, G.M. (1993). Insulin resistance and risk factors for coronary artery disease. *Clinical Endocrinology and Metabolism*, **7**, 1063–78.

Lebowitz, H.E. (1995). Diabetic ketoacidosis. *Lancet*, **345**, 767–72.

Nathan, D.M. (1993). Long-term complications of diabetes mellitus. *New England Journal of Medicine*, **328**, 1076–85.

Ratner, R.E. (1993). Gestational diabetes mellitus. *Journal of Clinical Endocrinology Metabolism*, **77**, 1–5.

Robertson, R.P. (1992). Pancreatic and islet transplantation for diabetes — cure or curiosities? *New England Journal of Medicine*, **327**, 762–6.

Selzer, H.S. (1989). Drug-induced hypoglycaemia: a review of 1418 cases. *Endocrinology Metabolism Clinics North America*, **18**, 163–84.

Service, F.J., McMahon, M.M., O'Brien, P.C., *et al.* (1991). Functioning insulinoma: incidence, recurrence and long term survival. A 60-year study. *Mayo Clinic Proceedings*, **66**, 711–19.

Yki-Jarvinen, H. (1995). The rôle of insulin resistance in the pathogenesis of NIDDM. *Diabetologia*, **38**, 1378–88.

12

The pancreas (2): other pancreatic peptides and their syndromes

PHYSIOLOGY

In addition to insulin and glucagon, the pancreas is the source of other hormones, as mentioned in the previous chapter. Prominent among these are somatostatin and pancreatic polypeptide, although other molecules, such as gastrin (only found in pancreatic tumours) and vasopressin, have been identified.

SOMATOSTATIN

Somatostatin is synthesized by the δ-cells of the islets and it clearly influences both glucagon and insulin from the α- and β-cells, respectively.

Somatostatin is a tetradecapeptide which is found in the central nervous system (e.g. the hypothalamic somatostatin is somatotrophin-inhibiting hormone, see Chapter 4) as well as in the pancreas, stomach, small and large intestines, and even in salivary glands and the thyroid. Somatostatin appears to be a general inhibitory substance and, in the pancreas, it inhibits the release of both insulin and glucagon.

Since somatostatin release may be stimulated by high blood glucose concentration, various amino acids (e.g. arginine and leucine), and the gastrointestinal hormones, secretin and PZ-CCK, the hormone has been implicated in the regulation of nutrient concentrations in the blood. Indeed, somatostatin has been postulated to retard the entry of nutrients into the portal blood by inhibiting various digestive events such as gastric emptying, acid, pepsin and gastrin secretions, monosaccharide and fat absorption, and duodenal motility. By delaying the absorption of nutrients, it is possible that a sudden rise in the blood metabolite concentration is postponed until the insulin–glucagon system has been appropriately mobilized.

PANCREATIC POLYPEPTIDE

Pancreatic polypeptide (PP) is a polypeptide of 36 amino acids located in specific F-cells of the pancreatic islets. An important stimulus for its release appears to be protein in the diet, and more specifically protein digestion in the small intestine. Acute hypoglycaemia also seems to stimulate its release, which appears to be dependent on the cholinergic innervation of the islets by vagal fibres (electrical stimulation of which increases pancreatic polypeptide production). The physiological role of PP is still unclear; indeed, its major effect appears to be an inhibition of gall bladder contraction and an inhibition of pancreatic enzyme secretion.

Gastrin

The production of pancreatic gastrin from a subgroup of the islet cells in the regulation of blood glucose has not yet been shown, and it may well be a product of abnormal cells in a pancreatic tumour.

Amylin

Amylin, a protein synthesized by the β-cells, has metabolic effects which are generally opposed to those of insulin. For example, it stimulates muscle and liver glycogenolysis and in this and other respects (such as a similarity in structure) it resembles the neuropeptide calcitonin gene-related peptide (CGRP). The physiological role of amylin is unclear, particularly since the effects on metabolism are only seen at concentrations far above those normally measured. However, it is possible that it might have a paracrine (or autocrine) role on islet cell secretion.

CLINICAL DISORDERS

As outlined earlier, the diffuse neuroendocrine system extends throughout the gastrointestinal tract. Individual cell representatives of this system all conform with criteria of the APUD concept; namely a capacity to demonstrate amine precursor uptake and decarboxylation. Among these, 16 separate cell types have been further characterized by immunohistochemistry, electron microscopy (EM), and *in situ* hybridization techniques: theoretically each can give rise to tumours in a variety of different sites. In fact, 20 per cent of islet cell tumours are non-functioning in terms of hormonal release, although even in these, immunohistochemistry and EM will identify hormone-specific granules. In addition, an apparently function-specific tumour often produces other peptides in clinically insignificant quantities: it is likely that the dedifferentiation process which characterizes APUD–cell neoplastic transformation permits the expression of otherwise repressed genes. A similar process is probably responsible for the 'ectopic' secretion of hormones from non-endocrine tumours such as bronchogenic carcinoma (see Chapter 16).

Although potentially hypersecreting neuroendocrine cells are distributed throughout the gastrointestinal tract, the majority of tumours arising from them do in fact occur within the pancreas, so that localization for surgical removal is rendered somewhat more straightforward than might appear likely at first consideration. Such tumours are also frequently associated with other components of the multiple endocrine neoplasia (MEN) syndromes which are discussed in Chapter 17. The mutations of cellular oncogenes and tumour suppressor genes which probably give rise to these tumours are also discussed in that chapter.

The challenge to diagnosis comes from two directions: first, an awareness of the identity of the rare clinical syndromes and secondly, the need to profile completely cases of MEN presenting with other non-pancreatic tumours. The diagnostic process requires access to assays to characterize completely any of the tumours described below. Also, a full knowledge of the non-neoplastic causes of serum peptide elevation is mandatory. Finally, localization techniques are needed. CT or MRI scanning are useful, but highest quality digital subtraction angiography (with or without CT) and probably isotope scanning are the two most important procedures. The therapeutic approach is limited by the malignant, multifocal, and metastatic nature of most of these tumours. Individual cases sometimes respond well to cytotoxic chemotherapy, while the somatostatin analogue, octreotide, has been useful in some cases of VIP-oma and glucagonoma.

The prevalence of all the tumours to be described is exceedingly low: overall less than 5 per 1 million population. Their major interest lies in the information that they provide about the normal physiology of the relevant hormones and both cellular and molecular biology.

Gastrinoma

The initial case description by Zollinger and Ellison in 1955 spawned a series of reports of severe ulcer dyspepsia, which is characteristically recurrent after repeated gastric surgery. Many cases also have diarrhoea, mediated by hyperacidic denaturation of lipolytic and proteolytic enzymes. True steatorrhoea is often seen. Serum gastrin levels are as expected very high, and further increments can be demonstrated in response to intravenous secretin, a response which is not seen with the many other causes of hypergastrinaemia. Pancreatic polypeptide (PP) and vasoactive intestinal peptide (VIP) are quite often co-secreted with gastrin, particularly in the MEN-I syndrome, with which gastrinoma is associated in about 30 per cent of cases. A mixed meal stimulus will provoke a rise of PP and VIP only in patients harbouring gastrinomas, and hence may be a more specific diagnostic tool.

The normal gastrin-producing cells of the stomach are negatively inhibited by a low pH of gastric contents and hence gastric acid secretion. Conversely, any reduction of gastric acid secretion will raise gastrin levels. Pernicious anaemia (characterized by extreme atrophic gastritis), H_2 receptor antagonists and proton pump inhibitors, vagotomy, and even high-dose antacids will accordingly induce hypergastrinaemia, although not usually to the levels seen in gastrinoma.

Experimental administration of high-dose omeprazole (a proton pump inhibitor) to rats has been shown to stimulate enterochromaffin cells within the gastric mucosa to undergo hyperplasia and subsequent autonomous tumour formation, with a morphology similar to spontaneous carcinoid tumours. These are largely reversible when the stimulus is removed. Such benign carcinoid tumours (also referred to as argyrophilic carcinoidosis) have also been reported in humans in in the context of Zollinger–Ellison syndrome and in pernicious anaemia. It seems likely that excess gastrin itself represents the oncogenic stimulus. Although theoretically possible, these carcinoid lesions have not been reported in the course of treatment with inhibitors of gastric acid secretion.

Most gastrinomas are situated in the pancreas, and can be localized by one of the techniques referred to earlier. In the context of MEN-I, the tumours are often multiple, malignant in 50 per cent, and already metastatic at diagnosis in 50 per cent of cases. Accordingly, long-term medical therapy with H_2-receptor antagonists or proton pump inhibitors is often required over and above initial excision of the most obvious tumour, most particularly with MEN-related tumours which are more likely to be multifocal.

Glucagonoma

The clinical features of this rare syndrome contain elements which do not immediately reflect hypersecretion of glucagon. Glossitis, venous thrombosis, and a variety of psychiatric disturbances have been reported. Characteristically, most patients have one or more prominent skin lesions in the lower limb-girdle area. Initially, the skin shows simple erythematous patches which blister, break down, and are often infected (because of their location). Referred to as necrolytic migratory erythema, the lesion is distinctive. There is no certain knowledge about its pathophysiology, although the skin problems resolve following tumour removal. The only clinical features which can be immediately attributed to glucagon itself are the weight loss (due to increased protein catabolism) and hyperglycaemia.

Serum glucagon is markedly raised, although high values are also seen in uncontrolled diabetes itself, pancreatits, trauma, and acute stressful illnesses. The immunologically distinct enteroglucagon (glicentin), a larger molecule which includes the 29-amino acid sequence of glucagon itself is consistently cosecreted with glucagonoma, but serum levels are not raised with other causes of raised serum glucagon. Treatment is by tumour resection, but in some instances the somatostatin analogue, octreotide, has been used, and will often cause resolution of the characteristic and sometimes disabling skin lesions.

Enteroglucagonoma is a particularly rare tumour of intestinal L-cells. Enteroglucagon, a 69-amino acid peptide is uniquely hypersecreted (without associated glucagon elevation). Vague abdominal symptoms and diarrhoea have been occasionally reported, and there is a characteristic hypertrophy and hyperplasia of small intestinal villi.

Somatostatinoma

First described in 1979, this syndrome conforms with most of the expected actions of somatostatin. Suppression of gastric acid and pancreatic exocrine function induce a variety of gastrointestinal symptoms, including dyspepsia and steatorrhoea: intestinal somatostatinomas may also cause small bowel obstruction because of their size, but are not usually endocrinologically active. Gallstones form due to inhibition of gall bladder motility. The dominant effect on insulin (rather than glucagon) secretion causes mild diabetes, sometimes with ketonaemia, and this is normally diet-controllable. The pancreatic somatostatinomas are often already metastatic at the time of diagnosis and neither surgical or medical (pharmacological) treatment is usually feasible. Although immunohistochemical staining for somatostatin has been noted in MEN-I-related tumours, as yet no case of somatostatinoma has been reported in this setting.

VIP-oma

This disorder, loosely described as pancreatic cholera was first characterized in 1958, and is sometimes known by its eponym of 'Verner–Morrison syndrome'. As previously described, vasoactive intestinal peptide (VIP) is widely distributed as a neuromodulator in central and peripheral nervous systems. VIP is known to be the causative agent of the severe and potentially fatal watery diarrhoea, which is accompanied by hypokalaemia and acidosis due to major losses of potassium and bicarbonate. VIP-mediated achlorhydria complicates the picture by inducing additional diarrhoea. Hypotension occurs as a consequence of vasodilatation and 50 per cent have hypercalcaemia, the mechanism of which remains unexplained. Hyperglycaemia is occasionally present and may be due either to the peptide itself or to the associated hypokalaemia, which impairs insulin release and decreases peripheral tissue insulin sensitivity. VIP-omas are often malignant and metastatic, and sometimes responsive to streptozotocin, an agent more usually employed in the treatment of insulinoma. Octreotide has been highly effective in a number of cases in reducing the severity of the gastrointestinal disturbance.

PP-oma

Neither a clinical nor even a physiological role has been found for pancreatic polypeptide (PP). However, it is frequently co-secreted with other tumours: even 25 per cent of so-called non-functioning islet cell adenomas in association with MEN-I have high circulating PP levels, and in all such cases PP can be identified by the appropriate immunohistochemical staining. Raised PP levels, hyperstimulable by secretin and a mixed meal may also be encountered in the premalignant islet hyperplasia of MEN-I. Random elevations of PP are also seen in inflammatory bowel disease, diarrhoea due to a variety of causes and chronic renal failure. In contrast to the neoplastic form, more benign PP elevation can be diagnostically suppressed by intravenous atropine administration.

Other tumours

Calcitonin, neurotensin, parathormone, corticotrophin, and GnRH have all been reported either alone or co-secreted with the above better-defined hypersecretion syndromes. However none produce a characteristic syndrome with the exception of GHRH (which can induce typical acromegaly) and ACTH (which causes Cushing's syndrome): the latter is found in approximately 5 per cent of patients with gastrinoma.

FURTHER READING

PHYSIOLOGY

Cooper, G.J.S. (1994). Amylin compared with calcitonin gene-related peptide: structure, biology and relevance to metabolic disease. *Endocrine Reviews*, **15**, 163–99.

CLINICAL

Adrian, T.E., Uttenthal, L.O., Williams, S.J., *et al.* (1986). Secretion of polypeptide in patients with pancreatic endocrine tumors. *New England Journal of Medicine*, **315**, 287–91.

Cherner, J.A., Doppman, J.L., Norton, J.A., *et al.* (1986). Prospective assessment of selective venous sampling for gastrin to localize gastrinomas. *Annals of Internal Medicine*, **105**, 841–2.

Hammond, P.J., Jackson, J.A., and Bloom, S.R. (1994). Localization of pancreatic endocrine tumours. *Clinical Endocrinology*, **40**, 3–14.

Stacpoole, P.W. (1981). The glucagonoma syndrome. Clinical features, diagnosis and treatment. *Endocrine Reviews*, **2**, 347–61.

Vinik, A.I., Strodel, W.E., Eckhauser, F.E., *et al.* (1987). Somatostatinomas, PPomas, neurotensinomas. *Seminars on Oncology*, **14**, 263–81.

Wynick, D. and Bloom, S.R. (1991). The use of long-acting somatostatin analogue octreotide in the treatment of gut neuroendocrine tumours. *Journal of Clinical Endocrinology and Metabolism*, **73**, 1–3.

13

Growth and development

PHYSIOLOGY

The processes of growth and development continue throughout life under various guises. The greatest growth and development occurs in the womb, the fetus reaching a peak growth rate of approximately 30 mm/day at around week 20. From birth to puberty, growth continues apace although growth velocity decreases steadily during this phase. Finally, at puberty, the growth spurt produces a transient acceleration in growth with the final height achieved at this stage. However, throughout the rest of life although linear growth ceases, the maintenance and regeneration of tissues (which can be included in the terms 'growth and development') continue.

FETAL GROWTH

Fetal growth is influenced by many factors, some of them determined by the fetus itself and some exerting an influence through the mother. The latter influences may be directly related to the mother while others are more environmental, and influence the fetus indirectly through the mother.

Fetal influences (fetal hormones)

The sex of the fetus is one factor which influences growth, and this is manifest by the general observation that boys are bigger than girls at birth. The fetal androgens are growth promoters but other fetal hormones are also important. Thus, fetal insulin has effects on growth, and its release can be stimulated by a raised blood glucose concentration. Indeed, if the mother becomes diabetic, the increase in her blood glucose concentration results in an increase in fetal blood glucose levels and this can then stimulate the fetal β-cells of the pancreatic islets to produce increased quantities of insulin. The growth-promoting effects of insulin in the fetus can result in a greater birthweight. Other important hormones for fetal growth and development, not just physical but also neural, are the thyroidal iodothyronines. In the absence of these hormones a physically and mentally impaired baby is born, and unless hormone replacement is begun within months the condition is irreversible (cretinism).

Interestingly, although somatotrophin and the somatomedins are produced by the end of the first trimester, there is no conclusive evidence that these hormones are vital for normal fetal growth and development. Finally, the role of various other growth factors in the fetus including the tissue-specific factors (such as nerve growth factor, epidermal growth factor, and platelet derived growth factor) and the more generally acting but locally produced insulin-like growth factors is relatively unknown.

Maternal influences (direct)

1. *Nutrition and diet.* The quantity of food and the nature of the diet can both influence birthweight. Restricted food intake, often associated with other influences such as economic and social factors (including cigarette smoking and drinking alcohol), is linked to a reduced birthweight. Regarding the nature of the diet, evidence suggests that a high protein diet is associated with increased linear growth of the fetus while a diet high in fats is associated with a greater birthweight.

2. *Specific drugs.* Cigarette smoking and drinking alcohol are two common habits which in excess are associated with a reduced birthweight when other factors are excluded. Contents of cigarettes, such as nicotine and tar, can influence fetal growth by reducing maternal appetite, decreasing placental blood flow, and causing structural changes to the placenta. The effects of excessive drug intake during pregnancy on physical and mental development of the child are still apparent at the age of 11 years, according to some surveys.

3. *Maternal age, social, and economic factors.* A direct relationship between the mother's age and birthweight appears to be present but this is likely to be due to other related factors such as the likely greater economic security and better nutrition in the older mother. Indeed, the social and economic factors are probably very important in determining the birthweight and well-being of the baby. The more obvious effects would be due to poor housing, poor nutrition, and other related factors.

Maternal influences (indirect)

Changes in the environment can indirectly influence fetal growth and development through the mother. One example is the well-documented famine which occurred in the Netherlands towards the end of the Second World War, in 1944, over a period of eight months. It was associated with a significant decrease in birthweight and a 25 per cent increase in premature (underweight) births.

Other changes in the environment, such as the increase in pollutants in the atmosphere, may well be shown to influence fetal growth and birthweight in due course. An interesting — and extremely worrying — pollutant which appears to have an important effect on the fetus (and thus on later stages of life) is the production of oestrogenic molecules from chemical effluents in water. Fish and aquatic reptiles are born as genetic, infertile males, or as females. The consequence for the survival of various species is of great concern. The possible involvement of such pollutants with the increased incidence of infertility in humans requires investigation.

PUBERTY

Puberty is the stage in life at which reproductive capability is achieved, and it is associated with the various physiological, morphological, and behavioural changes of adolescence. The maturation of the gonads is accompanied by the acceleration of growth (the growth spurt) and the development of secondary sex characteristics which are the most obvious physical changes during adolescence. In general, girls reach puberty earlier than boys (approximately between the ages of 10 and 16 in girls, and between the ages of 14 and 18 in boys). The clearest indication that puberty has been reached in girls is the first menstruation, or 'period', which is called menarche. The first indication that puberty has been reached in males is probably missed since the first spontaneous erection — and ejaculation — is likely to occur at night. These effects are related to the maturation of the hypothalamic– adenohypophysial–gonadal axis (see Figs 13.1 and 13.2).

Physical changes

The growth spurt

The acceleration of growth is mainly due to the increasing levels of sex steroids from the gonads acting with somatotrophin from the adenohypophysis. Other growth-promoting hormones (e.g. insulin) are probably necessary also for the normal growth spurt. Girls usually enter this phase, and reach peak height velocity, some two years earlier than boys who consequently experience accelerated growth from a greater initial height. Partly because of this, boys are generally taller at the end of the growth phase, and also because the peak height velocity is somewhat greater than in girls. The end of the growth spurt occurs when the epiphyses of the long bones have fused to the bone shafts (see Figs 13.3 and 13.4).

Secondary sex characteristics

In addition to the growth spurt, the increasing levels of circulating sex hormones induce development and growth of the genitalia and other sex characteristics such as the breasts and pubic hair.

Clearly identifiable stages in the development of the breasts and pubic hair have been described (Table 13.1). Breasts develop through five stages, primarily under the influence of the rising oestrogen levels. Pubic hair growth is controlled by adrenal and gonadal androgens. Other sex characteristics include the size of the hips (greater in females than in males) and the generally greater amount and distribution of body fat in females relative to males.

There are five classifiable stages in the development of the genitalia (penis, testes, and scrotum), and pubic hair in males (see Table 13.1). The various changes in the male are controlled by testosterone from the testes and the metabolite dihydrotestosterone formed by peripheral conversion. Other changes seen in the male at puberty are the growth of body and facial hair, and the voice which deepens ('breaking' voice). The latter change is due to androgens increasing the size of the larynx and the laryngeal muscles.

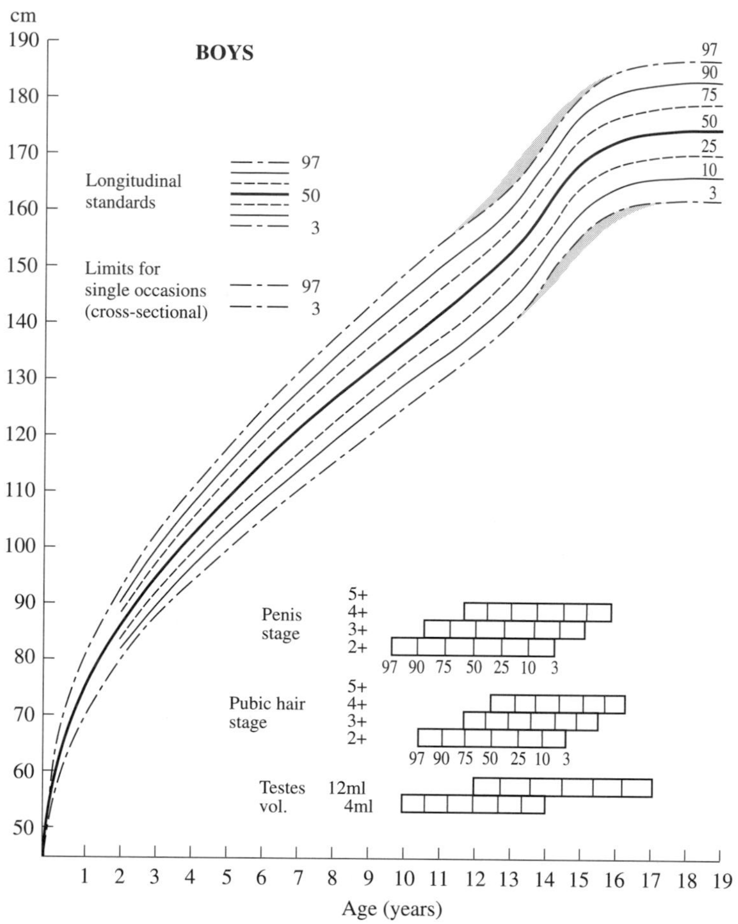

Fig. 13.1. Normal male growth chart. Testicular volume, penis and pubic hair stage centile distributions also shown e.g. 50% of boys reach pubic hair stage 2 by 12.5 yrs: 50% of boys have 12 ml testes by age 14.5 yrs.

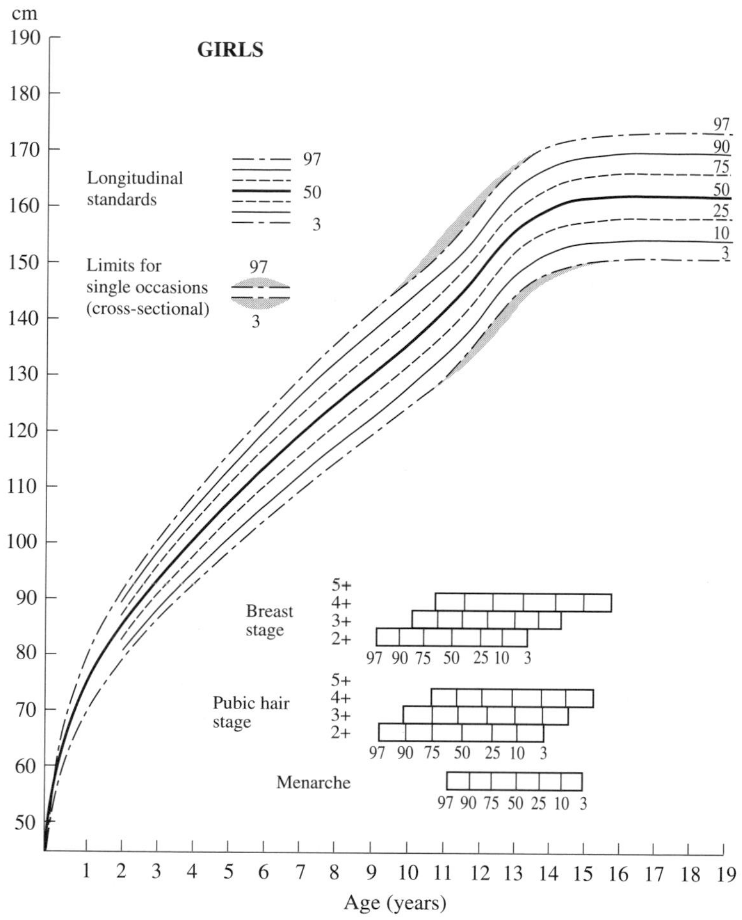

Fig. 13.2. Normal female growth chart. Menarche, hair and breast stage centile distributions also shown e.g. 97% of population has menarche by age 11 — 3% only have menarche beyond age 15.

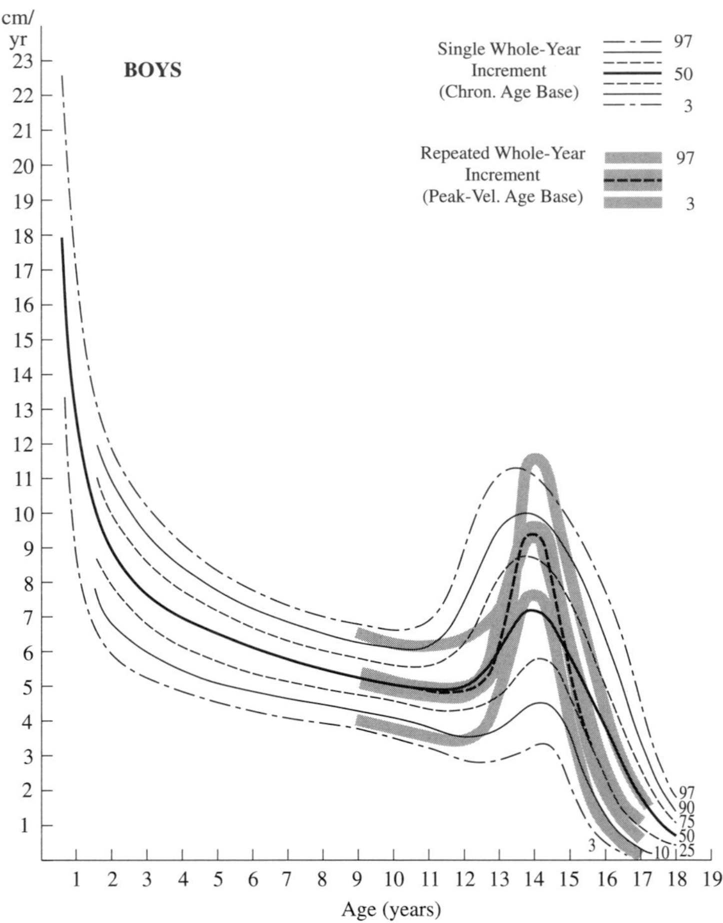

Fig. 13.3. Normal male growth velocity chart. For multiple within-year measurements, shaded norms are used.

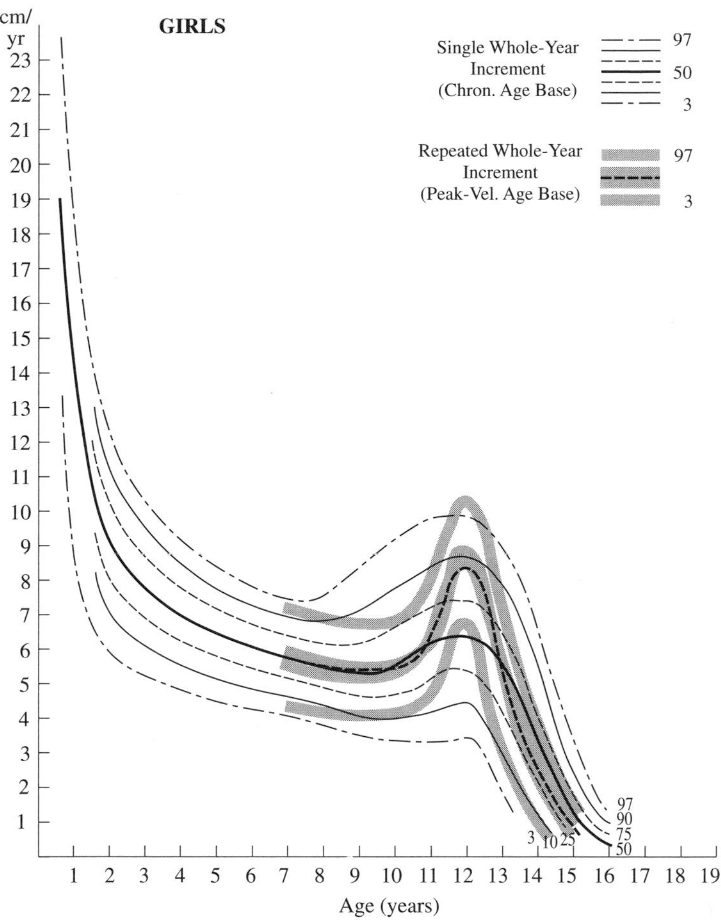

Fig. 13.4. Normal female growth velocity chart. For multiple within-year measurements, shaded norms are used.

Table 13.1. Stages of pubertal growth and development (after Tanner 1966)

A. *Pubic hair*: males and females	
Stage 1	Prepubertal: no pubic hair
Stage 2	Sparse growth of pubic hair chiefly around base of penis or along labia: hair long, either slighty curled or straight
Stage 3	Spread of hair which becomes darker, coarser, and more curled
Stage 4	Hair adult in type but is still restricted in area
Stage 5	Hair now has adult distribution and has spread to medial surface of thighs
Stage 6	This stage is associated with the spread of hair up the linea alba
B. *Breast development*: females	
Stage 1	Prepubertal: papilla elevated
Stage 2	Bud stage: breast and papilla develop as small mound; areolar diameter increased
Stage 3	Further enlargement of breast and areola
Stage 4	Areola and papilla develop to form a secondary mound above the breast
Stage 5	Adult stage: papilla projects out of the areola which becomes part of the breast contour
C. *Genital development*: males	
Stage 1	Prepubertal: testes, scrotum, and penis of size and proportion of early childhood
Stage 2	Scrotum and testes enlarge; scrotal sac becomes reddened and coarser
Stage 3	Penis enlarges, initially, mainly in length. Testes and scrotum continue to grow
Stage 4	Increased growth, in length and width, of penis: testes and scrotum enlarged and scrotal skin pigmented
Stage 5	Testes, scrotum, and penis, adult in size and shape

Hormone changes

Adenohypophysial hormones

Plasma gonadotrophins follicle stimulating hormone (FSH) and luteinizing hormone (LH) are present in low concentrations immediately after birth but then rise intermittently for the first one to two years of life before returning to low levels for the rest of childhood. Throughout adolescence, plasma FSH and LH levels then increase steadily, with increasing pulses of hormone release during the night, in the early stages. Adult concentrations are reached at puberty. Prolactin levels also increase at puberty, but in girls only.

Testosterone

Testosterone levels in the plasma of boys immediately after birth and for a period of a few months are as high as at puberty, but the level then falls and remains low until adolescence when it rises in conjunction with LH. In girls, the testosterone level is low until adolescence when the plasma concentration rises during the pubertal stages. The increase in the plasma androgen level in girls is nevertheless much less than in boys.

Oestrogens

The plasma oestrogen concentrations are very high in both males and females at birth because of placental conversions of C19 steroids from fetus and mother. The levels then drop markedly and remain low until adolescence when they begin to rise during the stages leading to puberty. The plasma oestrogen concentrations rise to much higher levels in girls than in boys in whom much of the oestradiol is derived from extraglandular testosterone aromatization.

Adrenal steroids

There is a progressive increase in the secretion of dehydroepiandrosterone and its sulphate from the adrenals which precedes, by some two years, the increases in gonadotrophin and gonadal steroid production. The time at which this increase begins in boys and girls is called adrenarche. The only clear effect of the adrenal androgen is to stimulate growth of pubic hair.

Control of puberty

While at present there is no single universally accepted hypothesis to account for the various endocrine changes which lead to puberty, it is probable that one important factor is the maturation of the hypothalamus and the gonadotrophin-releasing hormone (GnRH) neurones. A more controversial aspect of the pubertal mechanism is whether there is a change in the sensitivity of the adenohypophysis and/or hypothalamus to circulating gonadal (and/or adrenal) steroids. Thus, according to the proponents of this additional mechanism there is a gradual increase in the 'set point' at which the gonadal steroids exert their negative feedback on FSH and LH release (i.e. it becomes less sensitive to the feedback effect).

Puberty is initiated by a maturation of the central nervous system involving the gradual establishment of pulsatile GnRH release from the hypothalamic neurones. This may occur at the same time as the adenohypophysis (and perhaps the hypothalamus) becomes less sensitive to the negative feedback influence by gonadal steroids, and more sensitive to the GnRH pulses. The positive feedback effect of oestrogen on gonadotrophin release can only be elicited after puberty in women, and the LH surge effect must be a late pubertal development. The mechanism by which this cyclic effect of oestrogen can be elicited is not understood at present.

Maintenance of tissues in the adult

After the pubertal changes have occurred, tissue growth, maintenance, and, when necessary, regeneration continue to occur. Various growth factors are involved including the specific tissue factors, such as epidermal growth factor, and the various more general growth stimulators such as somatotrophin, the insulin-like growth factors, prolactin, and the thyroidal iodothyronines (see relevant chapters).

CLINICAL DISORDERS

Evaluation and management of growth problems

Introduction

Only in recent years have a number of issues regarding control of growth been resolved. Diagnosing abnormal growth has required an understanding of normal growth patterns, yielding the comparatively new speciality discipline of auxology. The physiological factors determining growth outlined in the earlier section of this chapter combine to produce a reasonably predictable range of growth curves when circumscribed normal populations are studied. Nevertheless, it is important to appreciate that even between individual Caucasian groups (i.e. US and UK whites), statistically different growth profiles have been documented, mainly reflecting minor ethnic/genetic variations as well as different nutritional patterns: for routine clinical applications such comparatively minor variations are of little significance. However, most published standard (normal) growth charts, which document linear growth as a function of age (together with derived age- and sex-specific growth velocity), in fact, describe Euripid populations, and such charts cannot be reliably used for Asian and Oriental populations, whose growth parameters are substantially lower.

Assessment of growth status

The standard growth charts shown in Figs 13.1–13.4 are those commonly used to identify growth status and velocity, and were derived from a population of 'normal' UK children and adolescents. The (per)centiles displayed represent probability distributions (e.g., 90th centile indicates that 90 per cent of the normal population will show stature or velocity below that figure). The almost Gaussian distribution of both stature and velocity also allows definition of growth in terms of standard deviations (SD) from the mean. Charts displaying plus or minus one, two, and three SD are also available; although derived differently. For clinical purposes, the range of plus-or-minus 2 SD corresponds broadly with the 3rd to 97th centile range.

Documentation of height requires care and precision: the simple and poorly engineered height-measuring apparatus often found in routine surgeries and clinics is inadequate except for very broad screening purposes. Documentation of growth changes should ideally be restricted to a constant operator using quality equipment. Such accurate and comparatively expensive stadiometers are mostly to be found in paediatric clinics. Accurate measurement also demands that the patient is physiologically 'stretched' to full length or height: muscular tone (even differing from morning to evening) is a critical variable. Pubertal status (see earlier) is a major determinant of normal growth and requires documentation at the time of height assessment, using the pubertal standards outlined earlier in this chapter. Puberty is responsible for the growth spurt shown in the centile charts

Since genetic factors are amongst the most important physiological variables, height expectation and prediction require knowledge of maternal and paternal (mature) heights. Each is expressed in centile status from the respective gender-specific charts, and then plotted on the patients own chart as a mid-parental height

(MPH). This may be used as one measure of 'expected' height for the patient under investigation. For example:

Short boy for evaluation.
Maternal height = 151 cm (3rd centile on female chart).
Plot 3rd centile on right ordinate of male chart (= 162 cm) .
Plot paternal height (170 cm) on ordinate.
MPH is midpoint = 166 cm.

Three more growth-related definitions are useful: chronological age (CA) represents actual age; height age (HA) is determined by horizontally extrapolating from actual height back to the 50th centile on the relevant growth chart; bone age (BA) is determined from radiology of the (usually) left hand and wrist using a standard reference manual which combines and collates data on appearance and fusion of epiphyses (Greulich and Pyle system or the rather more accurate Tanner-Whitehouse system which employs individual 'ageing' of 20 hand bones).

Criteria for defining 'short stature' vary. To some extent, the definition depends on a patient's (or their parents') perception of abnormality. However, both actual height or growth velocity below third centile (–2 SD) for age are commonly used indications for further evaluation. The principle of investigation is to identify those causes which are amenable to therapy in some form before epiphyseal fusion has occurred, and to provide a prognosis. Assuming that endocrine normality has been established, Bayley–Pinneau tables have been used to predict estimated or final mature height (EMH, FMH), although with accuracy that is limited to ± 3 cm.

Systematic application of clinical observation and appropriate biochemical and other tests are used to screen for the various conditions outlined below.

Causes and management of individual syndromes

1. *Familial short stature.* The majority of cases. Mid-parental height and family history reflect genetic trends. BA is similar to CA and puberty normal. No biochemical abnormality present. Treatment with growth hormone possible but expensive, and rarely justified by modestly low EMH.

2. *Simple delayed puberty/small delay syndrome/constitutional delay of growth and adolescence (CDGA).* Delayed growth beginning even prepubertally and mainly in boys. Family history of isosexual parent usually affected. Two- to four-year delay in pubertal onset. Endocrinologically normal except for low androgen, LH amd FSH levels. BA delayed, EMH normal. Androgen or gonadotrophin therapy possible, but final mature height unaffected by treatment (see also section on pubertal disorders, p. 334).

3. *Intrauterine growth retardation (IUGR).* Idiopathic or secondary retarded fetal development, with resulting low birthweight. Chromosomal abnormalities (10 per cent), maternal systemic disease (20 per cent), congenital infections (2 per cent), maternal malnutrition, alcohol excess, smoking, and addictive drugs. Also named primary growth failure syndromes of unknown cause including:

- *Silver–Russell syndrome:* small triangular face, syndactyly or clinodactyly and asymmetric limbs.

- *Seckel syndrome*: severe microcephaly and mental retardation.
- *Osteochondrodysplasias*: a variety of primary skeletal developmental anomalies.

Catch-up growth occurs in many cases. In others, FMH is low and a proportion will have demonstrable growth hormone deficiency, with low BA. In the latter group, growth hormone therapy may be appropriate.

4. *Psychosocial small stature (PSS).* Infantile or childhood varieties, involving a complex series of emotional and nutritional disturbances with consequent 'functional' (reversible) growth hormone deficiency. Parental rejection is a frequent underlying factor, but is readily overlooked. Adoption or parental counselling is sometimes successful in reversing delayed growth. Poor psychological prognosis.

5. *Turner's syndrome/gonadal dysgenesis*: Plates 13.1 and 13.2 (see Chapter 8).

6. *Underlying organic disease.* Malabsorption syndrome (including coeliac disease and cystic fibrosis), chronic asthma or other respiratory disease, congenital heart and chronic renal disease. Chronic corticosteroid therapy for any disorder.

7. *Juvenile hypothyroidism.* A readily overlooked cause of short stature, since the expected facial features are often absent. Auto-immune thyroid disease is usually responsible. BA is often markedly reduced compared with HA, and the biochemical profile diagnostic. Treatment is with thyroxine, carefully titrated to maintain a normal serum TSH (see Chapter 10).

8. *Growth hormone deficiency.* This is an uncommon but important disorder with many causes (see Table 13.2).

Clinical features are usually unremarkable with symmetrical and proportionate short stature and reduced growth velocity presenting at any age. BA is low compared with CA. Identification of growth hormone deficiency is initially by screening technique involving either exercise stress or, in some centres, sleep. If abnormal (maximum serum hGH < 20 mU/l), evaluation subsequently proceeds to definitive testing with sequential arginine infusion and insulin-induced hypoglycaemia (see Chapter 18). Serum IGF-I levels are low. Other endocrine deficiencies, especially gonadotrophin and TSH may be present, particularly in secondary causes. Such secondary causes referred to above are important to identify, since independent treatment may be indicated (e.g. removal of underlying craniopharyngioma may result in restoration of growth hormone secretion and subsequent spontaneous catch-up growth). Pituitary region CT or MRI scans are therefore essential.

Treatment with parenteral synthetic (recombinant DNA) growth hormone is expensive but effective and is usually self-administered. Growth velocity increases by 50–100 per cent and treatment is continued until epiphyseal fusion has occurred.

9. *Pseudo-growth hormone-deficient syndromes.* This represents a variety of uncommon syndromes including abnormalities of the hGH molecule (possibly due to mutation) which reduce its biological effectiveness. Abnormal hepatic growth hormone receptor activity also results in a variety of syndromes including the sporadic Laron-type dwarfism which manifests identical presenting features to

Table 13.2. Causes of childhood/adolescent growth hormone deficiency

Congenital
Rare syndromes involving multiple congenital abnormalities, including cleft face, Fraser's syndrome, Rieger's syndrome, septo-optic dysplasia, hypoplasia of the pituitary, arachnoid cysts

Acquired
1. Organic
   Middle cranial fossa tumours
   Craniopharyngioma
   Pituitary tumours (including prolactinoma)
   Granulomas (histiocytosis-X, sarcoidosis)
   Non-cephalic delivery
   Irradiation-induced
2. Functional (secondary reversible)
   Psychosocial deprivation
   Anorexia nervosa
   General acute and severe chronic illness (especially hepatic and renal disease)
3. Idiopathic (irreversible)
   Idiopathic growth hormone deficiency
   - sporadic
   - familial

   Prader–Willi syndrome

Pseudo-hypopituitary syndromes
Bio-inactive growth hormone
Impaired growth hormone receptor function
Laron-type dwarfism
African Pygmies, little women of Loja, Ecuador; Mountain Ok, New Guinea
IGF-I resistance syndromes

growth hormone deficiency. Serum hGH levels are normal or high to all stimuli, but IGF-I levels are low. The specific cause appears to be a complete absence of growth hormone-binding protein (GH-BP), which represents the extracellular domain of the growth hormone receptor. A similar partial resistance to hGH, mediated by reduced levels of GH-BP is responsible for the ethnic smallness of African Pygmies, and possibly other small stature populations such as the Loja of Ecuador and the Mountain Ok of New Guinea. Rare cases of insensitivity to IGF-I have also been reported.

10. *Other named syndromes of unknown aetiology.* A variety of rare, named multisystem disorders. Among these the more common are the Prader–Willi syndrome consisting of short stature, obesity, muscular hypotonia, microphallus, and hypogonadotrophic hypogonadism. Chromosome 15, region q11-13 deletions have been identified in some instances. Lawrence–Moon–Biedl syndrome includes short stature, hypogonadism, obesity, mental subnormality, polydactyly, and retinitis pigmentosa.

Disorders of puberty (see Plate 13.3)

Delayed puberty/constitutional delay of growth and adolescence (CDGA)

CDGA is the most common cause of pubertal delay and represents one end of the physiological spectrum of pubertal development. By definition, it is self-correcting in all instances, with both gonadal development and stature eventually reaching totally normal levels, although therapeutic intervention is sometimes required for largely social reasons. Deceleration of growth may occur as early as age 8 years, and a poor growth velocity (usually below 4 cm per annum) persists until pubertal development is initiated (usually not before the age of 15). It is more common in boys, with a frequent family history of identical but less striking problems in the isosexual parent. Height age and bone age (as defined earlier in this chapter) are almost identically delayed behind chronological age by up to 4 years. Spontaneous growth spurt and pubertal development occur once bone age is approximately 12–13 years. The precise mechanism for this extreme physiological variant is not known, and the diagnostic commitment is to exclude other causes of short stature and delayed sexual maturity.

The major differential diagnosis of CDGA is growth hormone deficiency (GHD) which is often associated with gonadotrophin deficiency. In both conditions, serum testosterone, LH, and FSH are low, and if IGF-I levels are normal, CDGA is the likely diagnosis. Some physicians prefer the proof of normal growth hormone secretory function (see Chapter 17). Other conditions to be considered are those outlined in the previous section on delayed growth: many patients in this group have at least some evidence of delayed pubertal development. Delay of sexual maturation without associated short stature raises other possibilities. In both males and females, hypogonadotrophic hypogonadism in all its forms and causes need to be excluded (see Chapter 4). In males, Klinefelter's syndrome, especially in its mosaic forms is quite common. In females, any of the causes of primary amenorrhoea need to be considered (see Chapter 8), together with functional hypothalamic anovulation/anorexia nervosa, gonadal dysgenesis, and polycystic ovarian disease.

Treatment for CDGA is never essential. However, the higher pitched voice, absence of shaving and immature appearance in boys are often socially detrimental, and confirmed male cases are now often treated. Treatment is provided either with testosterone oenanthate in a dose of 250 mg intramuscularly every 3 weeks for 3 months, or human chorionic gonadotrophin 2000 units twice weekly for 6 weeks. Even pulsatile GnRH can be used: although more physiological, it offers no advantages. Providing treatment courses are restricted to the above periods, there is no undue acceleration of bone age (with its risk of premature epiphyseal fusion): a growth spurt is initiated and usually maintained following a single course of treatment, with a 100 per cent increase in growth velocity commonly documented in the first post-treatment year. Treatment is not usually required for the less frequently encountered female cases of CDGA.

Precocious puberty (see Plate 13.4)

In both boys and girls, the appearance of secondary sexual characteristics before the age of 9 is considered abnormal, and therefore justifies consideration of underlying causes. Complete, true, or central sexual precocity indicates a pre-activation of the hypothalamic–pituitary–gonadal axis with demonstrably normal GnRH-dependent LH and FSH pulsatility. Incomplete or pseudo-precocious puberty results purely from an excess of androgens or oestrogens arising from adrenal and gonadal mechanisms. However produced, the clinical consequences common to all forms are an acceleration of general somatic development, most particularly an increase in growth velocity together with rapid skeletal maturation. If untreated, an above-average height in childhood is followed by stunting of mature height induced by premature epiphyseal fusion.

True precocious puberty

In addition to the above growth features, patients in this category develop all the secondary sexual characteristics seen in maturity. In girls, in whom this condition is more common, simultaneous onset of menstruation (the menarche) usually occurs. Although the most common 'cause' in both sexes is idiopathic sexual precocity, this cannot be confirmed without exclusion of underlying pathology: in boys, the likelihood of such pathology is greater. Investigations in all cases will invariably reveal pubertal levels of androgens or oestrogens, and LH and FSH concentrations are at levels expected for the stage of puberty. In contrast to pseudo-precocious puberty, GnRH provocation will induce a normal LH and FSH response. Bone age will be advanced compared with chronological age. Either MRI or CT scans are essential to exclude a wide range of pathologies.

The most common lesions are benign tumours termed hamartomas, which contain GnRH and release it in pulsatile fashion. They are not usually amenable to intervention, but are non-progressive. Other benign lesions are arachnoid cysts. Less benign are astrocytomas, gliomas, ependymomas, and germinomas, which are progressive, and may present as space-occupying lesions requiring treatment in their own right.

Treatment of this form of precocity involves surgery or radiotherapy (if appropriate) for the underlying lesion. Even if successfully dealt with, both idiopathic and secondary causes should all probably be treated pharmacologically as well: precociously pubertal girls are often attractive but psychologically immature and naïve, and therefore subject to abuse. Together with the embarrassment factor and the likelihood of ultimate short stature due to premature epiphyseal fusion, a strong case would have to be made for withholding treatment.

The disorder is amenable to treatment with any agent which inhibits gonadotrophin release. GnRH agonists in low (and particularly pulsatile) doses stimulate LH and FSH. However, in high doses they down-regulate pituitary GnRH receptors, inhibit gonadotrophin release, and accordingly androgen/oestrogen levels decline. Preparations are available for both intranasal and depot (monthly) intramuscular administration. Treatment is ideally continued until bone age and chronological age are similar, thereby ensuring a near-normal ultimate mature height.

Pseudo- (or incomplete) precocious puberty

Isosexual and contrasexual precocity are terms used to describe the clinical consequences of excess androgens and oestrogens in various gender settings described below. Both the statural and gonadal maturity will be clinically apparent, as in the cases of true sexual precocity. However, females will not be menstruating and are infertile, whatever the cause. In incomplete precocious puberty, investigations will reveal normal hypothalamic/pituitary anatomy by CT or MRI scanning (except in the rare hCG-producing hypothalamic hamartomas). Although either serum oestrogens or androgens are raised, FSH and LH concentrations are usually low in relation to pubertal status, and non-stimulable by GnRH testing. However, in hypothyroidism and the rare familial LH over-production syndromes, LH levels are raised.

Contrasexual precocity

This is almost exclusively seen in females. However, testicular feminization syndrome, due to defective tissue androgen receptors in the male may present as precocious puberty in a phenotypic female.

Congenital adrenal hyperplasia due to either 11- or 21-hydroxylase deficiency causes virilization in females. Raised serum androgens, 17-hydroxyprogesterone, and DHEAS are diagnostic, and cortisol therapy successfully reverses the clinical features. (see also Chapter 5).

Androgen-producing adrenal and ovarian tumours are rare in this age group. However, adrenal adenomas, either androgen-alone or combined androgen/cortisol-producing (Cushing's syndrome) are occasionally seen in girls, as are granulosa cell tumours and gynandroblastomas of the ovary (see also Chapter 6). Adrenal tumours also occasionally feminize males.

Isosexual precocity

Primary juvenile hypothyroidism is associated with precocity in both males and females, the hypothyroidism resulting in paradoxically delayed growth because of the thyroid deficiency. It is argued (but unproven) that the precocity is based on excess α-subunit which is common to both TSH and LH/FSH. The clinical features (also referred to as Van Wyk–Grumbach syndrome) are entirely reversible by thyroxine therapy (see also Chapter 10).

McCune–Albright syndrome is the combination of isosexual precocity with *café-au-lait* skin patches, polyostotic fibrous dysplasia, and occasionally other endocrine adenomas causing Cushing's syndrome or hyperthyroidism. It is more common in girls, and is probably due to mutations of the gene encoding for G proteins. Ultrasound may show cysts within enlarged ovaries, which are responsible for enhanced oestrogen secretion.

'Testotoxicosis' is a term used to desribe male-linked familial autonomous Leydig cell hyperactivity, possibly due to atypical LH secretion. The clinical effects of hyperandrogenism can be reversed either by the peripheral aromatase inhibitor, testolactone, which inhibits androgen to oestrogen conversion, or by the imidazole compound, ketoconazole, which inhibits conversion of 17-hydroxyprogesterone to androstenedione.

Tumours either of the testis (interstitial cell) or adrenal (adenomas or carcinomas) may cause precocity in males. Appropriate ultrasound or CT studies confirm the primary cause.

Gonadotrophin-producing tumours produce either LH (pituitary) or hCG (hepatomas. teratomas, germinomas). Appropriate assays and radiology are necessary to identify the source.

FURTHER READING

PHYSIOLOGY

Johnson, H.H. and Everitt, B.J. (1995). *Essential reproduction*. Fourth edition. Blackwell Science.

Rees, M. (1993). Menarche when and why? *The Lancet*, **342**, 1375–6.

Sinclair, D. (1984) *Human growth after birth*. Fourth edition. Oxford University Press.

Stanhope, R. and Brook, C.G.D. (1988). An evaluation of hormonal changes at puberty in man. *Journal of Endocrinology*, **116**, 301–5.

CLINICAL

Brook, C.D.G. (1995). Precocious puberty (investigation). *Clinical Endocrinology*, **42**, 647–50.

Bourguignon, J.P., Van Vleit, G.,Vandeweghe, M., *et al.* (1987). Treatment of central precocious puberty with an intra-nasal analogue of gonadotrophin releasing hormone (buserelin). *European Journal of Paediatrics*, **146**, 555–60.

Cara, J.F. and Johanson, J.A. (1990). Growth hormone for short stature not due to classic growth hormone deficiency. *Pediatric Clinics of North America*, **37**, 1229–38.

Costin, G., Kaufman, F.R., and Brasel, J.A. (1989). Growth hormone secretory dynamics in subjects with normal stature. *Journal of Pediatrics*, **115**, 537–42.

Devesa, J., Lima, L., and Tresguerres, J.A.F. (1992). Neuro-endocrine control of growth hormone secretion in humans. *Trends in Endocrinology and Metabolism*, **3**, 175–93.

Heinze, E. and Holl, R.W. (1992). Pseudo-hypopituitary syndromes. *Clinics in Endocrinology Metabolism*, **6**, 557–71.

Hindmarsh, P.C. and Brook, C.D.G. (1995). Short stature and growth hormone deficiency (investigation). *Clinical Endocrinology*, **43**, 133–42.

Holland, F.J., Kirsch, S.E., and Selby, R. (1987). Gonadotrophin-independent precocious puberty ('testotoxicosis'). *Journal of Clinical Endocrinology and Metabolism*, **64**, 328–33.

Lin, T.H., Kirkland, R.T., Sherman, B.M., *et al.* (1989). Growth hormone testing in short children, and their response to growth hormone therapy. *Journal of Pediatrics*, **115**, 57–64.

Rosenfield, R.L. (1990). Diagnosis and management of delayed puberty. *Journal of Clinical Endocrinology and Metabolism*, **70**, 559–64.

Stanhope, R., Brook, C.G., Pringle, P.J., *et al.* (1987). Induction of puberty by pulsatile gonadotrophin-releasing hormone. *Lancet*, **2**, 552–5.

Tanner, J.M. (1966). *Growth at adolescence*. Blackwell, London.

14

Disorders of lipid metabolism; and obesity

PHYSIOLOGY

The three principal dietary components of food are fats, proteins, and carbohydrates (excluding other important components such as vitamins and minerals). These components are all vital for the proper functioning of the body: for example, carbohydrates provide the principal source of readily available energy in the tissues, proteins provide many of the structural components of our cells, while fats are the chief storage form of energy substrate. The biochemical pathways which provide energy to the cells are associated with all three components. These are linked together so that, for example, some amino acids can be utilized directly in the tricarboxylic acid (TCA) cycle while carbohydrates can be converted to fats.

Lipid accumulation may be beneficial in conditions of food shortage, but in conditions where food is plentiful excessive fat deposition (obesity) can be harmful. This is particularly true for the accumulation of fatty deposits in the cardiovascular system because these atheromas can become the sites of vascular constriction and arterial 'hardening', or atherosclerosis. A particularly serious development can occur if it becomes the site of thrombus formation. Either the restriction of blood flow can result in tissue anoxia, or the thrombus can be dislodged, only to be carried to a smaller blood vessel such as a coronary or a cerebral vessel when a myocardial infarction or a cerebral stroke can occur, respectively.

Components of the Western diet perceived to be particularly associated with 'cardiovascular accidents' (CVAs) are the blood cholesterol level, the blood triglycerides and the proteins which carry these lipids in the blood called lipoproteins.

Absorption of lipids from the gastrointestinal tract

Relatively little happens to the fat in the diet until it reaches the duodenum, although the churning of the chyme in the stomach will promote the breakdown of large components to smaller globules. In the duodenum, the secretions of the gall bladder and the exocrine pancreas enter through the sphincter of Oddi and mix with the chyme. The gall bladder produces a concentrated bile which contains a mixture of bile pigments and various other excretory products, and bile salts. The latter are sodium salts of glycocholic and taurocholic acids, and they act like detergents, breaking down the fats to smaller globules, particularly in the presence of lecithin. This detergent action on fats increases the total surface area available to the actions of pancreatic lipase enzymes. The lipids are broken down mainly to their monoglyceride, glycerol, and fatty acid components by the action of these lipases. Subsequently, the bile salts and the various fat and steroid components aggregate to form micelles. These consist of small spherical structures composed of approximately 20 assorted molecules each, the non-polar lipophilic ends of the molecules facing the centre and the polar lipophobic ends facing outwards. The fatty acids, glycerol, and other lipid molecules, such as cholesterol in the lipophilic cores of the micelles, are thus transported to the intestinal walls. Here, the core contents are released to the brush borders of the intestinal mucosal cells which they enter by diffusion across the cell membranes. The bile salts are re-utilized many times before being absorbed themselves, further down in the ilium.

Transport of lipids in the blood

Small fatty acids (less than 12 carbon atoms) diffuse straight through the mucosal cells into the blood which transports them as free (non-esterified) fatty acids associated with plasma albumin. Larger fatty acids are re-esterified to triglycerides within the mucosal cells. These triglycerides, cholesterol esters, cholesterol, and phospholipids coalesce with proteins (called apoproteins) to form chylomicrons which are large lipoprotein complexes. These are released into the extracellular space by exocytosis, and from here they enter the lymphatics and, ultimately, the general circulation. The chylomicrons are removed from the circulation following the action of an endothelium-derived enzyme called lipoprotein lipase which catalyses the breakdown of triglyceride to free fatty acids and glycerol. These can enter the adipose tissue where they are re-esterified, or they can remain in the plasma bound to albumin. The cholesterol remnants of the chylomicrons continue to circulate in the blood associated with the lipoproteins. These are rapidly removed from the circulation by the liver which internalizes the cholesterol-rich lipoprotein by receptor-mediated endocytosis (Fig. 14.1).

In addition to the chylomicron-mediated transport system which links ingested lipids to the liver, there are various lipoprotein transport systems available for the general transport of these molecules which are also continually synthesized by the cells of the body. These systems consist of:

(1) very low density lipoproteins (VLDL) which are formed in the liver and which transport hepatic-synthesized triglycerides and other lipids to other tissues;

(2) intermediate density lipoproteins (IDL) which are formed from the VLDL after some of the triglyceride component has been removed by the action of lipoprotein lipase;

(3) low density lipoproteins (LDL) formed by the removal of even more of the triglyceride component but containing a much larger fraction of free cholesterol and its ester; and

(4) high density lipoprotein (HDL) which has a high protein and phospholipid content, and which takes up newly synthesized cholesterol leaving cells.

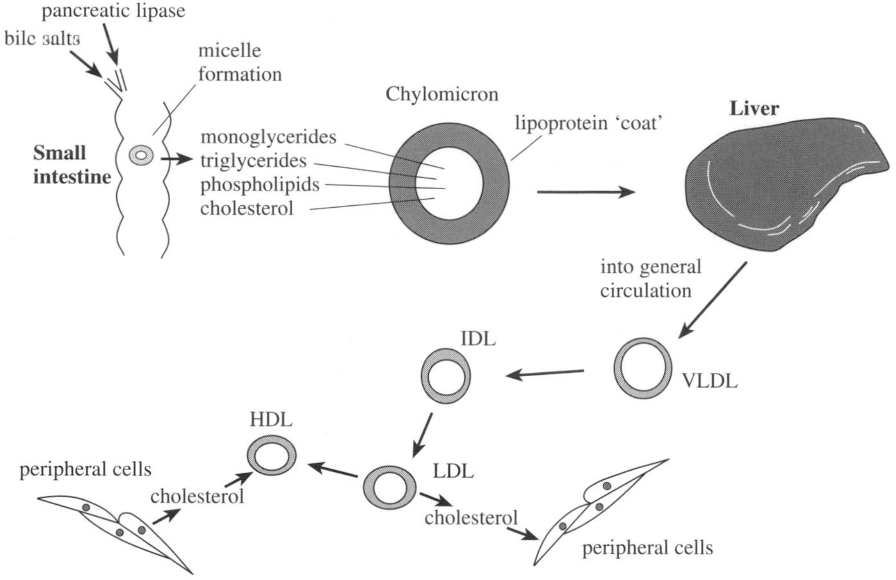

Fig. 14.1. Diagram showing the transport of lipids from the intestinal tract to peripheral tissues. (VLDL, very low density lipoproteins; IDL, intermediate density lipoproteins; LDL, low density lipoproteins; HDL, high density lipoproteins.)

The LDL component provides cholesterol to the tissues which require it for the synthesis of steroids and for membrane structure. It is taken up by cells through a receptor-mediated endocytosis which recognizes the apoprotein component. Inside the cells, the LDL is taken up by lysosomes which contain the enzymes necessary for the release of cholesterol within the cytoplasm. Intracellular cholesterol inhibits the cholesterol synthesis pathway (from acetate), stimulates esterification of any excess cholesterol, and inhibits the synthesis of LDL receptors, thereby exerting feedback control over the amount of cholesterol available to the cell.

Raised plasma cholesterol levels whether free or associated with LDL are associated with a higher incidence of atherosclerosis, myocardial infarction or strokes. Raised HDL levels, on the other hand, are associated with a 'protective' role and a decreased incidence of these disorders. Various hormones influence cholesterol metabolism. The thyroidal iodothyronines increase LDL receptor synthesis, hence decreasing the plasma cholesterol concentration. Oestrogens also decrease the plasma cholesterol concentration, a protective effect which is lost at menopause. Women also have a raised HDL concentration compared with men, and this correlates with a lower incidence of cardiovascular accidents until the menopause. The plasma level of cholesterol is also increased in untreated diabetes mellitus.

Various other factors influence plasma cholesterol and its transport lipoproteins. Exercise is associated with increased HDL levels and a decreased incidence of myocardial infarction, while smoking is associated with a decreased HDL concentration and an increased incidence of cardiovascular disease. Obesity and a sedentary life style are also known risk factors of heart disease.

CLINICAL DISORDERS

Obesity

Introduction and definitions

Obesity is found in all of the world's populations and ethnic groups. Its prevalence is, however, highly variable between races. In Western civilizations, between 10 and 20 per cent of the population is obese to an extent which increases morbidity and mortality. A definition of obesity is not easy for a variable which is continuously distributed within a population (although markedly skewed to the right). Over the years, insurance companies have been motivated to identify 'ideal weight' (IW) based on optimum morbidity and actuarially derived life-expectancy data. Accordingly, ideal weight tables have been contructed incorporating the major critical variables of height and gender, with further variables of age and 'frame' included in some instances. Having identified an individual's ideal weight (IW) in this way, excess can be defined in both absolute terms as well as in percentage departure of actual from ideal weight.

This system is still used, most particularly in lay publications, where simplified ideal weight tables enable the public to identify their own status: with 'overweight' carrying a significant social stigma, and with increased public awareness of the health significance of obesity, simple methods of self-evaluation are of increasing importance. However, ideal weight is not necessarily an appropriate concept when obesity presents as part of a clinical problem. For one thing, very few patients achieve, and even fewer can maintain their ideal weight, no matter what treatment is offered. Accordingly, a more arbitrary goal or target weight is clinically more useful and realistic, and accordingly more acceptable to most people.

Rather more recently, the concept of body mass index (BMI) was proposed, and has been universally accepted as a method of expressing body weight. It is very simply expressed as weight (in kilograms) divided by height (in metres) squared (i.e. a person with body weight 88 kg and height 1.68 m has a BMI of $88/1.68 \times 1.68 = 31$). The ranges set out below are generally accepted 'broad-brush' definitions of weight categories (and hence risk groups).

	Body mass index
Underweight	< 19
Normal weight	19–25
Overweight	26–30
Moderate obesity	31–35
Severe obesity	> 36

More importantly, since authorities have not always agreed on the definition of 'ideal weight', for both research and epidemiological purposes BMI has virtually superseded IW, and is now finding its way into lay publications as well.

The medical profession itself has been shown to have variable perceptions of obesity as a health problem: in various studies, it has been shown that doctors overlook 20–50 per cent of cases of obesity of a severity known to be associated with later morbidity. On the whole, doctors regularly identified obesity only when it represented an associated risk factor of another clearly defined condition such as diabetes or hypertension. Accordingly, most patients with obesity either initiate their own referral for opinion, or seek approaches through non-traditional medicine. Patients' own perception of their body image is also highly variable: studies using a range of stylized body-shape diagrams with which they are asked to identify, reveal a wide departure from the expected correlation.

In the very broadest terms, mortality risk rises proportionately to weight excess: using the older IW tables, per centage above ideal weight correlates roughly with excess mortality, a risk which is largely reversible by subsequent weight reduction.

Aetiology

In the simplest concept of energy balance, body weight should represent the net balance between energy intake and expenditure. It has been repeatedly shown, however, that individuals who are similar for these two variables may have widely differing weights. Some of the critical variables are discussed below.

1. *Endocrine factors.* These are mentioned first, largely because of the popular (but incorrect) lay notion that 'glands' and 'hormones' are the basis of common obesity. Only rarely does Cushing's syndrome present as obesity, and is then of characteristic truncal distribution. Although hypothyroidism is occasionally diagnosed in the overweight patient, restoration of euthyroidism rarely results in anything more than a few kilograms of weight loss. Endocrine factors are otherwise irrelevant.

2. *Genetic factors.* Studies have shown that identical twins of obese probands are more likely to be themselves obese than non-identical twins. This does not necessarily imply heritable metabolic factors: eating patterns are also probably genetically determined, and current studies have not adequately addressed this aspect. Certain named syndromes such as those of Lawrence–Moon–Biedl (obesity, hypogonadism, mental subnormality, polydactyly, etc.) and Prader–Willi (obesity, muscular hypotonia, microphallus, etc.) with the stated associated somatic defects suggest that at least in this small subset, genetic factors may be critical. It is tempting to propose, but as yet unproven, that minor degrees of such genetic factors are widely distributed in the population.

3. *Metabolic factors.* Metabolic rate is a variable which has aroused considerable interest. Many studies have shown that basal metabolic rate is, if anything, higher in the obese. However, the rise in oxygen consumption in response to eating and exercise has in some reports been shown to be significantly less in the obese. This has led to the suggestion that obesity is a state of metabolic hyperefficiency, and perhaps represents a genotype which may have had survival advantage in primitive man.

4. *Cellular factors.* Overall, fat cell mass can logically be increased by either adipocyte hyperplasia or hypertrophy. The fat cell mass has been shown to be particularly vulnerable to hyperplasia during childhood and adolescence: a net

positive energy balance whether achieved through overeating or inactivity during this period of development may therefore be expected to confer a comparatively non-reversible proneness to obesity, whereas a similar positive energy balance in adult life is more likely to result in hypertrophy of individual adipocytes, a phenomenon known to be reversible.

5. *Nutritional factors*. The calorie value of foods (4 per gram carbohydrate and protein; 9 per gram fat) are well known. Although certain foods (particularly proteins) are thought to be selectively 'calorigenic', there is no escaping the fundamental summative calorie value of foods based on their nutrient content. The pattern of eating, however, may be relevant in some individuals, with nibbling apparently conferring greater proneness to weight gain than regular meals, for reasons which have never been clarified.

6. *Activity factors*. That exercise increases metabolic rate is clear, and it has already been identified that the calorigenic response to exercise is variable. It has been further shown that exercise patterns in the obese tend to be 'efficient' in terms of energy conservation, whereas in the slim population, jerkier day-to-day movements and higher levels of incidental activity are observed using time-lapse photography techniques, thereby identifying a window of opportunity in treatment planning.

7. *Psychological factors*. These are arguably the most important variables, primarily conditioning behavioural eating and exercise responses to life events, and at the same time playing an important part in the clinical expression of obesity once it is present: reference has already been made to the highly diverse body images which people carry of themselves.

Clinical features and complications

Weight gain can occur in any period of life. Of particular note is the incremental weight gain suffered by some women during successive pregnancies, and for which no explanation is currently valid. The pattern of fat distribution also varies, and is relevant to cardiovascular morbidity and mortality: abdominal obesity (manifest by a high waist/hip ratio) is more significant weight-for-weight than the generalized obesity associated with lower waist/hip ratios. The mechanism for induction of this higher atherosclerosis risk in the obese is probably multifactorial. Hyperlipidaemia is more likely to be present in the obese (see later), and the nutritional and exercise profiles which are themselves responsible for the obesity are also more atherogenic, with higher fat content and lower activity patterns being the most relevant components. The hyperinsulinaemia which is regularly present in obesity is also a significant factor, although the precise mechanisms of insulin-induced atherogenesis are still under evaluation.

Aside from myocardial infarction and stroke (the two major clinical consequences of atherosclerosis), hypertension and diabetes, both possibly triggered by the phenomenon of obesity-related insulin resistance, are the two major medical complications of obesity. In addition, osteoarthritis, cholelithiasis, postoperative chest, and thrombotic complications, as well as pedestrian accidents, are all more common in the overweight. Psychological consequences have already been alluded to: anxiety and depression are both more frequent in the obese, and it is often difficult to identify whether these aspects are causative or resultant.

Treatment

The natural history of obesity presents a dismal picture. Furthermore, follow-up studies of almost every intervention also show a singular pattern of failure, most particularly when treatment is imposed by the medical profession, rather than emanating out of any natural desire of the patient to achieve anything approaching weight normality. Many treatments also fail because of unrealistic patient expectations both of the magnitude and rate of weight loss reasonably achievable. Thus, fat catabolism alone is unlikely to result in a weight loss greater than 0.5 kg weekly: a negative energy balance resulting in any greater weight loss than this is likely to stem either from additional loss of body water (a diuresis is common in the first 2 to 3 weeks of any weight loss programme) or more seriously from protein catabolism from within bone and muscle. Accordingly, in any obesity treatment programme, it is desirable to set a 'contract of expectations' with the patient, incorporating target weight and rate of weight loss: in this way, both customer and provider are less likely to be disappointed!

Medical approaches invariably involve a combination of diet and exercise. Restriction to less than 1000 calories daily is not usually sustainable long-term in patients continuing normal activity patterns. Fad and formula diets are not encouraged, since they are expensive and antisocial, and therefore also cannot be adhered to except in the short term. Incorporating as much fibre as possible improves the important feeling of satiety. Sympathomimetic drugs suppress appetite by a direct hypothalamic effect, but tolerance and habituation occur quite readily, and even substituted amines, such as dexfenfluramine, which may have additional lipolytic effects, are only licensed for short-term (3 month) courses.

Psychological elements are important. Approximately 30 per cent of the population respond to stress by overeating (so-called comfort eating), and a significant sector of the obese population accordingly come from within this subgroup. Furthermore visual, olfactory, and even auditory cues are more relevant than genuine hunger in triggering appetite surges and hence food intake. If one adds to this the psychosocial consequences of obesity, then it is clear that psychological approaches, including group therapy, behavioural modification, and hypnosis may all be of benefit in selected cases. Patients tend to be particularly receptive to this line of treatment once initial weight loss has been achieved.

Surgical approaches are being increasingly used. The rather crude approach of jaw-wiring was found to result in excellent weight loss, but rapid regain once wires were removed, and outcome was not benefited by concurrent behaviour modification techniques. Only slightly less crude was the operation of jejuno-ileal bypass, which induced an artificial malabsorption syndrome. The multiple deficiencies over and above fat malabsorption and the inevitable loose and offensive stools were significant factors in the discontinuation of this approach. Reduction of gastric volume by a variety of banding and stapling procedures has given good results, but do not allow normal eating patterns in most patients: reversal of the procedure sometimes proves necessary.

It is likely that the phenomenon of obesity will forever represent a treatment challenge: innovatory approaches would be expected to be matched by a spectrum of side-effects which would limit their usefulness.

Hyperlipidaemia

Introduction and definitions

Atherosclerosis, with its major consequences of occlusive vascular disease in the coronary, cerebral, and peripheral circulation represents the largest single cause of mortality in Western populations, and increasingly of developing nations as well. Diet, hyperlipidaemia, and atherogenesis are intimately connected with one another, and this section will deal with this interrelationship and the influences of the endocrine system on the expression of atherosclerosis.

Not to be overlooked are the dual phenomena responsible for vascular occlusion: the development of the atherosclerotic plaque, which both narrows the vascular lumen and presents an irregular surface for thrombogenesis, is well recognized as having a direct relationship to hyperlipidaemia of various types. However, the subsequent occlusive event itself, with platelet aggregation as one of the primary processes is also directly dependent on circulating lipids and fatty acids. It may well be that the benefits of lipid lowering demonstrated through intervention studies, whether achieved by diet or drugs, are mediated as much by the inhibition of this latter thrombotic process than by effects on the vessel wall.

Since the serum concentrations of cholesterol and its subfractions, as well as triglyceride and lipoproteins are continuously distributed in the population, definition of abnormality is necessarily arbitrary: most studies involving analysis of risk factors show curvilinear relationships between circulating lipid fractions and risk of vascular events such as myocardial infarction. However, this curvilinear regression approaches a plateau of minimum risk at cholesterol levels approaching 5.2 mmol/l (200 mg/100 ml), LDL cholesterol 3.4 mmol/l (130 mg/100ml), and triglyceride 2.3 mmol/l (200 mg/100 ml). Other variables known to predict atherosclerosis risk are a high total cholesterol/HDL cholesterol ratio, and the combination of raised triglyceride and reduced HDL cholesterol, as well as increased concentrations of more recently identified lipoprotein (a).

It is important to recognize that in the process of atherogenesis, hyperlipidaemia represents only one component of a multifactorial process. Other major risk factors include smoking, obesity, hypertension, and diabetes mellitus. The effective reduction of atherosclerosis and its sequelae demands multiple risk factor interventions: over-obsession with correction of hyperlipidaemia alone is not in the interests either of the individual patient or of populations in general. However, there remains no doubt about the wisdom of lowering cholesterol as a population phenomenon: for every 1 per cent reduction in serum cholesterol, there is a 2 per cent reduction in coronary risk. The biochemical basis of this reduction is not clear. Both halting of progression as well as actual regression of atherosclerotic lesions has been documented by a number of sophisticated techniques. Furthermore, there is good evidence to support an adverse influence of lipoproteins and lipids on platelet function, such that proneness to thrombosis is likely to be reduced by maintenance of a normal lipid profile.

The following analysis of hyperlipidaemia will focus on two broad categories. Secondary hyperlipidaemia introduces the concept of a broad range of abnormalities where diet extremes and a wide range of other medical disorders and drugs result in an abnormal serum lipid profile. Primary or genetic hyperlipidaemia is less common but arguably more important in the understanding of atherogenesis. In practice, both forms may coexist, particularly in the context of diet exacerbating an underlying genetically determined abnormality of lipoprotein metabolism.

An important classification of hyper-lipoproteinaemia was initially devised by Fredrickson & Levy and subsequently adopted by the WHO. Type definitions and relative atherogenic risks conferred by the abnormal lipoprotein patterns are shown in Table 14.1.

Table 14.1. WHO classification of hyper-lipoproteinaemia types, based on Fredrickson and Levy. Lipid abnormalities (normal = N) and relative atherogenicity (ATH) of lipoprotein patterns.

Type	Lipoprotein abnormity	Plasma lipid patterns			ATH
		CHOL	TG	CHOL/TG	
I	CHYLOMICRONS +++ (VLDL and LDL N)	N or +	++	<0.2	0
IIa	LDL + VLDL N	+	N	>1.5	+++
IIb	LDL + VLDL +	+	+	VAR	+
III	Abnormal LDL + (IDL)	+	+	0.3–>2.0	++
IV	VLDL + LDL N	N	+	VAR	+
V	CHYLOMICRONS + VLDL +	+	+	0.2–0.6	+

Secondary hyperlipidaemia

Nutritional and obesity related hyperlipidaemia

The importance of diet has been repeatedly emphasized in the genesis of raised serum lipid levels. Its importance is exemplified by the Ni–Hon–San study in which genetically similar Japanese were studied in three immigrant residential locations; Japan, Honolulu, and San Francisco. Diet was the significant variable, with higher body weight, total and saturated fat as well as cholesterol intake in the two American groups. These differences were paralleled by higher serum cholesterol and coronary heart disease event frequency in the American locations.

Cholesterol dietary excess is itself responsible for a rise in serum cholesterol, which is enhanced in individuals with a low polyunsaturated/saturated fat intake. At the same time, LDL receptors are down-regulated, and the number of LDL particles thereby increased.

Saturated fats, as commonly encountered in animal-derived and dairy products, all raise cholesterol levels, roughly in proportion to the number of double bonds in the fats concerned, also acting by down-regulating LDL receptors.

Mono- and polyunsaturated fats have a reducing effect on cholesterol. The major component of the monounsaturated group is oleic acid, as found in olive and rapeseed oil. Fish oils, which are rich in the omega-3 essential fatty acids, and leaf and seed oils rich in omega-6 fatty acids, such as linoleic and arachidonic, acids also lower serum triglyceride levels by a mechanism which currently defies explanation.

Total calories consumed directly relate to increased production of VLDL and reduced HDL. Triglyceride levels rise as body weight increases. This pattern is characteristic of the lipid profile in obesity, and is directly reversible by weight reduction. Alcohol is a potent cause of hypertriglyceridaemia, increasing hepatic synthesis of this lipid. This excess triglyceride is incorporated into VLDL. Any coexistent genetic or acquired defect in clearing VLDL (see later) will increase the likelihood of developing chylomicronaemia. In an extreme form, the so-called 'chylomicronaemia syndrome' develops, characterized by abdominal pain (pancreatitis), eruptive xanthomata, lipaemia retinalis, and neurological deficit in the form of dementia and peripheral neuropathy. Alcohol has no effect on LDL, but does increase HDL levels, possibly representing the mechanism for the significantly reduced prevalence of atherosclerosis in moderate drinkers.

Obesity, as indicated earlier, is logically the end result of positive energy balance. The resulting lipid profile will depend on the nutritional origins of the calorie excess, but the combination of high triglyceride and reduced HDL is typical, and is responsible for the substantial atherogenicity of obesity.

Diabetes mellitus

Lipid disturbances in diabetes are common and complex.

Insulin deficiency (as encountered in insulin-dependent diabetes) results in raised triglyceride and reduced HDL serum levels, and probably explains the demonstrated atherogenicity of uncontrolled diabetes. Restoration of normoglycaemia by adequate insulization corrects these changes. The subsequent development of diabetic nephropathy is associated with the acquisition of additional abnormalities also described later in this chapter: triglyceride, cholesterol, and LDL levels rise, and HDL levels fall, making this complication one of the most potent atherogenic settings. Non-insulin-dependent diabetes provides a higher prevalence of dyslipidaemia, with hypertriglyceridaemia and a reduced HDL level being encountered in up to 30 per cent of cases. The insulin resistance which is central to the aetiology of the hyperglycaemia promotes lipolysis in adipose tissue and increases delivery of free fatty acids to the liver. The reduced lipoprotein lipase activity also encountered in insulin resistance further reduces VLDL clearance. Thiazide or loop diuretics or the addition of beta blocking drugs with or without concomitant excess of alcohol can induce quite severe forms of chylomicronaemia syndrome. In contrast to insulin-dependent diabetes, quality of glycaemic control appears to have little bearing on the lipid profile. However, supervening nephropathy carries with it both deterioration in lipid profile as well as the additional cardiovascular risk outlined above.

Renal disease

Nephrotic syndrome is a potent cause of elevated VLDL with consequent hypertriglyceridaemia, and also LDL (with hypercholesterolaemia), but mostly a normal HDL. The mechanism is probably linked to hypoalbuminaemia which is thought to non-specifically activate hepatic protein production. Additional, as yet uncharacterized abnormalities may explain the dyslipidaemia seen even with normal serum albumin, and in which raised lipoprotein (a) may be a dominant feature.

Chronic renal failure is associated with quite striking reductions in hepatic lipase and postheparin lipolytic activity. Hypertriglyceridaemia is a result of raised VLDL triglyceride levels, with normal LDL and cholesterol levels. A distinct abnormal VLDL can be identified in some cases, with an unusual apolipoprotein composition. HDL levels are often low. Interest has recently focused on an apparent ability of hyperlipidaemia itself to accelerate deterioration of renal function: correction of hyperlipidaemia may therefore be important not only in the context of vascular protection, but also as a renoprotective manoeuvre.

Liver disease

Since the liver performs both synthetic and clearance roles in regard to lipoprotein metabolism, it is not surprising that dyslipidaemia is common in hepatic dysfunction.

Cholestasis occurs both as a consequence of extrahepatic obstruction, as well as with drug-induced cholestasis and primary biliary cirrhosis. In all these conditions serum cholesterol is markedly raised, sometimes sufficient to produce cutaneous xanthomata. The hypercholesterolaemia may be partly due to cholesterol 'back-diffusion' from bile into the hepatic parenchyma, but increasing evidence supports a lack of LDL clearance due to defective LDL receptors, as well as deficient activity of hepatic lipase and LCAT. An abnormal lipoprotein (LP-X) has also been identified in some cases. Triglyceride is raised but HDL commonly normal.

Hepatic parenchymal disease provides a confusing picture, since alcohol excess (a common cause of hepatic dysfunction) frequently coexists, with a profile alluded to earlier in this section. A wide range of abnormalities has been recorded, most commonly a raised total, but normal HDL, cholesterol. Advanced liver disease often results in uniformly low lipoprotein concentrations.

Endocrinopathies

Hypothyroidism has long been recognized as a cause of reversible hypercholesterolaemia: 5–10 per cent of patients with serum cholesterol above 7.0 mmol/l have raised serum TSH levels, and hypertriglyceridaemia is also seen in this situation. Reduced lipoprotein lipase and LDL receptor activity have been documented as the major causes of the abnormalities. The hypercholesterolaemia may cause xanthelasmata, and also represents a significant coronary risk factor, which is, of course, totally correctable. Depending on associated genetic traits the lipid profile can trigger the chylomicronaemia syndrome referred to earlier.

Hypo-androgenism is associated with increased longevity. Together with a reduction in atherosclerotic manifestations, this phenomenon may be lipid-mediated, since HDL levels are high and LDL levels low, changes which are promptly reversed by androgen administration. Androgens appear to exert their adverse effect by increasing hepatic lipase activity.

Hypo-oestrogenism results in opposite biochemical changes, with low HDL and raised LDL levels. These findings are in keeping with the accelerated atherosclerotic process which can be demonstrated in postmenopausal women, and which can be prevented by unopposed oestrogen administration. Higher-dose oestrogen administration causes an even greater fall in LDL, probably due to a reduction in hepatic lipase and a lesser reduction of lipoprotein lipase activity. The addition of progestogens has important consequences which need to be kept in mind, since progestogens are so commonly co-administered to the non-hysterectomized post-menopausal woman. The more commonly used androgenic (19-nortestosterone-derived) progestogens partially reverse the advantageous HDL and LDL changes consequent upon oestrogen replacement. In contrast, pregnane-derived progestogens, such as medroxyprogesterone, are virtually devoid of lipoproptein effects. Since hormone replacement therapy (HRT) has a promising role for long-term reduction in atherosclerotic risk (see Chapter 8), this finding has an important bearing on the formulation of HRT programmes. Glucocorticoids raise both VLDL and LDL levels. The mechanism of these changes is not clear.

Drugs

Several drugs commonly used in patients with complications of atherosclerosis, or in disorders which themselves represent vascular risk factors, have adverse effects on the lipid profile. Diuretics both of the loop and thiazide type elevate LDL and triglyceride and reduce HDL levels, with indapamide and spironolactone having the least effects.

Beta blockers of both the cardio- and non-selective types produce a similar profile of changes.

Alpha blockers, ACE inhibitors and calcium channel blockers have no lipoprotein effects, and for this reason may represent preferred drugs in the treatment of the younger patient.

Retinoids, as used in the treatment of refractory acne, raise VLDL and LDL cholesterol, with corresponding rises of cholesterol and triglyceride. HDL levels fall.

Oral contraceptives have effects which depend on the progestational agent used in the formulation. Those with progesterone-derived progestogens have very little effect on lipids on the low doses now used. In contrast, some increase in both LDL and triglyceride is seen when the progestogen is 19-nortestosterone derived.

Primary (genetic) hyperlipidaemia

A wide variety of abnormalities of lipid transport have been described, with differing modes of inheritance. The clinical expression of these disorders is often modified and complicated by nutritional status, or by one or more of the above secondary processes. The congenital nature of all these disorders, and the fact that many of the resulting lipid profiles are strikingly atherogenic has led to a critical appraisal of population screening programmes. With the potent drugs now available for treatment, cost–benefit and benefit–risk ratios need to be carefully considered. Only the major disorders of this group will be described in this book, and the reader is referred to the bibliography for more detailed discussion of the less common disorders.

Familial hypercholesterolaemia

The group of conditions which constitute this entity represent significant precursors of coronary artery disease, and come within the category of Fredrickson type IIa hyperlipidaemia. The biochemical changes are due to more than 10 discrete molecular defects of the LDL receptor, all of which are inherited as autosomal dominants. The heterozygote population frequency of any one of these genes is about 1:500, so that the frequency of either homozygote or double heterozygote is approximately 1:1 000 000. Heterozygotes have reduced, and homozygotes absent LDL receptor activity, with corresponding elevations of circulating LDL and cholesterol levels. The consequence is an acceleration of atherosclerosis, particularly of the coronary vessels, with clinical symptoms of angina and infarction occurring in the twenties and thirties in the homozygote, and as early as the forties in heterozygotes.

There is often abnormal deposition of lipid in the form of corneal arcus (see Plate 14.1) as well as tendon and tuberous xanthomata, even in heterozygotes. With diet and drugs, as outlined later, LDL and cholesterol levels can be largely normalized in heterozygotes, while regression of xanthomata can be expected in both heterozygotes and homozygotes. Reduced frequency of cardiovascular events has also been documented. Liver transplantation has been used to provide a source of effective LDL receptors, and plasmapharesis has been used as a method of removing the abnormal lipoproteins. In the future, gene therapy may prove feasible.

Familial hypertriglyceridaemia/combined hyperlipidaemia

This group of conditions also carry increased proneness to coronary artery disease, due to marked elevations of VLDL, and in the combined form with LDL as well. They come within the category of Fredrickson type IIb or IV hyperlipidaemia. Some patients are obese, some have corneal arcus, and some are hypertensive. Severe forms may have lipaemia retinalis, eruptive xanthomata, and hepatomegaly. Particularly in this group, differentiation from the acquired forms of mixed hyperlipidaemia can be difficult. They are inherited as autosomal dominants, but the genes have not been identified. Population prevalence is about 1:300. Whereas the individual lipid abnormalities can be effectively treated in most instances and cutaneous manifestations regress, the reversibility of coronary proneness has not been proven.

Familial chylomicronaemia

This represents a small group of rare, autosomal recessive disorders resulting from deficiencies of either lipoprotein lipase or apo C-II. Serum triglyceride concentrations are markedy raised, with chylomicrons imparting an opalescent or creamy character to serum stored at 4 °C. The syndrome corresponds with the

Fredrickson type I classification. Clinical features include hepatosplenomegaly, extensive eruptive xanthomas, and abdominal pain due to pancreatitis. Fat restriction, with or without fibrate therapy, is very successful in reversing the clinical features.

Strategic approach to the common hyperlipidaemias

Identification

Many cases of hyperlipidaemia encountered in clinical practice are, as outlined earlier, due to acquired causes. However, correction of these causes does not invariably restore circulating normality, suggesting additional sporadic genetic factors, which do not fall into the traditional familial patterns outlined above. In practice, most cases of hyperlipidaemia are identified by opportunistic or systematic screening programmes. In an adult population, about 50 per cent would be expected to have a serum cholesterol above 5.2 mmol/l (200 mg/100 ml), 25 per cent above 6.5 mmol/l (250 mg/100 ml), and 5 per cent above 7.4 mmol/l (285 mg/100 ml). Lipid profiles which include triglyceride, LDL, and HDL assays, as well as total cholesterol, have become commonplace, although possibly unnecessary. This is because the cardiovascular benefits of normalizing triglyceride and particularly HDL, although suggestive from present studies, are not yet conclusive. Restricting the 'full' profile to patients who have already shown serum cholesterol elevation might, at present, be more appropriate. In general, primary (i.e. general health) lipid screening may not be cost-effective, and indeed is potentially anxiety-provoking: diagnosis of hyperlipidaemia often leads to the use of lipid-lowering drugs which are expensive, and individual patients cannot be assured of beneficial effects either on morbidity or mortality, since treatment is usually initiated quite late in life. This has led to the alternative proposal that rather than primary screening, efforts should be concentrated on changing population trends in vascular risk factors, particularly in terms of smoking, exercise, body weight, and overall nutritional profile. Even with this approach, selective screening of those with past or family history of ischaemic cardiac events would remain entirely appropriate. Further research in the next few years will probably clarify the respective roles of these two major management strategies.

Nevertheless, there is now ample evidence that lowering abnormally raised serum cholesterol in patients who have already sustained a myocardial infarct (secondary screening and intervention) is beneficial in terms or reducing subsequent cardiovascular events, although this approach is far from universally practised. Furthermore, recent research now suggests similar reduction of coronary mortality in previously healthy but hypercholesterolaemic subjects treated with statins.

Management

Achievement of a serum cholesterol less than 5.2 mmol/l (200 mg/100 ml) cannot be assured, whatever treatment is employed. Between 5.2 and 7.4 mmol/l, the intensity of approach depends on the presence of other risk factors and age: comparative youth and a 'strong' family history would justify more vigorous intervention.

Diet remains the fundamental treatment of all hyperlipidaemias, and probably at all ages, although above a cholesterol level of 7.4 mmol/l, it is unlikely that diet alone will suffice. Weight reduction to a BMI of less than 25 is essential, and needs to be linked to increased exercise and abolition of smoking. Total fat calories are reduced to less than 30 per cent and saturated to less than 10 per cent of total calories. Dietary cholesterol is limited to a maximum 300 mg daily. For hypertriglyceridaemia, restriction of refined carbohydrate and alcohol is also advised.

Following 6 months of diet, persistent cholesterol elevation above 7.4 mmol/l (285 mg/100 ml) without, and 6.5 mmol/l (250 mg/100 ml) with other risk factors, is an indication for drug therapy using one of the HMG-CoA reductase inhibitors (statin) group of drugs, except in the elderly. At lower cholesterol levels, previous or family history of myocardial infarction may prompt use of statins.

As referred to earlier, normalization of triglyceride and HDL concentrations, although logical, is not yet universally recommended. However, particularly with either hereditary or acquired mixed hyperlipidaemia, the fibrate group of drugs are very effective. They increase LDL receptor activity (and hence lower LDL and cholesterol levels) and also stimulate lipoprotein lipase activity (hence lowering VLDL and triglyceride levels). HDL levels also rise, although the precise mechanism is unclear. If the current data suggesting a reduction of 3–4 per cent in coronary risk for every 1 per cent rise in HDL is confirmed, fibrates will be far more frequently used. Serum triglyceride levels approaching 10 mmol/l indicate a risk of pancreatitis and chylomicronaemia syndrome (see earlier). Hypertriglyceridaemia of this degree should therefore be treated by diet in the first instance, and subsequently by using a fibrate.

Other drugs which are sometimes used in hyperlipidaemia are the nicotinic acid derivatives (which inhibit VLDL synthesis and hence are very useful in hypertriglyceridaemia), bile acid sequestrants (which both increase LDL receptor activity and stimulate cholesterol oxidation), and fish oils (which inhibit synthesis of VLDL).

FURTHER READING

Bray, G.A. (1987). Overweight is risking fate: definition, classification prevalence and risks. *Annals of the New York Academy of Science*, **499**, 14–28.

D'Allessio, D.A., Kavle, E.C., Mozzoli, M.A., *et al.* (1988). Thermic effect of food in lean and obese men. *Journal of Clinical Investigation*, **81**, 1781–9.

Durrington, P.N. (1995). Lipoprotein (a). *Clinical Endocrinology and Metabolism*, **9**, 773–96.

Jiang H., Kryger, M.H., Zorick, F.J., *et al.* (1988). Mortality and apnea index in obstructive sleep apnea. *Chest*, **94**, 9–14.

Kopelman, P.G. (1994). Investigation of obesity. *Clinical Endocrinology*, **41**, 703–8.

Schonfeld, G. (1990). The genetic dyslipoproteinemias. *Atherosclerosis*, **81**, 81–90.

Packard, C.J. (1995). The rôle of stable isotopes in the investigation of plasma lipoprotein metabolism. *Endocrinology and Metabolism*, **9**, 755–72.

Thompson, G.R. (1993). Treatment of hyperlipidaemia. *Clinical Endocrinology*, **38**, 337–42.

15

Ectopic hormone syndromes: production of hormones by non-endocrine tumours

INTRODUCTION

Polypeptide hormones can be secreted by many tumours which arise in organs not normally associated with endocrine activity. These frequently malignant tumours of non-endocrine tissue may induce clinical syndromes which are similar to that of hypersecretion of the appropriate endocrine gland. When this occurs, it is usually referred to as 'ectopic' secretion, or a paraneoplastic endocrine syndrome.

Even when an obvious endocrine syndrome is not clinically apparent, the assay for certain hormones in patients with malignant disease reveals elevated values in many subjects. It is assumed that either the hormone has been secreted over an insufficient period of time, or in insufficient quantities to produce the clinical syndrome in question. Alternatively, the hormone secreted, although assayable, may be biologically inactive in the patient, because of very minor variation in amino acid sequence. Confusion has also arisen from the reciprocal situation: biological activity in the absence of assayability, again due largely to variation in molecular configuration.

The finding of an elevated hormone level in association with a tumour does not, of course, imply that the tumour in question is producing it. Thus, in order to characterize an entity justifying the title of an 'ectopic hormone syndrome', it was considered incumbent on a researcher to satisfy a number of criteria:

1. Association of hormone excess with a tumour cell type not normally associated with hormone production.
2. Association with a defined clinical endocrine excess syndrome.
3. An increased concentration of the relevant hormone in blood.
4. Identification both of the relevant hormone in tumour cells, and establishment of an arteriovenous concentration gradient across the tumour circulation (implying that the tumour is actually producing the hormone).
5. Reversal of the clinical syndrome and elevated hormone levels by tumour removal.
6. Ability to demonstrate autonomous hormone production when the relevant tumour cells are cultured *in vitro*.

The frequency of various syndromes in patients with neoplastic disease is not easy to define, since the full clinical picture may only occur terminally, and may be submerged by other manifestations of malignant disease. Furthermore, since it is clearly not feasible or indeed justifiable to satisfy all the criteria-listed above in an individual patient, there is a tendency for mere identification of one elevated hormone level to be immediately classified as 'ectopic'. This is particularly relevant to cortisol, whose random level is frequently elevated in advanced or terminal malignant disease, reflecting a stress state rather than any ectopic secretion process.

Nevertheless, continued awareness of the syndromes is essential for a number of reasons: (1) they may antedate appearance of the tumour, and thus masquerade as a primary endocrine problem; (2) they may be responsible for a significant proportion of the disability of malignant disease and be independently readily treatable; (3) they may represent appropriate tumour markers for judging the activity of the disease in response to therapy.

It should also be remembered that not all peptides produced by tumours are in fact hormones; carcinoembryonic antigen (CEA) and alpha-fetoprotein (AFP) are tumour markers in their own right without known metabolic activity.

Pathogenesis

The recognition that tumours may secrete a comparatively wide range of hormones has naturally led to a great deal of speculation on how this might arise. The most probable explanation appears to be that when a cell becomes neoplastic, sections of the genome which are normally repressed may become available for transcription. This explains why only polypeptide hormones have so far been conclusively shown to be produced ectopically: the production of a steroid, for instance, would require a complex enzymatic pathway to be developed, which seems an extremely improbable consequence of random de-repression. As it is also debatable whether prostaglandins can be synthesized by tumours, the theory is still tenable.

One problem with the de-repression theory is that it does not explain why certain types of tumour preferentially secrete particular hormones. If de-repression were random, one might expect the type of hormone produced to be also random, apart from being polypeptide in structure.

A possible explanation for this specificity of hormone production by tumours is given by the theory that the cells which produce such hormones when they undergo neoplastic change have a common embryological derivation, and in particular that they are APUD cells. These cells have the potential for amine precursor uptake and decarboxylation (APUD), (e.g. of the neurotransmitters dopamine and serotonin) and have specific staining activities that identify APUD cells in whichever tissue they are present. The APUD cells, embryologically derived from the neural crest, are responsible not only for the formation of the central nervous system and sympathetic ganglia, but are known to migrate into the mucosa of the gastrointestinal tract, and into various endocrine organs as well as the lung. When appropriate histological stains are used, the amazing ubiquity of these cell types can be readily demonstrated.

The physiological hormones produced by APUD cells are either amines or peptides. Benign or malignant tumours of APUD cells (colloquially referred to as 'apudomas') depending on their site, induce well-recognized clinical syndromes. For example, the carcinoid syndrome is produced by enterochromaffin cells in various parts of the gastrointestinal tract (and occasionally lung). The syndrome consists of diarrhoea (due to serotonin and histamine) and sweating (due to catecholamines). The diagnosis can be easily confirmed by measuring the 24-hour excretion of 5-hydroxyindole acetic acid, a urinary metabolite of serotonin.

These features do not, strictly speaking, represent an ectopic syndrome. However, in some cases, particularly in bronchial carcinoid tumours, adrenocorticotrophin is produced (with the corresponding symptoms and signs described in Chapter 5) in addition to the substances mentioned above: it is postulated that in this case de-repression of the APUD cell has occurred. A further specific example of probable APUD cell de-repression is seen in medullary carcinoma of the thyroid, where the characteristic cell type is the thyroid parafollicular C-cell of APUD cell origin. In almost all cases of primary and metastatic tumour, C-cell-derived calcitonin production has represented a tumour marker, useful both for diagnosis and for monitoring response to therapy. Other peptides (e.g. bradykinins) and amines (e.g. serotonin) are produced in varying amounts by this tumour, and are probably responsible for the diarrhoea and flushing which form the particular features of the metastatic syndrome. Presumed de-repression is also responsible for the ectopic adrenocorticotrophin production seen in the high proportion of the metastatic cases.

In summary, at the present time the process of gene de-repression both of the APUD cells as well as a variety of other cell types is considered to be the more likely link between the neoplastic process and the excess hormone syndrome. Summaries of the major ectopic syndromes are outlined below.

Ectopic corticotrophin syndrome (see Plate 15.1)

The most common tumour is a small-cell carcinoma of the lung, but carcinoid and C-cell tumours (particularly in patients with multiple endocrine neoplasia: MEN-II) as well as thymoma and phaeochromocytoma are quite frequently the cause. The clinical syndrome is characterized by a rapidly developing form of Cushing's syndrome, where the mineralocorticoid effects of fluid retention (causing oedema and hypertension) and hypokalaemia (producing gross weakness) often dominate the clinical picture. The more glucocorticoid-related obesity and facial plethora are less frequently seen except in slower growing tumours (particularly C-cell), because these latter features take longer to develop.

Investigations show very high levels of urinary and plasma cortisol which are non-suppressible by exogenous steroid in the conventional dexamethasone suppression tests. Plasma corticotrophin levels are often, but not necessarily, extremely high. Accordingly, diagnostic confusion with pituitary-dependent Cushing's syndrome can still occur. Other POMC-derived peptides, such as β-MSH, γ-lipotropin, and corticotropin-like intermediate lobe peptide, are usually also present in high concentration in contrast to the pituitary-dependent variety of

Cushing's disease, and thus may be used for diagnostic definition in difficult cases. Corticotrophin-releasing hormone (CRH), which produces a normal or exaggerated ACTH response in pituitary-dependent cases, usually has no effect in the ectopic ACTH syndrome.

Correction of the syndrome is not usually feasible by treatment of the underlying tumour since most cases are already metastatic at the time of diagnosis, but adrenal blocking drugs such as metyrapone (2 g daily) or ketoconazole (600–1200 mg daily) with or without aminoglutethamide (750–1500 mg daily), can be used to provide satisfactory clinical benefit in many cases. Occasionally, even bilateral adrenalectomy is justified.

A small number of cases of ectopic CRH syndrome have been reported. Clinical features and management are identical to the ectopic ACTH syndrome.

Ectopic vasopressin (AVP) syndrome

The most common tumour responsible for this syndrome is again the small-cell bronchial carcinoma as well as a wide variety of less common tumours, including liver, colon, prostate, and adrenal cortex; Hodgkin's disease has also been recorded. As many as 40 per cent of subjects with oat-cell carcinoma have elevated AVP levels. It has been shown that elevated AVP levels may in some cases be derived from resetting of the hypothalamic osmostat rather than being of tumour origin. However, if thirst control mechanisms are intact there is insufficient AVP to necessarily induce either clinical or even biochemical consequences. The full syndrome is characterized by nausea and vomiting, with lethargy and headache, confusion, and coma leading directly to death in some cases. All these symptoms and signs can be attributed to water retention, consequent on fluid overload which may be readily induced during various therapeutic procedures.

The biochemical hallmark is a dilutional hyponatraemia with serum sodium levels occasionally as low as 105 mmol/l. The differential diagnosis of causes of this clinical and biochemical picture of SIADH is considered in greater detail in Chapter 4.

Fluid restriction to 500 ml daily is the immediate therapeutic approach followed by surgical removal of the tumour if at all possible. Various drugs, such as demeclocycline or lithium, have been used with the purpose of inducing a nephrogenic form of diabetes insipidus, and are usually effective and well tolerated.

Ectopic hypercalcaemia

Bone metastases are clearly a possible cause of hypercalcaemia seen in association with extensive malignant disease. Cases of haematological malignancy, such as multiple myeloma, induce hypercalcaemia by elaborating cytokines and prostaglandins, and as such qualify as causes of ectopic hypercalcaemia of a specific type. The fact that immunoreactive parathormone (PTH), when measured by the newer specific assays for 'intact' PTH, is clearly suppressed in most cases of tumour-associated hypercalcaemia provided difficulties in understanding the syndrome, until PTH-related peptide (PTHRP) was identified. This 139-amino acid peptide is now acknowledged to be the major hypercalcaemic tumour product. It has actions identical to native parathormone since its 1–34 sequence is homologous with native PTH (but does not react in the intact molecule PTH assay) and stimulates urinary cyclic AMP secretion in an identical manner to parathormone. A few cases of malignancy-associated hypercalcaemia have been shown to be due to high 1,25 dihydroxy-vitamin D levels, presumably synthesized in tumours analogous to the behaviour of sarcoid granulomas.

Clinically, the hypercalcaemic features are often severe (see Chapter 11) and are often associated with an unexplained hypokalaemic alkalosis rather than the hyperchloraemic acidosis seen in primary hyperparathyroidism. Almost all malignant tumours have been at least occasionally reported in association with hypercalcaemia, although by their very frequency, bronchogenic carcinoma is the most likely to be encountered in clinical practice.

Immediate and maintained rehydration using normal saline or occasionally sodium sulphate represents the central point of therapy, since patients are often dehydrated. This may be due to the underlying disease, with or without the additional effect of renal water loss due to hypercalcaemic renal tubular damage. Pamidronate (30 mg by slow infusion in one litre of saline) almost predictably lowers serum calcium by 1–2 mmol/l, and can be repeated as necessary. Phosphate supplementation is also useful as a therapeutic tool: many patients with less progressive forms of malignant disease can by symptomatically helped by the administration of 1–1.5 g of elemental phosphate daily, given as effervescent tablets. Long-term use, however, risks the development of ectopic (soft tissue) calcification.

Ectopic hypoglycaemia

The classical associations are with mesenchyme-derived tumours such as mesotheliomas, fibromas, and sarcomas. These are characterized by being very large tumours averaging 2.5 kg. It was postulated that insulin was being synthesized, but although tumour extracts may have insulin-like activity in bio-assay systems, insulin itself has not been identified except in rare cases. Subsequently, IGF-II has been sometimes found in both serum and tumour extracts, with reduced serum IGF-I. The hypoglycaemia is likely to be induced either by excessive glucose metabolism by the tumour, or more commonly by IGF-II-mediated enhanced glucose utilization, possibly coupled to suppressed somatotrophin production. Treatment with diazoxide has been successful in some cases.

Ectopic gonadotrophin

Tumours of trophoblastic cells, both choriocarcinoma as well as teratoma frequently secrete gonadotrophins; whether this is truly 'ectopic' is semantic. Gynaecomastia in males and menstrual irregularity in females may be seen. Furthermore, since TSH shares the α-subunit of hCG, hyperthyroidism is quite often also apparent. Small quantities of chorionic gonadotrophin (CG) can be identified in most non-malignant cell systems. Tumours associated with high detectable levels are thought to preferentially glycosylate CG, also rendering it biologically more active. Hepatoma and oat-cell carcinoma appear to be particularly capable of synthesizing gonadotrophin and late-onset gynaecomastia should always raise the suspicion of one of these diagnoses.

Ectopic thyrotrophin

This is rare, but most frequently reported with choriocarcinoma, since gonadotrophin shares an α-subunit with thyrotrophin (see above). In the extreme concentrations encountered in trophoblastic tumours, sufficient α-subunit is secreted to stimulate the thyroid. Biochemical hyperthyroidism is quite common, but the clinical manifestations are less readily apparent, being occasionally submerged by the general 'toxic' clinical picture of metastatic disease. Once again bronchogenic and also ovarian carcinoma has been occasionally reported in association with thyrotrophin excess.

Ectopic somatotrophin and GHRH syndromes

Bronchial carcinoid tumours have been reported in association with acromegaly. Both hGH and GHRH have been isolated from tumours, and acromegalic features have been shown to regress as a result of successful tumour therapy. Ectopic hGH has also been reported with non-carcinoid bronchogenic carcinoma.

Ectopic erythropoietin

Polycythaemia as a consequence of erythropoietin excess is encountered most commonly with renal cell carcinoma and hepatoma, and to a lesser extent with certain benign renal lesions and cerebellar haemangioblastomas. Occasionally, reversal of polycythaemia is encountered with successful treatment of the tumour, although the syndrome may be metastatic by the time the ectopic syndrome is clinically apparent.

Other ectopic syndromes

A variety of tumours (especially of prostate and mesenchyme) have been reported in association with hypophosphataemic osteomalacia, often associated with low 1,25-dihydroxy-vitamin D levels. Calcitonin, typically a product of parafollicular C-cells, has also been reported in association with bronchial, colonic, breast, and gastric tumours. Various neurological paraneoplastic syndromes have been reported: although it has been proposed that some humoural agent is responsible, proof has not been forthcoming. There is rather more evidence that these syndromes are antibody-mediated.

FURTHER READING

Daughaday, W., Emanuele, M.A., Brooks, M.H., *et al.* (1988). Synthesis and secretion of insulin-like growth factor II by a leiomyosarcoma with associated hypoglycaemia. *New England Journal of Medicine*, **319**, 1434-40.

Goldberg, M.A., Glass, G.A., Cunningham, J.M., *et al.* (1987). The regulated expression of erythropoeitin by two human hepatoma cell lines. *Proceedings of the National Academy of Sciece*, USA, **84**, 7972–6.

Gutierrez, G.E. Poser, J.W., Katz, M.S., *et al.* (1990). Mechanism of hypercalcaemia of malignancy. *Clinical Endocrinology and Metabolism,* **4**, 119–38.

Hirata, Y., Matsukura, S., Imura, H., *et al.* (1976). Two cases of multiple hormone producing small cell carcinoma of the lung: co-existence of tumor ADH, ACTH and B-MSH. *Cancer*, **38**, 2575–82.

White, A. and Clark, H.A.L. (1993). The cellular and molecular basis of the ectopic ACTH syndrome. *Clinical Endocrinology*,. **39**, 131–42.

16

Multiple endocrine syndromes

MULTIPLE ENDOCRINE NEOPLASIA

Introduction

Several decades after the initial description of this interesting group of familial disorders, it is becoming clear that they also provide a unique insight into the natural history of endocrine disorders resulting from single gland hyperfunction of the sporadic type. Previous understanding was limited by the fact that at the time of initial clinical diagnosis, sporadic hyperfunctioning endocrine tumours have almost certainly been present for many years. Of even greater application is the molecular biology of MEN syndromes. This introduces opportunities for genetic screening, earlier diagnosis and treatment, and ultimately even gene therapy. This again allows speculation on the mechanisms of oncogenesis in the more prevalent sporadic endocrine tumours. (See Table 16.1 for the components of four MEN syndromes.)

Multiple endocrine neoplasia type I

Although the gene responsible for this syndrome has not yet been identified, it has been shown to reside on chromosome 11, and the condition is inherited as an autosomal dominant with almost complete penetrance. Prevalence is of the order of 1:5000. Even in the absence of gene identity, considerable knowledge has accrued, and it is likely that mutant oncogenes (which are the basis of proliferative and stimulated cell function) and/or deleted tumour suppressor genes (which can be inactivated as a consequence of mutations) are fundamental to the pathophysiology of this tumour syndrome. The potentially related retinoblastoma suppressor gene has been shown to be inactivated in the abnormal parathyroid tissue taken from some MEN-I cases. Studies using linked polymorphic DNA sequences from affected probands have made it possible to identify gene carriers. This approach to the kindred of MEN-I probands is just as important as the management of the probands themselves, and creates a major diagnostic and management challenge.

Clinical features

As indicated above, three organ systems are potentially involved, but not necessarily simultaneously. Hyperparathyroidism eventually develops in over 90 per cent of probands, but islet cell tumours are the presenting feature in about 60 per cent of newly diagnosed patients. Autopsy data reveal pituitary adenomas in more than

Table 16.1. Components of the four MEN syndromes

MEN type I
Parathyroid adenoma or hyperplasia (hyperparathyroidism)
Pancreatic islet tumour (insulinoma, gastrinoma, somatostatinoma)
Pituitary adenoma (non-functioning, prolactinoma, acromegaly or ACTH-dependent Cushing's syndrome)*
Small bowel tumours (carcinoid syndrome)*
Differentiated thyroid carcinoma*
Non-functioning adrenal adenomas*
Lipomas*
MEN type IIa
Parathyroid hyperplasia (hyperparathyroidism)
Adrenal medullary tumour (phaeochromocytoma)
C-cell tumours (medullary thyroid carcinoma)
MEN type IIb
C-cell tumours (medullary thyroid carcinoma)
Adrenal medullary tumour (phaeochromocytoma)
Marfanoid features, multiple cutaneous and mucosal neuromas, neurofibromas, and gastrointestinal ganglioneuromas
FMTC
Familial medullary thyroid carcinoma (alone)

*These disorders are rare.

two-thirds of cases, but biochemical hypersecretion is only identifiable in about half this number during life. The clinical diagnosis in probands is usually made by the age of 50, while as a consequence of family screening, affected individuals within the kindred are usually diagnosed 20–30 years earlier.

The parathyroid lesions are initially mostly asymptomatic. However, in contrast to the sporadic forms of hyperparathyroidism, where serum calcium can remain remarkably stable for many years, serum calcium rises progressively in MEN-I cases, with quite rapid evolution of hypercalcaemic manifestations identical to those seen in sporadic cases: fatigue, nephrolithiasis, myopathy, and arthralgia. Dyspepsia is often present, and may in part be due to a coexistent gastrinoma. Histologically, the hyperparathyroidism is usually caused initially by parathyroid hyperplasia, with multifocal adenomas being superimposed over a period of time. The diagnosis is confirmed by simultaneously demonstrating hypercalcaemia and raised levels of serum PTH, ideally by intact molecule assay (see also Chapter 10).

The pancreatic islet lesions are also usually multifocal. The initial hyperplastic process within the islets is referred to as nesidioblastosis, in some cases appearing to be a re-differentiation of duct epithelium. Although the tumours often secrete multiple hormones, one (most frequently gastrin) predominates with severe and sometimes drug-resistant ulcer dyspepsia as seen in sporadic cases of gastrinoma. The hyperacidity can induce diarrhoea to complete the clinical picture of the Zollinger–Ellison syndrome. Insulinoma is the next most frequent hypersecretory syndrome, with classical symptoms of hypoglycaemia as outlined in Chapter 11. Both of the above tumour types often cosecrete pancreatic polypeptide (PP), glucagon, somatostatin and/or vasoactive intestinal peptide (VIP). In fact, hyper-responsiveness of serum PP and gastrin to a standard mixed meal can be used as a diagnostic procedure to identify early pancreatic tumours. At the time of surgery, more than 50 per cent of gastrinomas but considerably fewer insulinomas are found to be malignant, of which a proportion will already be metastatic.

The pituitary lesions may take the form of non-functioning adenomas, producing symptoms only by their mass effect (see Chapter 4): cases identified from kindred screening may have quite substantial tumours by the age of 20, with no apparent secretory activity. Ultimately, the biochemical and clinical features characteristic of prolactinoma, ACTH (Cushing's disease) or growth hormone (acromegaly) excess become apparent in about 50 per cent of cases. The diagnosis is made using the previously described basal and dynamic function tests, coupled to high-quality MRI scanning.

Management

Once hypercalcaemia is present, there is little point in deferring surgery. In contrast to sporadic cases, all four parathyroids are identified and removed, a small amount of parathyroid tissue being auto-grafted back into sternomastoid or forearm muscles to maintain normocalcaemia. Should such residual tissue remain or subsequently become hyperfunctioning, its retrieval from these sites is simpler and safer than re-exploration of the thyroid/parathyroid bed (with its inherent danger of recurrent laryngeal nerve damage). Of interest is the reduction in both gastrin and (possibly independently) acid secretion which follows successful correction of hyperparathyroidism in MEN-I with coexistent gastrinoma, even in malignant cases. The mechanism of this relationship is not clear. With sometimes confusing pre-operative localization studies, identification and excision of the multiple pancreatic lesions is often difficult. Pancreaticoduodenal resection is sometimes resorted to, or more conservatively simple blockade of acid production with the proton pump inhibitor, omeprazole. Management of pituitary tumours in MEN-I falls broadly into line with the approach outlined in Chapter 4 for sporadic tumours.

Screening philosophy

Given the high penetrance of the gene, some form of family screening programme is mandatory: early diagnosis and treatment will clearly reduce morbidity and mortality. Until recently, all first degree relatives required screening for life in the certain knowledge that only 50 per cent would prove to be affected. Currently, RFLP analysis of DNA from two affected members of a MEN-1 kindred allows subsequent identification of carriers in other apparently unaffected members with more than 99 per cent accuracy, so that only the 50 per cent who are genetically positive require follow-up. Shortly, identification of the gene will allow simple probing at birth.

Serum calcium, PTH, PP, and gastrin (with provocative meal), prolactin, glucagon, and insulin/glucose ratio are likely to continue as the necessary 'basket' of screening tests, which need to be instituted in childhood and continued for life at 2- to 3-yearly intervals. Theoretically, modifying genes might in future be identifiable, and could give a clue to the expected pattern of organ involvement.

Multiple endocrine neoplasia type II

The basic components of the MEN syndrome are listed in Table 16.1 and were originally described by Sipple in 1961 as the syndrome now referred to as MEN-IIa. Some years later, Williams described a syndrome in which parathyroid abnormalities were rare: instead somatic (Marfanoid) features and a unique type of gastrointestinal ganglioneuromatosis were recorded, and this syndrome is now identified as MEN-IIb. Type II MEN in both forms, as well as a lone familial medullary thyroid carcinoma (FMTC) are transmitted as autosomal dominants with almost complete penetrance. The gene(s) for MEN-IIb appear to be more completely expressed than in MEN-IIa. The causative genes for these variants reside in close proximity to each other near the centromere of chromosome 10, a locus which is highly relevant to the growth, development, and migration of primitive neural crest cells to their ultimate destinations in the thyroid, adrenal, and gastrointestinal tract. A mutation activating a specific (RET) proto-oncogene is now known to be the basis of MEN-IIa and FMTC; unrelated MEN families show evidence of separate mutations. It seems likely that other activating mutations of the same oncogene are likely to be the basis of MEN-IIb.

Clinical features

MEN-IIa

Only 50–70 per cent of genetically predisposed individuals develop medullary thyroid carcinoma (MTC), 30 per cent phaeochromocytoma, and approximately 20 per cent parathyroid disease: thus MEN-IIa is less completely expressed than MEN-1. Nevertheless, clinically inapparent thyroidal C-cell hyperplasia is the hallmark of MEN-IIa, only later progressing to multifocal MTC changes.

The parathyroid lesions are similar to those seen in MEN-I, with underlying parathyroid hyperplasia. However, the clinical pattern of presentation of hyperparathyroidism is usually less progressive than in MEN-I and closer to the behaviour of the sporadic forms. Despite the apparent rarity of hyperparathyroidism in MEN-IIa, calcium infusion, which suppresses serum PTH in normal individuals, often fails to do so even in normocalcaemic MEN-I subjects. This confirms the relative autonomy of the parathyroids even in the earliest stages.

The thyroid lesions are those of C-cell hyperplasia or tumour (MTC), with corresponding rising levels of serum calcitonin. Early cases may have normal basal calcitonin, but show hyper-responsiveness of serum calcitonin to injection of the peptide pentagastrin. Clinical presentation as in the sporadic case (see Chapter 9) may be as a thyroid swelling, with 50 per cent of cases already metastatic to liver or lymph nodes at the time of initial diagnosis. Severe diarrhoea is present in about 30 per cent of cases, but neither calcitonin nor the associated hypersecreted peptides (calcitonin gene-related peptide, ACTH, somatostatin) are responsible: an as yet unidentified peptide is clearly involved. The hypersecreted ACTH is responsible for (ectopic) Cushing's syndrome which coexists clinically in about 30 per cent of cases. It was initially suggested that the consistently elevated levels of calcitonin, acting through a reduction in serum calcium were responsible for the induction of a secondary/tertiary form of hyperparathyroidism: there is no evidence to support this connection.

The adrenal lesions are bilateral: although only a unilateral phaeochromocytoma may be identified, the contralateral adrenal will show nodular or diffuse medullary hyperplasia. A small minority of cases are malignant (invasive and/or metastatic). The clinical features are those of the sporadic case (see Chapter 6), although some cases have raised urinary catecholamines (dominantly epinephrine) without symptoms or hypertension.

MEN-IIb (see Plate 16.2)

Almost 100 per cent of patients in this subtype show Marfanoid features. Only occasional families have been described where mucosal neuromas and ganglioneuromas have been absent. The endocrine markers of this subtype are phaeochromocytoma and MTC, each eventually present in about 80 per cent of cases. Hyperparathyroidism is rare.

The somatic features include those characteristic of Marfan's syndrome (tall stature, arched palate, and arachnodactyly) but without the lens or aortic pathology seen in classical Marfan's syndrome. In addition, other skeletal characteristics may be present such as kyphoscloiosis and hyperextensibility of joints.

The mucosal neuroma syndrome is manifest by variable size nodular swellings in eyelids, and most characteristically on lips and tongue. These so-called ganglioneuromas extend throughout the length of the gastrointestinal tract, producing various combinations of vomiting, diarrhoea, and constipation in most individuals.

The thyroid lesions are qualitatively similar to those of MEN-I and MEN-IIa, but in some patients are more aggressive and occur at an earlier age.

The adrenal lesions are identical to those in MEN-IIa.

Management

Because of the universality of eventual C-cell hyperplasia and the almost invariable malignant and metastatic potential in MEN-IIb, total thyroidectomy is now considered mandatory even in the neonatal period in those patients who show the phenotypic characteristics referred to above. In MEN-IIa, the lower prevalence of MTC has sometimes allowed a deferral of surgery until either the basal or pentagastrin-stimulated calcitonin level is raised (although calcitonin levels are occasionally elevated in a number of other conditions). Debate exists over the virtues of bilateral versus unilateral adrenalectomy when only a unilateral phaeochromocytoma is identified pre-operatively. No treatment is possible for the mucocutaneous features, although isolated larger tumours have been removed endoscopically when symptomatic.

Screening philosophy

With the availability of a genetic marker, the number of kindred members requiring subsequent follow-up immediately falls by 50 per cent.

In this predisposed subgroup, the following screening tests are usually carried out at yearly intervals: random calcitonin (and if normal, pentagastrin stimulated); serum calcium and PTH; 24-hour urinary adrenaline and noradrenaline.

MULTIPLE ENDOCRINE DEFICIENCY SYNDROMES

In the course of this book, repeated reference has been made to the auto-immune nature of endocrine deficiency syndromes, and to the association of such a process in one endocrine gland with the same process in another. The importance of poly-endocrine immune syndromes is twofold: (1) an awareness that between 5 and 10 per cent of patients with any one such disorder either has, or will develop one or more further disorders. (2) the familial occurrence of any one disorder probably approaches 20 per cent. The awareness of this fact raises important issues in preventive medicine policy and practice, and is relevant to both primary care and hospital/specialist health service delivery.

Pathogenesis

All these disorders represent defects in cell and antibody-mediated immunity. One component is a B-lymphocyte phenomenon: the formation of antibodies against normal cell components. These antibodies are almost invariably nothing more than markers of the immunological disorder. Only in the case of anti-acetylcholine (myasthenia gravis) and TSH receptor (Graves' disease) antibodies is there evidence of a significant effect of the antibody on the disease process. Similarly, first degree relatives more frequently show abnormal antibody titres than the general population, without necessarily developing the relevant clinical syndrome(s), although, in general, the likelihood of doing so is greater in relatives who manifest the abnormal antibodies than those who do not.

The T-lymphocyte abnormalities include functional defects and certain alterations in cell-surface markers, with a reduction in suppressor T cell activity being the most frequent abnormality. A characteristic lymphocytic infiltrate, usually followed by fibrosis in the organs concerned together represent the histological hallmarks of this group of disorders, highlighting the fact that it is these T-cell phenomena that are directly responsible for the dysfunctional state.

The genetic factors that predispose to auto-immune pathology have already been alluded to in earlier chapters. Thus, histocompatibility antigens HLA-B8, and HLA-DR3 and 4 are much more commonly found in these disorders. However, there is no particular genetic marker associated either with strongly familial cases or with multiple gland involvement. HLA associations are only a partial explanation of susceptibility. They probably relate only to a permissive component of the disorder, as reflected by a maximum concordance rate of 50 per cent in identical twins, one of whom (for example) has auto-immune thyroiditis. The fact that an identical twin is significantly more likely than an HLA-identical sibling to have such a disorder highlights the existence of additional, as yet uncharacterized genes outside the HLA region which clearly influence the active process which initiates auto-immune events, and may determine patterns of multiple gland involvement and the age of onset.

As with the MEN syndromes, the chronology of development of the individual disorders appears to be quite random, but with one or two patterns of interest: for example, a disorder such as Hashimoto's disease occasionally follows the onset of type I diabetes by as long as 30 years, but still with a likelihood of not more than 10 per cent. Yet Addison's disease is followed in almost 50 per cent of cases by another auto-immune disorder (usually thyroid) within a 10-year period. Finally, the clinical features of individual endocrinopathies are no different when occurring as part of the familial or polyglandular syndromes than when sporadic. (See Table 16.2 for the components of multiple endocrine deficiency syndromes.)

Specific associations

Type II/type I classification

A separation has been proposed, in which type I grouping is characterized by a high incidence of mucocutaneous candidiasis and low incidence of IDDM. This

Table 16.2. The components of multiple endocrine deficiency syndromes*

Endocrine
Hashimoto's thyroiditis
Graves' disease
Primary hypothyroidism
Idiopathic adrenal insufficiency (Addison's disease)
Type I (insulin-dependent) diabetes
Premature gonadal (especially ovarian) failure
Idiopathic hypoparathyroidism
Hypophysitis (pan- or monotrophic hypopituitarism)

Non-endocrine
Vitiligo
Chronic mucocutaneous (occasionally systemic) moniliasis
Pernicious anaemia
Alopecia totalis
Idiopathic thrombocytopenia purpura, diabetes insipidus, gluten-sensitive enteropathy, Sjögren's syndrome (kerato-conjunctivitis sicca), myasthenia gravis, chronic active hepatitis and rheumatoid arthritis are additional components of the syndrome which are less frequently encountered

*Note that non-endocrine associations are included for comprehensiveness.

grouping appears to have no HLA associations and affects only siblings. In com parison, type II has classical HLA associations, affects multiple generations with a high incidence of IDDM and does not include candidiasis. Both types can include the other disorders listed above. There are probably lessons to be learned from this classification, but it is probably wiser to assume that the possibility exists of any one disorder being superimposed on any other, either within an individual or the family members.

Schmidt's syndrome

The combination of Addison's disease and hypothyroidism was described in 1926. Either disorder can occur first, and increasingly the association has extended to hyperthyroidism, which coexists almost as frequently as hypothyroidism. When hypothyroidism presents concurrently with Addison's disease, thyroid function often reverts to normal spontaneously when physiological steroid replacement is initiated. This phenomenon remains unexplained.

Chromosomal syndromes

Patients with Down's syndrome (trisomy-21) have a markedly higher prevalence of auto-immune thyoid disease of all types as well as IDDM. They show T-lymphocyte abnormalities of varying types. Patients with Turner's syndrome (46 XO gonadal dysgenesis) and Klinefelter's syndrome (47 XXY) also have a higher prevalence of these disorders. A satisfactory explanation of the association has not been arrived at.

Vitiligo (see Plate 16.1)

The patchy skin depigmentation which characterizes this disorder has long been recognized to be associated with Addison's disease. Anti-melanocyte antibodies have been identified which lyse cultured melanocytes *in vitro*, and which are present in many patients with the disorder. It has recently been identified that the antigen is a 69 kDa protein, almost certainly the enzyme tyrosinase, which plays a key role in melanin synthesis.

DIDMOAD syndrome

This syndrome probably does not have an auto-immune basis. The cause of the association of cranial diabetes insipidus, diabetes mellitus, optic atrophy, and deafness is not known. Partial forms have been often described.

Screening philosophy

From the clinical viewpoint a high index of suspicion is necessary with regard to any individual patient with one of these disorders. Antibodies are readily assessed for pernicious anaemia (gastric parietal cell and intrinsic factor), thyroid disorders (microsomal/thyroid peroxidase and thyroglubulin components), insulin-dependent diabetes (islet and insulin antibodies) and Addison's disease (adrenal antibody). A more specific steroid cell antibody relevant to premature gonadal failure is also being evaluated. The extent to which these antibodies should be screened for in families with a proband affected by a single auto-immune disorder is not known. Even in those with a specific antibody identified, it is similarly uncertain how often biochemical screening should be carried out.

FURTHER READING

Lairmore, T.C., Ball, D.W., Baylin, S.B., *et al.* (1993). The management of phaeochromocytoma in patients with multiple endocrine neoplasia type II syndromes. *Annals of Surgery*, **217**, 595–603.

Larsson, C., Shepherd, J., Nakamura, Y., *et al.* (1992). Predictive testing for multiple endocrine neoplasia type 1 using DNA polymorphisms. *Journal of Clinical Investigation*, **89**, 1344–9.

Molligan, L.M. and Ponder, B.A. (1995). Multiple endocrine neoplasia Type II. *Journal of Clinical Endocrinology*, **80**, 1989–95.

Pozzilli, P., Carotenuto, P., and Delitala, G. (1994). Lymphocytic traffic, homing into target tissue, and the generation of endocrine auto-immunity. *Clinical Endocrinology*, **41**, 545–554.

Rizzoli, R., Green, J., and Marx, S.J. (1985). Primary hyperparathyroidism in familial multiple endocrine neoplasia type I. *American Journal of Medicine*, **78**, 467–72.

Samaan, N., Quais, S., and Ordonez, N.G. (1989). Multiple endocrine syndrome type I: clinical, laboratory findings and management of 5 families. *Cancer*, **64**, 741–8.

Thakker, R.V. (1993). The molecular genetics of the multiple endocrine neoplasia syndrome. *Clinical Endocrinology*, **38**, 1–14.

Weetman, A.P. (1995). Autoimmunity to steroid-producing cells and familial polyendocrine immunity. *Clinical Endocrinology and Metabolism*, **9**, 157–76.

17

Specific tests and procedures for evaluating endocrine function

INTRODUCTION

Many tests of endocrine function are expensive, time-consuming, and uncomfortable for the patient, so that it is often logical to perform an initial screening test, and to proceed with more definitive testing only if the screening test proves abnormal. Where such an approach is appropriate, the tests will be listed in this manner. Excessive reliance should never be placed on a single test result; sampling, administrative, and laboratory errors may occur, and all results must be carefully interpreted in conjunction with the clinical features of the patient.

Neurohypophyseal function

Diabetes insipidus

Random measurements of vasopressin, serum, or urine osmolality are not diagnostic, and should therefore not be performed. In patients in whom there is a comparatively low index of suspicion, the simplest test is to provide 18 hours of (ideally overnight) dehydration: the patient may eat solid foods but no semi-liquids or liquids. Serum and urine osmolality are measured at the end of this period. Where suspicion is higher, the test is commenced in the morning, and 2-hourly samples of urine and blood are collected together with simultaneous body weight measurement. A reduction in weight of greater than 5 per cent is an indication for immediate discontinuation of the test (rapid decreases in weight from dehydration occur in severe diabetes insipidus and can be dangerous). Otherwise the test is concluded in 24 hours. Typical responses are shown in Table 17.1.

Although normal subjects maintain serum osmolality less than 295 mmol/kg and urine osmolality rises above 600 mmol/kg, in diabetes insipidus (DI), serum osmolality exceeds 300 mmol/kg while urine osmolality remains hypo-osmolar compared to serum. As shown, it is sometimes useful to immediately follow the above procedure with a subcutaneous or intramuscular injection of 2 μg desmopressin (DDAVP). Failure of urine osmolality to rise from a subnormal value demonstrates that the DI is nephrogenic in origin: in cases of cranial DI, the percentage increment in urine osmolality following DDAVP is an broad indication of the severity of vasopressin deficiency. Psychogenic polydipsia, although usually giving normal responses to the above tests, can in some instances produce a picture suggestive of nephrogenic DI: prolonged polyuric syndromes of whatever cause appear to (reversibly) impair tubular water reabsorption.

Table 17.1. Findings in a 38-year-old woman with diabetes insipidus due to a hypothalamic tumour (fluid deprivation was commenced at time 0)

Time (h)	Weight (kg)	Serum osmolality normal 285–295 (mOsm/kg)	Urine osmolality min. norm value (mOsm/kg)
0	60.0	290	205
2	59.1	292	208
4	58.6	298	210
6	58.0	305	240
8	56.9	312	225
(i.e. 3 kg weight loss (5%): DDAVP 0.1 ml given intranasally.)			
10	57.5	300	440
12	57.0	292	720

Direct assay of vasopressin in serum can now be performed in some centres: failure of serum vasopressin to rise in response to the osmotic stimulus of fluid deprivation would be further confirmation of the diagnosis. Vasopressin can also be assessed after the infusion of hypertonic saline, an alternative method of inducing hyperosmolarity.

Syndrome of inappropriate ADH (SIADH)

Measured plasma sodium concentrations are invariably subnormal (and are often lower than 120 mmol/l). Plasma potassium and protein concentrations are also decreased by the haemodilution process. The diagnosis cannot be made in the absence of normal renal function; thus plasma urea and creatinine must be within the normal range. The ultimate criterion is a demonstration of an elevated urine osmolality in the face of serum hypo-osmolality. (See Table 17.2.)

Adenohypophyseal function

Short synacthen test

If only the pituitary–adrenal axis requires to be tested, the short synacthen test is normally employed: a basal sample of cortisol is followed by the intramuscular injection of the aqueous ACTH analogue, tetracosactrin (Synacthen) 250 μg.

Table 17.2. Findings in a 65-year-old man with SIADH secondary to an oat cell bronchogenic carcinoma

Serum osmolality (mmol/kg)	(Normal range)	Urine osmolality (mmol/kg)
264	285–295	615
Serum Na = 110; K = 3.0; Cl = 89 mmol/l		

Thirty minutes later a repeat plasma cortisol sample is taken. A normal rise represents an elevation by a minimum of 300 nmol/l from a basal level of not less than 250 nmol/l.

Failure to respond is seen in hypopituitarism unless it is of less than 3 weeks standing (i.e. postoperative for pituitary tumour), due to the atrophy of the adrenal which follows prolonged non-stimulation by ACTH. An abnormal result is also seen in patients recently treated with corticosteroids, and more typically in adrenocortical deficiency (Addison's disease) which is dealt with later in this chapter.

Combined pituitary function test

This procedure is costly, sometimes uncomfortable, and occasionally dangerous. In children, it should be performed with particular care, and avoided altogether where there is a history of fits, and only in exceptional circumstances in the elderly (in view of the risks imposed by cerebrovascular or cardiovascular disease). It should not generally be performed unless there is a high level of clinical suspicion, supported either by some biochemical evidence of hypopituitarism on basal endocrine function testing (e.g. a low serum thyroxine with normal or low serum TSH, low androgen or oestrogen levels with low LH or an elevated serum prolactin).

The recommended procedure includes the simultaneous administration of thyrotrophin-releasing hormone, TRH (which stimulates both TSH and prolactin release) and gonadotrophin-releasing hormone (GnRH), together with the induction of insulin-induced hypoglycaemia (which stimulates somatotrophin and corticotrophin secretion).

Procedure

The patient is fasted overnight, allowed free access to water, and should be lying down comfortably throughout the procedure. An indwelling venous catheter, such as a G19 Butterfly with a three-way tap, is inserted: the catheter can be kept patent with heparinized saline. After an initial rest period of 30 minutes, a basal blood sample is taken. Soluble (actrapid) insulin is then administered in a bolus dose, usually of 0.15 U/kg body weight. In patients already suspected of hypopituitarism the dose can be reduced to 0.1 U/kg, while in patients with confirmed acromegaly (see later), it can be increased to 0.3 U/kg. A syringe of 20 ml of 50 per cent dextrose is prepared for use in the event of severe hypoglycaemia. The two hormones, GnRH and TRH, are given simultaneously as an intravenous bolus in doses of 100 μg and 200 μg, respectively. A blood sample is then taken every 15 minutes for the first hour and every 30 minutes for the second hour.

Hypoglycaemia occurs 20–50 minutes after injection, the symptoms and signs being mainly sweating, headaches, raised blood pressure, and increased heart rate. Blood glucose concentration should decrease to below 2.2 mmol/l with the hypoglycaemia ideally uncorrected for 15–20 minutes. At the end of the test the patient should receive a full meal.

If hypoglycaemia has not occurred within one hour, the same dose of insulin can be repeated. Some patients may suffer severe hypoglycaemic symptoms and in these circumstances it is advisable to give 20 ml of 50 per cent dextrose solution.

Even if severe hypoglycaemia has occurred, and dextrose is given, the appropriate blood samples should still continue to be taken.

The various blood samples are then analysed and the concentrations of glucose and various hormones are estimated. In Table 17.3, values obtained for a normal person given the combined pituitary function test are presented as an example.

Results

In order to interpret the results it is necessary to know the normal basal values for the concentration of the various substances estimated. In the example of the normal patient (Table 17.3), hypoglycaemia occurred within 15 minutes, and produced various symptoms 30 minutes after the intravenous injection, lasting for approximately 30 minutes.

In response to hypoglycaemia there should be:

1. An increase in cortisol concentration of more than 250 nmol/l from the basal value (at 60–90 minutes postinjection).
2. A rise in the somatotrophin (hGH) level to above 20 mU/l (at 60–90 minutes postinjection).

In response to the 200 μg TRH there should be:

1. An increase in thyrotrophin (TSH) concentration up to 3–15 mU/l should occur some 20 minutes after injection.
2. An increase in serum prolactin to at least 1800 mU/l.

In response to 100 μg GnRH, there should be:

1. An increase in LH levels to within an expected range of 15–42 U/l, approximately 20 minutes after injection.
2. An increase in FSH levels to within an expected range of 10–30 U/l.

Table 17.3. Example of normal combined pituitary function test in a female weighing 70 kg in the follicular phase of the menstrual cycle*

Time (min)	Glucose (mmol/l)	TSH (mU/l)	PRL (mU/l)	Cortisol (nmol/l)	LH (mU/l)	FSH	hGH (mU/l)
0	4.3	1.5	210	350	1.6	2.6	0.5
10 U soluble insulin, 200 μg TRH; 100 μg GnRH given as IV bolus at 0 time							
15	1.3	4.9	1080	355	10.9	6.0	0.5
30	1.4	3.5	1800	390	16.7	10.2	13.0
45	1.7	2.5	2000	480	11.4	8.3	60.0
60	2.1	2.5	1800	640	9.7	8.0	84.0
90	2.5	2.0	1200	640	8.5	6.7	54.2
120	3.0	1.8	702	460	4.6	3.0	24.5

*Serum-free T_4 = 15.5 pmol/l (N = 12–24).
Serum oestradiol = 465 nmol/l (N = 180–640). (N, normal range.)

Table 17.4. Example of pituitary function test in a man with a pituitary adenoma prior to trans-sphenoidal removal

Time (min)	Glucose (mmol/l)	TSH (mU/l)	PRL (mU/l)	Cortisol (nmol/l)	LH	FSH (mU/l)	hGH
0	4.7	2.2	1480	405	5.5	5.9	0.5
Insulin, TRH, and GnRH given at 0 time							
15	2.4	5.0	2000	335	4.9	9.7	0.5
30	1.7	5.0	1940	235	21.2	9.6	0.5
45	1.6	4.3	1760	420	21.7	10.7	0.5
60	3.0	4.1	1700	600	19.7	9.2	1.0
90	3.5	2.8	1440	550	12.1	5.9	0.9
120	3.9	2.4	1120	350	6.8	4.8	0.5

*Serum free T_4 = 18 pmol/l (N = 12–24).
Serum testosterone = 21 nmol/l (N = 13–40). (N, normal range.)

In contrast, Table 17.4 gives the values found in a patient with a non-functioning chromophobe adenoma before hypophysectomy.

In this example, the interpretation of the results is:

1. In the basal blood sample (0 time) the only abnormality detected is the high prolactin level (due to pituitary 'disconnection').
2. The insulin hypoglycaemia induced a normal cortisol response but there was no somatotrophin (hGH) response.
3. The TRH induced a normal thyrotrophin (TSH) response, and prolactin increased.
4. GnRH: both LH and FSH responses were normal.

Table 17.5 shows the results of the combined pituitary function test in the same patient after hypophysectomy. Note the loss of normal cortisol response to hypoglycaemia, the flatter LH/FSH response to GnRH (with a subsequent but typically delayed fall in serum testosterone), and the similarly slow fall in free T_4 indicating the development of hypothyroidism. The diagnosis of panhypopituitarism was thereby confirmed and appropriate replacement therapy instituted.

Hypersecretion of somatotrophin (acromegaly)

IGF-I (screening) measurement is neither 100 per cent specific nor sensitive. Accordingly, a modified glucose tolerance test (GTT) is carried out in a patient with a borderline raised value. The patient is fasted overnight. Between 8 a.m. and 10 a.m. a basal sample is taken and 75 g of glucose given orally. Blood samples are then taken every 30 minutes for 2 hours. Glucose and somatotrophin concentrations are estimated in each sample. A normal subject has a normal GTT curve and somatotrophin is suppressed to less than 3 mU/l after glucose administration.

Table 17.5. The pituitary function test in the same patient as Table 17.4 performed 10 days following surgery*

Time (min)	Glucose (mmol/l)	TSH (mU/l)	PRL (mU/l)	Cortisol (nmol/l)	LH (mU/l)	FSH (mU/l)	hGH (mU/l)
0	3.3	3.1	1000	90	3.7	4.1	0.5
Insulin TRH and LHRH given at 0 time							
15	2.0	6.1	1160	150	6.4	5.5	0.5
30	1.0	4.1	1500	180	6.0	4.4	0.5
45	1.8	3.5	1400	190	4.7	5.1	0.7
60	1.9	2.7	1160	290	3.5	4.8	1.0
90	2.0	2.9	1120	280	3.4	2.6	1.0
120	3.1	2.3	1040	170	3.1	2.7	0.8
Serum-free T_4 level 1 month later had fallen to 6.8 pmol/l, and serum testosterone to 8 nmol/l							

*Serum free T_4 = 14 pmol/l (N = 12–24).
Serum testosterone = 13 nmol/l (N = 12–40). (N = normal range.)

An example of the type of response found in acromegaly is given in Table 17.6. In this patient, there is not only failed suppression, but also a paradoxical rise in the somatotrophin concentration, an observation found in about 30 per cent of acromegalics. Note that mild glucose intolerance has also been demonstrated (2-hour blood glucose normally < 7.0 mmol/l).

In non-acromegalics, intravenous TRH does not raise somatotrophin levels: in acromegaly there is usually a diagnostic 100–300 per cent rise: in this patient, a TRH test on the following day demonstrated a rise of serum hGH from a basal value of 15.1 mU/l to a peak of 38.5 mU/l at 60 minutes after injection.

Hyposecretion of somatotrophin

The diagnosis of growth hormone deficiency arises in the diagnosis of patients with suspected hypopituitarism and is revealed by an absence of rise in the somatotrophin level after insulin-induced hypoglycaemia.

In children with short stature, somatotrophin deficiency often requires exclusion. Prior to doing any form of testing, it should be first confirmed that the child's

Table 17.6. Example of the results of a glucose tolerance test in a patient with acromegaly

Time (min)	Glucose (mmol/l)	hGH (mU/l)
0	7.4	15.3
75 g glucose given orally at 0 time		
30	14.2	19.5
60	14.9	20.0
90	15.1	52.0
120	12.9	24.0

height is below the 3rd centile for his or her age. The screening test of choice involves intense exercise, preferably on a bicycle ergometer for a period of 15–20 minutes, almost to the point of exhaustion. Stair-climbing for a similar period of time is a less satisfactory alternative. Samples are taken for somatotrophin assay immediately after conclusion of the exercise and again 20 minutes later: 90 per cent of normal subjects produce a serum growth hormone concentration at either of these points which exceeds 20 mU/l.

Should this value not be reached, insulin hypoglycaemia (0.1 μ/kg) is used as the appropriate test stimulus, usually preceded by an additional growth hormone release stimulant, arginine hydrochloride (0.2 g per kg by intravenous infusion over 15 minutes). Once again in children, the augmented stimulus should result in a maximum growth hormone response exceeding 20 mU/l).

Adrenal medullary function

Hypersecretion of catecholamines

To diagnose a patient with phaeochromocytoma, urinary vanillyl mandelic acid (VMA) concentration is traditionally measured. However, it only has a sensitivity of 60–75 per cent, even with repeat consecutive 24-hour analyses. Urinary metadrenaline is more sensitive, but assay of the separate catecholamines (noradrenaline and adrenaline) in the urine is the only worthwhile assay. Extramedullary phaeochromocytomas preferentially secrete adrenaline, since they lack the enzyme *n*-methyltransferase required for conversion of adrenaline to noradrenaline.

Dynamic function testing aiming to stimulate (tyramine. histamine) or suppress (phentolamine) blood pressure have now been discontinued except in most unusual cases, since these procedures may be both unreliable and dangerous.

Adrenal cortical function

Hypersecretion of cortisol (Cushing's syndrome)

A screening test should always be performed first: 2 mg of dexamethasone is given orally between 10 p.m. and midnight. Between 9 a.m. and 11 a.m. the following morning a single plasma sample is taken for a cortisol assay. A normal response is represented by a suppression of plasma cortisol to below 250 nmol/l while in Cushing's syndrome (as well as in a proportion of patients with depression and acute or chronic anxiety, or hospitalized for acute illness) cortisol concentration is above this level.

Alternatively, a 24-hour urinary cortisol estimation can be carried out, but care should be taken to ensure that the collection is accurate. Lack of diurnal cortisol variation and high random measurements of serum cortisol are often seen in Cushing's syndrome, but their lack of specificity means that they are of no diagnostic value.

Table 17.7. Findings in three typical patients with different causes of Cushing's syndrome

	Urinary cortisol (N 100–340 nmol/24 h)	Plasma ACTH (N <50 ng/l)
Pituitary-dependent Cushing's disease	480	65
Cushing's syndrome (adrenal adenoma)	540	< 20
Ectopic ACTH syndrome	1510	385

Definitive diagnosis is achieved by confirming elevated levels of urinary cortisol on a second 24-hour specimen and by assessing plasma ACTH by radioimmunoassay. Typical examples of urinary cortisol and plasma ACTH in the three major varieties of Cushing's syndrome are indicated in Table 17.7.

In some borderline cases, a dexamethasone suppression test can be performed. 24-hour urinary cortisol measurements are performed consecutively over a period of five days. On days 3, 4, and 5, dexamethasone 2 mg is given 6-hourly. All normal subjects and the majority of patients with pituitary-dependent Cushing's syndrome suppress 24-hours urinary cortisol to below 200 nmol per 24 hours, and in some cases, to less than 100 nmol per 24 hours. In contrast, patients with ectopic ACTH syndrome or adrenal cortical adenoma or carcinoma have either non- or partially suppressible urinary cortisol levels. Imaging is also used for diagnosis and localization (see Chapter 5).

Hypersecretion of aldosterone (Conn's syndrome)

This test should not normally be performed unless the hypertension which is being investigated is accompanied by at least borderline hypokalaemia (serum potassium less than 3.2 mmol/l).

The simplest screening procedure is to sit the patient quietly for 15 minutes, then taking a single serum sample for renin and aldosterone assay. It is important to correct any hypokalaemia before performing the test, since this may inhibit aldosterone release even in patients with an adenoma. A sample result from a patient with an ultimately confirmed adenoma is shown in Table 17.8.

Alternatively, 2 litres of normal saline can be infused intravenously over 4 hours and plasma aldosterone level assayed before and after. Suppression to less than 200 pmol/l (80 pg/ml) excludes the diagnosis.

Table 17.8. Findings in a patient with primary hyperaldosteronism, presenting with hypertension, muscle fatigue, and a serum potassium of 2.3 mmol/l (corrected to 3.7 mmol/l before testing)

Serum aldosterone	= 1640 pmol/l	(N = 200–800)
Plasma renin	= < 0.3 pmol/h/ml	(N = 0.5–2.5)

Further tests can then be performed to localize the tumour using selective catheterization as described in Chapter 5.

Hyposecretion of cortisol (Addison's disease)

This diagnosis will be considered in many patients in whom asthenia and weight loss is present. However, it is important to realize that a diagnosis may be made in the absence of any typical blood pressure or electrolyte changes, and with minimal symptomatology.

Screening test

The short synacthen test is performed, as described earlier. Criteria for interpretation are identical. It follows that this test only identifies cortisol deficiency to be of either primary adrenal or pituitary origin, and further investigation is therefore essential.

The screening short synacthen test can be performed even once treatment has been commenced for a presumed Addisonian crisis, providing rehydration is initiated and a synthetic corticosteroid such as dexamethasone is used for repletion. This will not interfere with the assay for cortisol referred to above. Normal subjects should reach a maximum serum cortisol greater than 550 nmol/l.

Definitive test

If the screening test is abnormal, it must be followed by a definitive test. Plasma ACTH is invariably and markedly raised in Addison's disease and adrenal antibodies are found in 90 per cent of cases. This suffices to confirm the diagnosis. Alternatively, daily injections of tetracosactrin depot 1 mg intramuscularly are given on 3 consecutive days or a continuous infusion of aqueous synacthen 500 μg in 500 ml normal saline over 6 hours. In either case, a normal response is indicated by an increment of serum cortisol to more than 650 nmol/l from the minimum of 250 nmol/l. Normal subjects and patients whose hypoadrenalism is secondary to hypopituitarism show a 'normal' response to this test.

Thyroid function

Suspected hyperthyroidism

Measurement of total T_4 does not suffice and is often misleading. Elevated values occur even in the absence of hyperthyroidism as a result of increased protein binding induced by oestrogens as well as in the uncommon hereditary dysalbuminaemic hyperthyroxinaemia. Misleadingly normal levels of serum T_4 (potentially leading to a falsely rejected diagnosis) are obtained in situations which reduce serum proteins or their binding potential (phenytoin administration). Furthermore, early hyperthyroidism, especially in iodine-deficient areas, is associated with normal total (and even free T_4) levels. Free T_3 measurement represents the best quantification of hyperthyroidism, in association with a serum thyrotrophin concentration which is suppressed below normal, and elevated thyroidal

Table 17.9. Example of hormone levels in a patient with hyperthyroidism (Graves' disease)

Levels in patient		(Normal range)
Serum T_4	190 nmol/l	(60–145)
Serum-free T_4	38 pmol/l	(12–24)
Serum-free T_3	21 pmol/l	(4.3–8.4)
Serum TSH	< 0.1 mU/l	(0.5–3.5)

isotope uptake, which is essential to exclude thyroiditis or thyrotoxicosis factitia.(See Table 17.9.)

Table 17.10 gives an example of the blood levels in a pregnant patient thought also to be thyrotoxic. In these circumstances, free hormone levels and serum TSH were normal.

Table 17.10. Example of hormone levels in a pregnant woman thought to be thyrotoxic on the basis of a raised serum thyroxine level.

Levels in patient		(Normal range)
Serum T_4	195 nmol/l	(60–145)
Serum-free T_3	5.6 pmol/l	(4.3–8.4)
Serum TSH	2.4 mU/l	(0.5–3.5)

It is important to re-state that the measurement of serum TSH is fundamental to any assessment of thyroid function, whether the presence of either hypothyroidism or hyperthyroidism is being probed.

Suspected hypothyroidism (myxoedema)

Measurements of total T_4 and thyrotrophin levels are made. In most primary hypothyroid patients the serum T_4 is less than 60 nmol/l and serum thyrotrophin is greater than 10 mU/l. A TRH test would show an exaggerated TSH response but does not add to the diagnosis of overt cases. Table 17.11 gives an example of values found in primary hypothyroidism

A subgroup of patients has been shown to have normal total T_3 and T_4 levels but raised thyrotrophin levels, and this group of patient has been classified as having

Table 17.11. Example of hormone levels in a patient with primary hypothyroidism (thyroid antibodies were positive, TMA 1:6400)

Levels in patient		(Normal range)
Serum T_4	35 nmol/l	(60–145)
Serum TSH	62 mU/l)	(0.5–3.5)

premyxoedema or compensated hypothyroidism. These patients may have a history of thyroid surgery, a biosynthetic block, or have positive thyroid antibodies. They usually show an exaggerated response to the TRH test. Some of this group of patients have serum free T_4 concentrations which are low, so that subclinical hypothyroidism is then a preferable term. Subjects with isolated raised serum TSH levels (with normal free hormone concentrations) undergo a transition to clinical hypothyroidism at the rate of approximately 5 per cent per annum.

In patients with low TBG concentration (e.g. with nephrotic syndrome, chronic liver disease, or in the rare instance of hereditary deficiency of TBG) total T_3 and T_4 levels will be low but the free hormone concentrations will be normal: thyrotrophin levels and the response to TRH test will again be normal.

Hypothyroidism due to hypopituitarism

Thyroid function (together with adrenal cortical function) is often one of the last functions to be affected in hypopituitarism. The total and free T_4 levels are low, but serum thyrotrophin is usually (paradoxically) normal rather than being low, as might be expected: there is sometimes a diminished response to the TRH test. Hypopituitarism is usually indicated by other evidence.

In hypothyroidism due to hypothalamic disorder, a similar spectrum of thyroid function tests is seen. However, TRH often induces an exaggerated and progressive rise of TSH between 20 and 60 minutes.

Hypothalamic or hypopituitary-type biochemical profiles of thyroid function are also confusingly encountered in the entity of the ‘sick euthyroid syndrome’. As previously mentioned, this situation is seen in some patients with severe acute or lower grade chronic disorders. It is due to a combination of hypothalamic ‘turn-off’ and impaired binding of thyroid hormones.

If possible, tests should be repeated when the underlying condition has been treated: sometimes, other investigations are required to identify or refute other pituitary hormone deficiencies since it is unusual for solitary TSH deficiency to be encountered in hypothalamic/pituitary disease.

Gonadal function

One cause of decreased gonadal function is hypopituitarism, which has been considered earlier in this chapter. It is useful to remember that gonadal function is frequently affected quite early in the course of a developing pituitary tumour.

Serum oestradiol, gonadotrophins, and prolactin are the basic hormonal tests performed.

Primary and secondary amenorrhoea (see Chapter 8)

Benign androgen excess

This condition, of which polycystic ovary syndrome represents a subgroup, is occasionally associated with normal androgen and gonadotrophin levels. However, in most cases, serum testosterone level is raised, serum sex-hormone-binding

Table 17.12. Example of hormone levels in a patient with polycystic ovary syndrome

Serum testosterone	4.4 nmol/l	(N = 0.6–2.6)
Serum SHBG	22 nmol/l	(N = 35–75)
Free androgen index	4.4 : 22 = 20	
Oestradiol	368 pmol/l	
Progesterone	1.0 nmol/l	
LH	28.6 U/l	
FSH	5.8 U/l	

globulin is decreased (implying an elevated free testosterone level: T/SHBG in normal women is < 4.5 units) and LH and FSH concentrations may be either normal or high. (See Table 17.12.)

Prolactinoma

Secondary amenorrhoea may be caused by either a micro- or macroadenoma hypersecreting of prolactin. Table 17.13 shows an example of the hormone profile of a female patient who had secondary amenorrhoea for 9 years, and more recently galactorrhoea. A 12 mm pituitary adenoma was identified by MRI scanning.

Table 17.13. Example of hormone levels in a patient with secondary amenorrhoea due to pituitary prolactinoma

T_4	60 nmol/l
Serum TSH	2.0 mU/l
Prolactin	36 500 mU/l (N = < 500)
Oestradiol	166 pmol/l
Testosterone	1.6 nmol/l
Progesterone	< 1.0 nmol/l
LH	1.7 U/l
FSH	0.4 U/l

The prolactin level was very high, while the LH and FSH concentrations were low, together with a resulting low oestradiol by the short prolactin feedback loop. Furthermore, there was no LH or FSH response to GnRH. Treatment of this patient consisted of bromocryptine which resulted in restoration of normal prolactin levels and the resumption of normal menstruation and radiologically confirmed shrinkage of the pituitary adenoma.

Premature ovarian failure

In these patients, as in gonadal dysgenesis (Turner's syndrome), serum oestradiol concentration is low, while LH and FSH levels are high.

Decreased gonadal function in the male

When hypogonadism is suspected in males, serum testosterone, gonadotrophins, and prolactin should be measured.

In hypopituitarism or hypothalamic disease, both serum testosterone and gonadotrophin levels are low. Prolactin-producing or non-functioning pituitary adenomas must always be considered as a possible cause. Hypothalamic and pituitary causes can be differentiated, by GnRH stimulation test (as above). However, a false negative response is sometimes seen in longstanding hypothalamic disorders. Further specificity is achieved by infusing GnRH at the rate of 100 μg over 4 hours daily for 3 days: LH is measured basally, and 24 hours after each infusion. Patients with hypothalamic disease demonstrate 'recruitment': a progressive increment in LH which is not seen in pituitary disease.

Kallman's syndrome is a selective form of hypogonadotrophic hypogonadism. Patients do not demonstrate normal pulsatility of LH. Although a variety of other tests have been proposed, none are absolutely diagnostic, and the syndrome must be diagnosed on the basis of combined clinical and biochemical features. (See Table 17.14.)

Table 17.14. Example of findings in a male patient with Kallman's syndrome

Basal hormone levels:	
Testosterone	1.3 nmol/l
LH	2.2 mU/l
FSH	0.7 mU/l
LHRH test	
20 minutes post LHRH test:	
LH	4.1 mU/l
FSH	1.5 mU/l
60 minutes post LHRH test:	
LH	4.7 mU/l
FSH	2.0 mU/l
(After 3 days of GnRH 100 ug; serum LH rose to 16.8 mU/l)	

Delayed puberty is essentially a form of hypogonadotrophic hypogonadism, but serum prolactin is always normal, GnRH responsiveness developing as puberty becomes imminent. The diagnosis is again made on the combination of typical biochemical findings, often coupled to exclusion of other causes.

Klinefelter's syndrome represents the principal diagnostic possibility if gonadotrophin levels are markedly elevated. A karyotype should be performed to confirm the diagnosis. (See Table 17.15.) Other varieties of primary hyper-gonadotrophic hypogonadism are uncommon, and have been dealt with in Chapter 7.

Table 17.15. Example of hormone levels in a male patient with Klinefelter's syndrome (karyotype 47-XXY)

Basal plasma concentrations:	
Testosterone	2.9 nmol/l
LH	34.5 mU/l
FSH	29.5 mU/l

Parathyroid gland function

Hypoparathyroidism

This condition is relatively rare, and is usually confirmed by the finding of hypocalcaemia, hyperphosphataemia, and a serum PTH level at or below the sensitivity of the assay (all other causes of hypocalcaemia are associated with elevated levels of PTH).

Hyperparathyroidism

Serum calcium levels which are persistently elevated without other obvious explanation may often be the key factor leading to further investigation. The simplest confirmation consists of estimating serum parathormone. The intact molecule assay is the most useful for diagnosis, although even here, in mild hypercalcaemia serum parathormone levels may be at the upper limit of the normal range. Additional features of some use include a demonstration of hyperchloraemia and low serum bicarbonate which contrasts with the hypochloraemia and high serum bicarbonate often associated with the hypercalcaemia of malignancy. Urinary calcium and phosphate measurements are rarely of diagnostic value.

Pancreatic function

Insulinoma

1. If the patient is seen during a spontaneous hypoglycaemia episode, simultaneous sampling for plasma glucose and insulin may be all that is necessary to establish a diagnosis. This should be accompanied by demonstration of the patient's clinical response to intravenous dextrose. A plasma glucose less than 2.2 mmol/l together with plasma insulin of greater than 10 mU/l is diagnostic of inappropriate hyperinsulinism. Plasma C-peptide concentrations are similarly raised in insulinoma. This investigation also helps to identify surreptitious administration of insulin (where C peptide is suppressed). Serum pro-insulin levels can also be measured and add some diagnostic certaintly to borderline values of insulin or C-peptide.

2. Prolonged fasting (16–48 hours) may be necessary to provoke an episode of hypoglycaemia. Plasma glucose and insulin samples are taken 2-hourly, the test being terminated when hypoglycaemia occurs clinically and biochemically (blood

glucose less than 2.2 mmol/l). Only if hypoglycaemia occurs, need plasma insulin samples be assayed. The criteria referred to above are used in interpreting the results.

3. Intravenous injection of pork or beef insulin is given at a dose of 0.15 units/kg, with a basal, 30-, 60-, 90-, and 120-minute sample for blood glucose and C- peptide assay. In normal subjects, the induction of hypoglycaemia suppresses C-peptide concentration to less than 0.1 pmol/l. In insulinoma, plasma C-peptide concentration usually remains higher than 0.5 pmol/l.

It should be noted that surreptitious or accidental administration of oral sulphonylurea drug may cause similar abnormalities to that of insulinoma. Serum assay for sulphonylurea can be performed, usually by HPLC methods.

Diabetes mellitus

1. A blood glucose level taken preferably 2 hours after the end of a meal, and exceeding 11 mmol/l is diagnostic of diabetes; no further tests need be performed.

2. More reliably, a single plasma glucose level taken exactly 2 hours after a 75 g oral dextrose load can be measured (the patient need not be fasting). The same diagnostic criteria referred to above apply.

3. Only if blood glucose is between 7 and 11 mmol/l in test 2 (above) need a standard glucose tolerance test be performed.

4. Excessive reliance is often placed on the fasting blood sugar level in the diagnosis of diabetes. Clearly, a markedly raised fasting level exceeding 11 mmol/l is definitive. However, as indicated below, although 6.7 mmol/l represents the diagnostic cut-off point between normality and abnormality, so many factors, including oral contraceptives, smoking, alcohol, drugs, stress, and previous nutritional status can produce minor (but measurable) effects particularly on the fasting level of glucose, that it should not be relied on to provide an accurate or definitive diagnosis.

5. *Oral glucose tolerance test.* Patients should be fasting and at rest during the whole procedure. A minimum 150–200 g carbohydrate diet should have been consumed during the preceding three days (dieting during this period may produce falsely elevated blood glucose levels even in normal subjects). Oral dextrose 75 g is given, with blood glucose levels measured basally and at 30-minute intervals for 2–3 hours, ideally sampled through an indwelling cannula. Measurement of plasma insulin level does not add to the diagnostic specificity.

Preparation for the glucose tolerance test is essential, with appropriate dietary precautions clearly outlined. In addition. smoking and a variety of drugs including thiazide diuretics, nicotinic acid, phenytoin, β-adrenergic blocking drugs, oestrogen, corticosteroids, and phenothiazine drugs all adversely affect glucose tolerance.

Interpretation

For epidemiological purposes, agreement has been reached for the diagnostic categories shown in Table 17.16.

Table 17.16. Diagnostic criteria (WHO) for diabetes categories using oral glucose tolerance. Ranges are quoted for venous whole blood and a 75 g glucose load (for capillary blood, figures in parentheses). For serum or plasma add 1 mmol/l

	Blood glucose (mmol/l)	
	Fasting	2 hours
Normal glucose tolerance (NGT)	< 6.7	6.7
Impaired glucose tolerance (IGT)	< 6.7	6.7–10.0 (11.1)
Diabetes mellitus	> 6.7	> 10.0 (11.1)

Excessive significance has been attributed both to a lag response glucose tolerance test (peak blood glucose at 1 hour greater than 11 mmol/l but normal at 2 hours), and to a 'flat' glucose response. However, a small but significant proportion of patients with lag curves subsequently develop diabetes. A very small proportion of subjects with a flat glucose tolerance curve are subsequently found to have intestinal malabsorption.

Impaired glucose tolerance (IGT) responses should be interpreted with care. Under the age of 50, this 'abnormality' should probably be followed by repeat testing, although the frequency with which this should be done is not clear: between 20 and 50 per cent of these patients may develop diabetes later in life. Over the age of 50, a progressively increasing proportion of an apparently normal population will show IGT responses, and because of the necessarily shorter follow-up periods, the interpretation of this phenomenon is uncertain. Nevertheless, it has been shown that macrovascular disease (coronary, cerebral, and peripheral) is more common in subjects with this glucose profile than in the general age-matched population, and in some series is equivalent to the risk in clinical diabetes mellitus.

A 'reactive' fall of blood glucose as low as 2.5 mmol/l at 90–120 minutes is found in 10–20 per cent of the normal population. Although the syndrome of 'reactive hypoglycaemia' is a popular concept used to explain diverse symptoms of weakness, faintness, and sweating in otherwise healthy individuals, the attribution of such symptoms to this fall is usually ill-founded.

It is customary to perform 30-minute urine collections coincident with the oral glucose tolerance test. This is of value in determining the renal threshold for glucose, which is important when monitoring a patient with diabetes with urine glucose testing methods. Glycosuria, in the absence of hyperglycaemia (renal glycosuria), is not a prediabetic manifestation, and represents either increased glomerular filtration rate (due to a number of causes) or a renal tubular defect, which may be solitary or associated with amino-aciduria (Fanconi syndrome).

Intravenous glucose tolerance test. This is rarely used as a diagnostic procedure for diabetes mellitus, since it is occasionally normal with proven oral glucose tolerance. However, it is of some value in small-scale epidemiological studies, for assessing insulin resistance (when insulin levels are simultaneously measured) or for assessing the action of drugs on carbohydrate metabolism where it is intended that the component of intestinal glucose absorption should be excluded from the study. Details of this test should be sought in reference texts. (e.g. see Further Reading.)

Glycosylated haemoglobin (HbA_{1c}) has been previously described as a monitoring method for diabetic control. However, its use in the diagnosis of diabetes has been shown to be unreliable. Sensitivity is low, so that less marked but nevertheless diagnostic levels of glucose intolerance would be missed. Because it can be assayed by a wide variety of methods, normal ranges vary considerably, with upper limits for normal subjects ranging from 5.9 per cent to 8.5 per cent. For long-term monitoring, it is therefore desirable that the same laboratory is used. It is important to note that for most assay methods, the presence of an abnormal haemoglobin variant (i.e. sickle cell) reduces, and therefore effectively invalidates Hb A_{1c} measurements. Haemolysis, acute blood loss, and pregnancy also lower values, while the presence of haemoglobin F, alcoholism, renal failure, and hypertriglyceridaemia can produce falsely elevated Hb A_{1c} levels in most assay methods. Serum fructosamine assay is the logical alternative in these situations (see Chapter 11).

FURTHER READING

Bouloux, P.-M.G. and Rees, L.H. (1994). *Diagnostic tests in endocrinology and diabetes.* Chapman and Hall, London.

Appendix. Normal ranges of commonly measured hormone concentrations

(Normal ranges may vary between laboratories due to methodology)

Hormone		Normal Value	Some useful conversions from SI units
Blood			
Aldosterone	Recumbent:	100–450 pmol/l	
	Ambulant:	200–800 pmol/l	1 pmol/l = 0.38 pg/ml
	Normal Na^+, K^+ diet		
	(Na^+:100–200 mmol/24 h;		
	K^+: 50–80 mmol/24 h)		
Calcitonin		< 0.08 μg/l	
Cortisol	0900 h	200–700 nmol/l	1 μg/100 ml = 28 nmol/l
	2400 h	up to 250 nmol/l	
Corticotrophin (ACTH)	0900 h	< 25 ng/l	
	2400 h	< 10 ng/l	
Follicle-stimulating hormone	Children		
(FSH)	(1 year to puberty)	< 2.5 U/l	
	Adult males	1–7 U/l	
	Adult females:		
	Follicular	4–10 U/l	
	Mid-cycle peak	6–25 U/l	
	Luteal	2.5–10 U/l	
	Postmenopausal	30–120 U/l	
Luteinizing	Male	1.5–10 U/l	
hormone (LH)	Female:		
	Follicular	2.5–15 U/l	
	Mid-cycle peak	13–80 U/l	
	Luteal	up to 13 U/l	
	Postmenopausal	> 25 U/l	

Continued

Hormone		Normal Value	Some useful conversions from SI units
17β-Oestradiol	Male	< 175 pmol/l	1 pmol/l = 0.27 pg/ml
	Female:		
	Follicular	75–300 pmol/l	
	Mid-cycle	750–1800 pmol/l	
	Luteal phase	350–1100 pmol/l	
	Postmenopausal	< 200 pmol/l	
Androstenedione	Female/male	4–10 nmol/l	
Dehydroepiandrosterone sulphate	20–40 yrs	0.5–11.5 μmol/l	
(DHEAS)	40–60 yrs	0.5–7.0 μmol/l	
Progesterone	Follicular	1–4 nmol/l	1 nmol/l = 0.32 ng/ml
	Luteal	30–80 nmol/l	
17α-hydroxy-progesterone	Morning sample	up to 15 nmol/l	
Prolactin		up to 425 mU/l	
Parathyroid hormone (PTH)	(intact molecule assay)	10–50 ng/ml	
Testosterone	Male	13–30 nmol/l	
	Female	0.5–2.5 nmol/l	1 nmol/l = 0.29 ng/ml
Sex hormone binding globulin (SHBG)	Female	35–100 nmol/l	
Testosterone: SHBG ratio	Female	1.3–4.5	
Insulin	Fasting	up to 17 mU/l	
Growth hormone	Resting	< 2 mU/l excludes acromegaly	
		> 20 mU/l excludes growth hormone deficiency	

Continued

Hormone		Normal Value	Some useful conversions from SI units
Renin activity (PRA)	Recumbent:	0.5–2.0 pmol/ml/h	
	Ambulant: Normal Na^+, K^+ diet (Na^+: 100–200 mmol/l per 24 h K^+: 50–80 mmol/24 h)	0.5–3.1 pmol/ml/h	
Thyrotrophin (TSH)		0.2–4.0 mU/l	
Thyroxine (T_4)		60–145 nmol/l	1 nmol/l = 0.8 ng/ml
Free thyroxine (FT_4)		10–25 pmol/l	
Free triiodothyronine (FT_3)		5.4–9.3 pmol/l	
25-Hydroxycholecalciferol (25-Hydroxy vitamin D)		15–100 nmol/l	1 nmol/l = 0.4 ng/ml
Vasopressin (AVP)		1–2 mU/l	1 mU/l = 2.5 pg/ml
Somatomedin-C (IGF-I)	< 5 yrs	3–36 nmol/l	
	6–10 yrs	4–90 nmol/l	
	11–16 yrs	11–125 nmol/l	
	17–20 yrs	19–101 nmol/l	
	21–60 yrs	13–64 nmol/l	
	> 60 yrs	6–30 nmol/l	

Continued

Hormone		Normal Value	Some useful conversions from SI units
Urine (24-h collection)			
Aldosterone	Normal Na^+, K^+ diet (Na^+: 100–200 mmol/l/24 h; K^+: 50–80 mmol/l/24 h)	10–25 nmol	
Free cortisol		< 340 nmol	
Pregnanetriol	Male	3–6 μmol	1 μmol = 0.33 mg
	Female:		
	Follicular	0.5–5.0 μmol	
	Luteal	2.5–6.5 μmol	
Dehydroepiandrosterone (DHA)	Male	0.35–7 μmol	
	Female	0.7–1.75 μmol	
Vanillyl mandelic acid (VMA)		less than 40 μmol	

Index